EVALUATING THE
HEALTHCARE
SYSTEM

EVALUATING THE HEALTHCARE SYSTEM

Effectiveness, Efficiency, and Equity

LU ANN ADAY

CHARLES E. BEGLEY

DAVID R. LAIRSON

CARL H. SLATER

AHSR

Health Administration Press
Chicago, Illinois

02 01 00 99 98   5 4 3 2 1

Library of Congress Cataloging-in-Publication Data
Evaluating the health care system : effectiveness, efficiency, and
   equity / submitted by Lu Ann Aday . . . [et al.]. — 2nd ed.
      p.   cm.
   Rev. ed. of: Evaluating the medical care system / Lu Ann Aday . . .
[et al.]. 1993.
   Includes bibliographical references and index.
   ISBN 1-56793-079-4
   1. Medical care—United States—Evaluation.   2. Medical care—
Research—United States.   3. Medical policy—United States—
Evaluation.   I. Aday, Lu Ann.   II. Evaluating the medical care
system.
   [DNLM: 1. Health Services Research—United States.   2.   Health
Policy—United States.   3. Delivery of Health Care—United States.
W 84.3 E92 1998]
RA399.A3E95   1998
362.1'068'5—dc21
DNLM/DLC
for Library of Congress   98-12225
                                                                  CIP

The paper used in this publication meets the minimum requirements of American National Standard for Information Sciences—Permanence of Paper for Printed Library Materials, ANSI Z39.48–1984. ⊗ ™

Contents

List of Figures and Tables vii

Foreword by Stephen M. Shortell ix

Preface xiii

Acknowledgments xvii

1 Introduction to Health Services Research and Policy
   Analysis 1

   Appendix 1.1 Progress on Healthy People 2000
                 Sentinel Objectives 41

   Appendix 1.2 Age-Adjusted Death Rates by Selected
                 Cause, Race, and Sex, United States,
                 1990 and 1980 43

2 Effectiveness: Concepts and Methods.................. 45

3 Effectiveness: Policy Strategies, Evidence, Criteria, and
   an Application 73

4 Efficiency: Concepts and Methods 105

5 Efficiency: Policy Strategies, Evidence, Criteria, and an
   Application 131

6 Equity: Concepts and Methods 173

7 Equity: Policy Strategies, Evidence, Criteria, and an
   Application 207

   Appendix 7.1 Highlights of Selected Indicators of
                 Equity of Access to Healthcare 242

8 Integrating Health Services Research and Policy
   Analysis 247

9 Applying Health Services Reseach to Policy Analysis 277

Index 319

About the Authors 333

List of Figures and Tables

Figures

1.1	Continuum of Health Services	5
1.2	Comparison of Focus of Health Services Research with Other Types of Research	5
1.3	Comparison of Objectives of Health Services Research with Other Types of Inquiry	8
1.4	Framework for Classifying Topics and Issues in Health Services Research	10
2.1	Factors Contributing to Population Health	47
4.1	Production Possibility Frontier	111
4.2	Individual Demand Curve	115
4.3	Individual Supply Curve	116
4.4	Market Demand and Supply	116
6.1	An Expanded Conceptual Framework of Equity	179

Tables

1.1	Levels of Analysis in Health Services Research	13
2.1	Dimensions of Effectiveness	51
2.2	Framework for Effectiveness Research	53
3.1	Health Policy Strategies Related to Factors Contributing to Population Health	75
3.2	Health Status Indicators, United States, 1993	82
3.3	Criteria for Assessing Health Policies in Terms of Effectiveness	95
4.1	Comparisons of Cost-Effectiveness, Cost-Benefit, and Cost-Utility Analysis	121

5.1   Public Coverage against Cost of Medical Care and
      Average Percentage of Bill Paid by Public Insurance:
      Selected Countries, 1995 143
5.2   Use of Inpatient Healthcare in Selected Countries 144
5.3   Healthcare Expenditures in Selected Countries 145
5.4   Comparative Expenditures and Health Indicators for
      Seven Industrialized Countries 147
5.5   Criteria for Assessing Health Policies in Terms of
      Efficiency 157
6.1   Contrasting Paradigms of Justice 175
6.2   Criteria and Indicators of Equity 186
7.1   Criteria for Assessing Health Policies in Terms of
      Equity—An Application to Socially Responsible
      Managed Care. 230
8.1   Stages of Policymaking, Relevant Information, and
      Type of Research. 256
9.1   Dimensions of State Health Reform 280
9.2   Inclusiveness of Public Coverage 286
9.3   Comprehensiveness of Public Benefits 290
9.4   Regulatory versus Voluntary Methods to Expand
      Private Coverage 292
9.5   Regulatory versus Pro-Market Methods to Contain
      Costs. 294
9.6   Regulatory versus Pro-Market Methods to Ensure
      Quality 297
9.7   Summary of Effectiveness, Efficiency, and Equity
      Performance Criteria 299
9.8   Evaluation of State Health Reform Options 302

Foreword

(The U.S. healthcare system is in the midst of a major transition as private market and public policy forces collide and coalesce producing increased consolidation of providers and purchasers, and new demands for accountability in regard to both cost and quality of care. There is a new search for value defined as the combination of cost and quality attributes (service quality and technical quality) that satisfies purchasers. Those providers that can deliver greater quality as desired by the purchasers of health services for a given price, or conversely, a given quality of services for a lower price relative to competitors are adding value. There is growing evidence that in selected areas across the United States purchasers and consumers alike are making healthcare decisions based on value and not cost alone.)

Concern about the potentially harmful impact of managed care has also led to increased demands of accountability. This is reflected in the development of healthcare "report cards" such as those represented by the health employer data and information system (HEDIS) developed by the National Committee for Quality Assurance (NCQA), the work of the Foundation for Accountability (FAACT), and the new outcome-oriented approach taken by the Joint Commission on Accreditation of Healthcare Organizations (JCAHO). It is reflected as well in the growing demand for patient self-protection legislation.

Along with the increased search for value and demand for evidence-based accountability has come the realization that many health problems have their root in the community—domestic violence, teenage pregnancy, and substance abuse representing a few examples. Through prevention, health promotion practices, and community building activities the hope is that these issues can be effectively addressed before they make costly demands on the medical care system. This will require healthcare organizations and providers to work with community agencies, schools, local businesses, and religious organizations in new ways that emphasize the population epidemiological perspective and the need for community-wide collaboration.

This revised second edition of *Evaluating the Medical Care System: Effectiveness, Efficiency, and Equity* provides a much needed conceptual and empirical road map for understanding the new dynamics associated with value, accountability, and community emerging from our healthcare system. Organized around the core concepts of effectiveness, efficiency, and equity, Aday and colleagues provide a holistic, integrative examination of our healthcare system. In considering effectiveness, the second edition is strengthened by the increased attention given to community-wide health issues and the population-based approach to healthcare delivery. Issues of efficiency are considered from both an allocative social welfare perspective and a production theory of the firm perspective. Equity of access issues are addressed from multiple perspectives addressing distributive justice, social justice, and deliberative justice. Particularly informative is the application of the equity criteria to managed care initiatives. Drawing on the effectiveness, efficiency, and equity paradigm, data are marshaled to enable readers to understand the current state of knowledge regarding relevant health issues.

The authors are to be particularly commended for their discussion of the types of health services research that can best influence different stages of the policy process. The strengths and limitations of the rational-comprehensive, satisficing, mixed-scanning, and political models of policymaking are also duly noted. The utility of the overall framework of effectiveness, efficiency, and equity is illustrated in the application to state Medicaid managed care initiatives. The authors examine the extent to which these initiatives are likely to be successful based on the effectiveness, efficiency, and equity criteria developed in the book. Among their findings: (1) there is no evidence of a population-based approach to delivery; (2) the market alone is not likely to be effective in containing costs; and (3) whether or not equal treatment norms prevail will be highly dependent on implementation issues across the states.

Superbly organized and clearly written, this revised edition will be of considerable value to researchers and policymakers, as well as those involved in the direct provision and management of health services delivery. It will also serve as an extremely useful text for graduate and doctoral students in health services research and policy analysis. This book makes a significant contribution toward the development of a common framework and knowledge base for those interested in improving the delivery of health services to the American public.

Stephen M. Shortell
A. C. Buehler Distinguished Professor of Health Services
Management and Professor of Organization Behavior
J. L. Kellogg Graduate School of Management
Center for Health Services and Policy Research
Northwestern University, Evanston, Illinois

Preface

This book defines and integrates the fundamental concepts and methods of health services research as a field of study, and illustrates their application to policy analysis. A model of health policy analysis is linked to a framework for classifying topics and issues in health services research. The book provides a historical perspective and applies the concepts and methods of epidemiology, economics, sociology, and related disciplines to illustrate the measurement and relevance of effectiveness, efficiency, and equity as criteria for evaluating healthcare system performance. Specific examples of the application of health services research in addressing contemporary health policy problems at the national, state, and local levels are presented.

The primary audiences for the book are practicing professionals and graduate students in public health, health administration, and the healthcare professions; and federal, state, and local policymakers and program planners charged with the design and conduct of policy-relevant health services research. Professionals and students in medical sociology, the behavioral sciences, and public administration interested in conducting applied or policy-oriented health and healthcare research will also find the book of considerable interest. The authors developed and applied the perspective presented in the book in a course they have offered to graduate students in public health since 1986.

Revisions to the first edition of the book, *Evaluating the Medical Care System: Effectiveness, Efficiency, and Equity*, were primarily as follows: (1) the introduction of an expanded definition and continuum of *health services*, encompassing prevention-oriented and long-term as well as acute medical care, as the focus of *health services research*; (2) an expansion and application of the conceptual framework for the book to accommodate a consideration of community (environmental and population) factors in influencing the design and impact of health services delivery on *health*; (3) an explication of the development and application of data systems to evaluate the performance of the health services delivery system at the community, system, institution, and patient levels; (4) providing examples of the application of health services research to policy analysis based on contrasting the major features of state health reform strategies; and (5) revising the core chapters on the effectiveness, efficiency, and equity concepts to reflect the expanded conceptualization of the predictors and dimensions of health as the ultimate focus of health policy.

In general, the revised edition of the book is intended to encompass a broader and more integrative look at the role of both population (or public) health and personal (or medical) care services in enhancing community and individual well-being; the design of health services research to assess the effectiveness, efficiency, and equity of service delivery; and the normative and empirical application of the effectiveness, efficiency, and equity criteria in evaluating specific health policy alternatives.

Chapter 1 presents a framework for classifying the major topics and issues addressed by health services research as a field of study. This framework is then used to provide an integrative overview of the contributions of health services research to describing and evaluating the performance of the healthcare system with respect to the objectives of effectiveness, efficiency, and equity. This chapter defines the relationship between health services research and the major objectives and methods of policy analysis. The historical role of health services research in the formulation of health policy is highlighted.

Chapters 2, 4, and 6 introduce the concepts and methods of effectiveness, efficiency, and equity research, while Chapters 3, 5, and 7 review the policy strategies that have emerged to accomplish these objectives, as well as the criteria and evidence regarding their success in achieving them, with a particular focus on Medicaid managed care.

The effectiveness chapters (Chapters 2 and 3) introduce and apply a conceptual framework based on Donabedian's classical triad of structure, process, and outcome, as well as the associated methods for assessing the effectiveness of medical and non-medical interventions from both the population and clinical perspectives.

The efficiency discussion (Chapters 4 and 5) examines the concepts of production and allocative efficiency, and the major findings regarding the performance of the U.S. and other countries' healthcare systems with respect to these objectives.

The equity chapters (Chapters 6 and 7) introduce an expanded conceptual framework of equity, grounded in emerging and expanded theoretical dimensions of deliberative, distributive, and social justice, and apply it to assessing the progress of the U.S. healthcare system in achieving equity along each of these dimensions.

Chapter 8 analyzes the interrelationships between and among the objectives of effectiveness, efficiency, and equity, and the role of health services research in conceptualizing and measuring the trade-offs among them in formulating health policy. Chapter 9 discusses these trade-offs in the context of evaluating specific state healthcare reform alternatives.

This book makes a number of unique contributions: (1) it presents and applies an organizing framework for defining health services research as a field of study, in the context of the major system performance dimensions of effectiveness, efficiency, and equity; (2) it reviews and integrates the conceptual, methodological, and empirical contributions of health services research to addressing these issues; (3) it illustrates how the perspectives and methods of effectiveness, efficiency, and equity research can be used to anticipate and pose relevant questions to inform both current and future health care policy debates; and (4) it provides a primer and point of reference at a time when both the support for and demands upon health services research and policy analysis are increasing.

Lu Ann Aday
Charles E. Begley
David R. Lairson
Carl H. Slater

The syllabus for the University of Texas School of Public Health course PH5110: Health Services Delivery and Performance, which is taught by the authors and organized around this text, can be found at http://www.sph.uth.tmc.edu/www/res/outcomes/ph5110syl.htm.

Acknowledgments

The authors gratefully acknowledge colleagues who provided thoughtful and constructive comments on earlier drafts of the manuscript: Ronald M. Andersen, Judith D. Kasper, Stephen H. Linder, Miriam Orleans, John C. Ribble, and J. Michael Swint, as well as the anonymous Health Administration Press reviewers.

Special thanks go to Anne-Marie Broemeling, who served as the Teaching Assistant for the course in which the manuscript was developed, and who also located, copied, and entered many of the sources cited in the book. We gratefully acknowledge the contributions of Gloria Tzuang as well in compiling and editing the references for the book, and to Regina Fisher and Linda Matthews, who assisted with typing the manuscript.

We are grateful for the flexible environment at the University of Texas School of Public Health, which supported the rewarding task of writing the book as a routine component of faculty roles and responsibilities.

We owe a special debt to the students in our course on health services delivery and performance throughout the years, as well as to students in Carl Slater's medical outcomes assessment class, who stimulated and challenged us to sharpen our mastery of the ideas put forth in the book.

Each of us feels that our understanding of the concepts of effectiveness, efficiency, and equity has been broadened and deepened in the process of writing the book. Our hope is that those who read it will be similarly rewarded.

Chapter 1

Introduction to Health Services Research and Policy Analysis

"The goal of health services research is to provide information that will eventually lead to improvements in the health of the citizenry" (U.S. National Library of Medicine 1997). This book provides guidance for applying the concepts and methods from health services research on the effectiveness, efficiency, and equity of healthcare in assessing the performance of health policies and programs in contributing to this goal.

Definitions

Health services research *produces* knowledge about the performance of the healthcare system, and policy analysis *applies* this knowledge in defining problems and evaluating policy alternatives. This book delineates and defines the working partnership between health services research and policy analysis in assessing the performance of the U.S. healthcare system with respect to the objectives of effectiveness, efficiency, and equity, where

1. *effectiveness* examines the benefits of healthcare measured by improvements in health;
2. *efficiency* relates these health improvements to the resources required to produce them; and
3. *equity* is concerned with health disparities and the fairness and effectiveness of the procedures for addressing them.

Effectiveness focuses on the benefits produced by healthcare, as measured by improvements in people's health. Improvements in health include not only the sum of the individual benefits, that is, reduced mortality rates, increased life expectancies, and decreased prevalence of disease, but also reference to a distribution of disease and health in a way that maximizes overall economic productivity and well-being. The *clinical perspective* on effectiveness assesses the contribution of medical care to improving the health of individuals, while the *population perspective* assesses the contribution of medical and non-medical (e.g., environmental and behavioral) factors to the health of communities as a whole.

A second major objective of the healthcare delivery system is the drive for *efficiency*. Where healthcare is viewed as an output, the focus is on *production efficiency* (producing services at least cost), and where healthcare is viewed as an input in the production of health improvements, the emphasis is on *allocative efficiency* (maximizing health given constrained resources).[1] Allocative efficiency depends on the relative cost and effectiveness of medical and non-medical investments in improving health. Ultimately, maximization of health requires both production and allocative efficiency.

Equity is concerned with health disparities and the fairness and effectiveness of the procedures for addressing them. The ultimate test of the equity of health policy is the extent to which disparities or inequalities in health persist among subgroups of the population. *Substantive equity* is reflected in minimizing subgroup disparities in health. *Procedural equity* refers to the extent to which the structure and process, or procedures, for achieving these outcomes may be judged to be fair. The normative relevance of variations in the structure and process of care ultimately, however, can be judged empirically by the contributions of these variations to predicting inequalities in health across groups and communities.

The three objectives are often complementary. Improving healthcare effectiveness while holding resources constant increases efficiency. Increases in efficiency create opportunities for improved effectiveness and equity. However, the objectives may also be in conflict. Maximizing effectiveness by allocating additional resources to improve health may conflict with efficiency if the cost of the resources is high relative to their effectiveness. Maximizing effectiveness and efficiency by distributing resources to persons who would gain the most may be deemed unfair in terms of procedural equity if the policy leads to a very uneven distribution of these resources.

Identifying appropriate trade-offs among the three objectives is an important product of health services research. Assuming that all three are important objectives, a key question for decision makers in comparing policy alternatives is the degree to which one objective must be sacrificed to achieve the others.

The chapters that follow review the conceptual, methodological, and empirical foundations for the effectiveness, efficiency, and equity objectives, show how they are applied in policy analysis, and examine the health services research questions posed in analyzing the trade-offs between these objectives in formulating health policy.

In this chapter, the fields of health services research and policy analysis are compared and contrasted with other types of inquiry. We present a framework for classifying topics and issues in health services research and use this framework to provide a descriptive overview of the U.S. healthcare system. Historical contributions of health services research to the development of health policy are highlighted, and selected applications in terms of current U.S. policy debates are introduced.

Definition of Health Services Research

A 1979 Institute of Medicine panel charged with defining and evaluating the field of health services research offered the following definition of the enterprise: "Health services research is inquiry to produce knowledge about the structure, processes, or effects of personal health services" (Institute of Medicine 1979, 14). A study could be classified as health services research if it dealt primarily with "personal health services" and drew upon a conceptual framework other than that of applied biomedical science, which primarily focuses on the fundamental life processes of the human organism. Personal health services were defined as transactions between providers and clients for the purpose of promoting the health of the clients. These transactions largely fall within the domain of the *medical care* system, in contrast to *public health*, which focuses on interventions to promote the health and well-being of the community or the population as a whole rather than that of particular individuals within it.

A later Institute of Medicine (1995, 17) report offered the following revised definition of health services research: "Health services research is a multidisciplinary field of inquiry, both basic and applied, that examines the use, costs, quality, accessibility, and delivery, organization, financing, and outcomes of health care services to increase knowledge and understanding of the structure, processes, and effects of health services for individuals and populations." The newer definition differs from the former primarily in acknowledging that health services research serves to make contributions to basic, as well as applied, research in selected areas (e.g., the operation of medical care markets in health economics theory) and that it is concerned with studying a broader continuum of healthcare services, focusing on population-based as well as personal services.

The array of programs and services that would be encompassed in such a continuum is displayed in Figure 1.1. The continuum implies continuity and integration over time and between components in the context of promoting and protecting the health of individuals and populations through primary prevention to inhibit the onset of health problems, secondary prevention to restore a person who is already affected to maximum functioning, and tertiary prevention to minimize the deterioration of function for those with problems that are essentially not curable. The provision of ambulatory and acute institutional care within the conventional medical care system encompasses the treatment-oriented center of the continuum. Community social and economic and public health programs and policies define the primary prevention-oriented beginning of the continuum, and long-term institutional, home, and community-based care extend the continuum to enhancing the quality of life and maximizing the functioning of the chronically ill or disabled. The prevention-oriented and long-term care poles encompass an array of non-medical, as well as medical, programs and services directed toward promoting or protecting the health of the public and individuals.

Health services research is inherently interdisciplinary in focus, in that it draws on and applies theories and methods from an array of disciplines, including sociology, political science, epidemiology, demography, economics, law, and medicine, among others (Choi and Greenberg 1982; Ginzberg 1991). Basic disciplinary research is

Figure 1.1 Continuum of Health Services

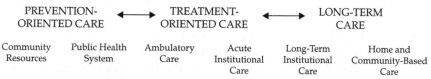

Source: Used with permission from Aday, L. A. 1993. *At Risk in America: The Health and Health Care Needs of Vulnerable Populations in the United States.* San Francisco: Jossey-Bass. Figure 5.1, 117.

primarily concerned with the development and testing of theories to explain social or biological phenomena, while health services research applies the theories and methods that have evolved within these disciplines to investigating problems related to the operation and performance of the healthcare delivery system. Further, whereas clinical research is principally concerned with medically related services and outcomes for individual patients, health services research more broadly acknowledges the array of non-medical (i.e., social, economic, and organizational) factors that may help to promote health or prevent illness (see Figure 1.2).

Definition of Policy Analysis

Policy analysis is defined in terms of two principal objectives: (1) the production of information relevant to policymaking; and (2) the

Figure 1.2 Comparison of Focus of Health Services Research with Other Types of Research

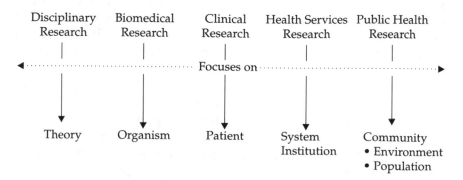

development of reasonable arguments translating the information into recommendations for governmental action (Dunn 1994). The distinction between health services research and policy analysis is that the first objective—the *production* of knowledge—defines the primary contributions of health services research, and the second—the *application* of knowledge—represents the primary contributions of health policy analysis to governmental decision making.

The first objective most directly mirrors the goal of health services research that is concerned with generating knowledge about the implementation and effects of specific health services programs and policies. The principal questions and issues being addressed are factual or objective: to document the scope or origins of a problem (e.g., the proportion of the population and subgroups without insurance coverage) and the probable consequences of alternatives for addressing it (cross-national comparisons of alternative systems of financing medical care).

The second objective extends somewhat beyond the role traditionally assumed by health services research. This objective attempts to justify the relevance of particular types of research, to weigh existing evidence and competing values, and finally, to construct a logical case for policymakers regarding the significance of a problem or the utility of specific programs or policies in addressing it. The primary emphases of this objective are normative and prescriptive: to provide a logical, well-documented rationale for evaluating the adequacy of existing policies (e.g., in providing insurance coverage) and to prescribe the choice of one (health insurance reform) alternative over another in the light of competing health policy goals (effectiveness, efficiency, and equity).

These objectives assume a rational, problem-solving process of policymaking that does not take into account the nature of political institutions and the processes that determine those issues that actually come to be acknowledged and addressed. These political elements include the attitudes, concerns, and opinions of the public at large and of special interest groups; their respective and relative ability to influence decisions; the institutions and processes for making these decisions; and the nature and content of competing items on the policy agenda. Health services research and policy analysis influence policymaking by providing information and analysis for documenting the policy problem of concern (e.g., the limited willingness of providers to see Medicaid patients), the development of possible solutions (increased provider fees, extended medical liability coverage, or Medicaid managed care), and evaluation of alternative policy proposals. The political will to apply this information to the policymaking process is not always forthcoming. Attempts at national healthcare reform in the early 1990s provide evidence on the uses of information and analyses to enrich as well as distort policy debates (Peterson 1995).

At the end of the chapters presenting the policy strategies and the evidence regarding the effectiveness, efficiency, and equity of healthcare that follow (Chapters 3, 5, and 7), criteria for assessing policies from each of these perspectives will be identified and then applied to evaluating a specific policy alternative, Medicaid managed care. The final chapter illustrates the integrative application of these perspectives in a policy analysis of different models of state healthcare reform.

Differences from Other Types of Inquiry

Figure 1.3 contrasts health services research and policy analysis with other types of basic and applied scientific inquiry in terms of the primary research objectives of each. Disciplines (e.g., economics) provide useful theories (of demand and supply) to explain biological or social phenomena (the operation of consumer and provider behavior in the medical care marketplace). These theories underlie the ways in which health services research describes and assesses the performance of the healthcare system—in terms of efficiency, for example. Health program evaluation is concerned with assessing the effect of specific policies and programs (e.g., Medicaid managed care, physician reimbursement schemes, or consumer cost-sharing provisions) on a defined policy outcome of interest (e.g., cost containment), and applies the concepts and methods of health services research in evaluating these alternatives. Evaluating the implementation and effect of healthcare programs such as neighborhood health centers, hospital-based group practices, or immunization outreach efforts has been a major activity of health services research (Shortell and Richardson 1978). To the extent that such evaluations are directed toward assessing specific governmental policies or programs, they may provide direct input to related health policy analysis efforts. Policy analysis draws on the fund of knowledge generated by disciplinary and health services research to (1) define and analyze current problems (e.g., cost, access, or effectiveness of care for Medicaid eligibles); and (2) compare and evaluate health policy alternatives (different Medicaid managed care models).

Health services research has been criticized historically for not being sufficiently involved in the conduct of research that directly informs difficult health policy decisions (Anderson 1991; Choi and Greenberg 1982; Flook and Sanazaro 1973; Ginzberg 1991; Institute of Medicine 1979, 1991, 1995). Compilations of the contributions of health services research to health policy and management do clearly

Figure 1.3   Comparison of Objectives of Health Services Research with Other Types of Inquiry

Type of Inquiry	Objective
Disciplinary Research	To explain biological or social phenomena $$X \longrightarrow Y$$
Health Services Research	To describe and assess the performance of the healthcare system

$$\textit{Structure} \quad \textit{Process} \quad \textit{Outcome}$$
$$X \longrightarrow Y$$

Health Program Evaluation   To evaluate the effect of health policies and programs

$$x_0 \longrightarrow y_0$$
$$x_1 \longrightarrow y_1$$
$$x_2 \longrightarrow y_2$$
$$x_3 \longrightarrow y_3$$

Health Policy Analysis   To analyze and compare alternative (1) problem definitions, and (2) health policy solutions

(1) Problem Analysis

$$x_1$$
vs.
$$x_2 \longrightarrow x$$
vs.
$$x_3$$

(2) Solution Analysis

$$y_1$$
vs.
$$y_2 \longrightarrow y$$
vs.
$$y_3$$

indicate, however, that the lines between health services research and policy analysis are more aptly characterized as diffuse, rather than distinct. Health services research has been directly used in evaluating a variety of policy options, such as the cost, quality, and access implications of alternative universal health insurance proposals and of enrolling Medicaid- and Medicare-eligible individuals in managed care (Altman and Reinhardt 1996; Brown 1991; DeFriese, Ricketts, and Stein 1989; Ginzberg 1991; Shi 1997; Shortell and Reinhardt 1992; White 1992).

Topics and Applications of Health Services Research

Framework for Classifying Topics and Issues in Health Services Research

A framework for classifying topics and issues in health services research is provided in Figure 1.4. The shaded boxes represent revisions or additions to the framework introduced in the first edition of this book (Aday et al. 1993), influenced by a conceptual framework focusing on the social and individual determinants of health developed by Evans, Barer, and Marmor (1994) and extended by Roos et al. (1996). The revised framework acknowledges the important role that physical, social, and economic environments, and their associated health risks, play in producing health. It also sets the stage for the arguments and evidence to be presented in subsequent chapters regarding the importance of encompassing the role of both medical care and non-medical factors in evaluating the effectiveness, efficiency, and equity of the U.S. healthcare system and associated policies.

As implied in the framework (Figure 1.4), the design and conduct of health services research is often motivated by questions related to the formulation or evaluation of health policy. The access, cost, and quality dilemmas faced by governmental and private policymakers and institutions at the national, state, and local levels in providing and paying for healthcare serve as invitations to investigators to contribute to the knowledge and expertise needed to address those dilemmas. The availability of support

Figure 1.4   Framework for Classifying Topics and Issues in
Health Services Research

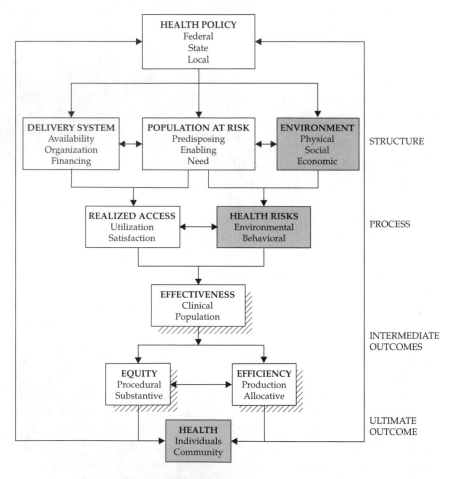

through government contracts, investigator-initiated studies, and
foundation-sponsored research and demonstration projects provides direct incentives for developing research projects, consultative
arrangements, or conferences and task forces to study these issues.

The concepts and methods of health services research provide
guidance by *describing, analyzing,* and *evaluating* the *structure, process,*
and *outcomes* of the healthcare system.

Structure refers to the availability, organization, and financing
of healthcare programs; the characteristics of the populations to be

served by them; and the physical, social, and economic environments to which they are exposed. *Process* encompasses the transactions between patients and providers in the course of actual care delivery, as well as the environmental and behavioral transactions exacerbating health risks.

One may view effectiveness, efficiency, and equity as intermediate *outcomes* of the healthcare delivery process that ultimately is concerned with enhancing the health of individuals and communities. The U.S. Public Health Service Healthy People Year 2000 Objectives and World Health Organization (WHO) Year 2000 Health Objectives, both of which are discussed later in this chapter, provide benchmarks for assessing the extent to which selected health goals are reached (National Center for Health Statistics [NCHS] 1995b, 1996b; WHO 1994). Improving the health of individuals and communities is best viewed, however, as a dynamic and ongoing process. Effectiveness, efficiency, and equity research provide intermediate, evaluative indicators of this process.

Clinical effectiveness, production efficiency, and procedural equity focus on healthcare services: clinical effectiveness addresses the impact of medical care on health improvements for individual patients; production efficiency is concerned with the combination of inputs required to produce these and related services at the lowest costs; and procedural equity assesses the fairness of care delivery.

Population effectiveness, allocative efficiency, and substantive equity focus on the ultimate outcome of interest, community-wide health improvements: population effectiveness addresses the role of medical and non-medical factors in influencing the health of populations as a whole; allocative efficiency analysis attempts to pinpoint and address the combination of inputs that produce the greatest health improvements given available resources; and substantive equity is judged ultimately by the extent to which those health benefits are shared equally across groups in the community.

Effectiveness—or the production of health benefits—is placed before efficiency and equity in the framework (Figure 1.4) to indicate the central role it plays in assessing the cost of producing health benefits (i.e., efficiency) as well as the distribution of these benefits and costs across groups (i.e., equity). Comparison of health indicators at the national, state, or local level with desired normative endpoints such as those defined by the U.S. Public Health Service or WHO provides an indication of whether the health goals of health policy have been achieved. Effectiveness, efficiency, and equity research can assist policymakers in deciding, given constrained resources, the fairest and most effective ways to do so.

Health services research provides basic descriptive data on the organization and operation of the healthcare system, such as the number and distribution of providers, the percentage of population uninsured, and the rates of service utilization. It also analyzes likely relationships between and among components (reflected in the arrows in Figure 1.4), examining the impact of health policy on the delivery system and the individuals and populations affected by these initiatives; on the effectiveness, efficiency, and equity of the delivery system; and, ultimately and most importantly, on the health of the population the delivery system was intended to serve.

Macrolevel versus Microlevel of Analysis

The structure, process, and outcomes of healthcare can be studied at the macrolevel or microlevel of analysis (see Table 1.1). The macrolevel refers to the population perspective on the determinants of the health of communities as a whole, and the microlevel represents a clinical perspective on the factors that contribute to the health of individuals at the system, institution, or patient level. The community level encompasses the population in a defined area and the physical, social, and economic environment in which they reside. System level refers to the healthcare system, including " . . . the resources (money, people, physical infrastructure, and technology) and the organizational configurations used to transform these resources into health care services" either for the country as a whole or within a specific region (Longest 1994, 2). Institution level refers to a specific organizational entity such as a hospital, clinic, or health maintenance organization. The patient level refers to the microcosm of clinical decision making and treatment.

Information from each of these levels is required to fully understand and interpret the effects of health policies and programs. Commitments to developing medical technologies or procedures to optimize individual patient outcomes may fail to consider whether, in the light of limited resources, these are the best investments to enhance the health and well-being of the population as a whole.

Table 1.1 Levels of Analysis in Health Services Research

	Level of Analysis[1]				
	Community		System	Institution	Patient
Data Sources	Environment	Population			
Census	X	X			
Public health surveillance systems	X	X			
Vital statistics		X			
Area resource files			X		
Market area inventories			X		
Surveys					
Population		X			
Organizations			X	X	
Providers			X	X	
Patients			X	X	X
Records					
Enrollment		X	X	X	X
Encounters			X	X	X
Claims			X	X	X
Medical records			X	X	X
Qualitative studies					
(Non)participant observation	X	X	X	X	X
Case studies			X	X	
Focus groups		X			X
Ethnographic interviews		X			X

[1]The denominator for population-level analyses are individuals residing in a designated geographic area. The denominator for patient-level analyses are individuals who have utilized healthcare services. Data collected at one level can be aggregated to other levels of analysis in which these units are nested (e.g., patient-level data can be aggregated to the institution or system level). Patient-level data, and estimates based on aggregating them to the system or institution level, may be used as the numerator, but not the denominator, for population-level analyses.

Treatments that have been demonstrated to be efficacious at the individual patient level may not be applied similarly across institutions, or even within the same institution. System-level outcomes may be influenced by organizational and financial incentives that influence the patterns of healthcare provision. Community-level outcome studies allow exploration of the variations in care that may result from differential access to healthcare and from different styles of practice not detectable by outcomes research at the institutional or system levels alone. A focus on the role that personal lifestyle practices (e.g., smoking) and attitudes (e.g., toward regular physical activity) play in affecting individuals' health status may not fully reveal the array of social structural and environmental factors (e.g., poverty, lead paint, toxic wastes) that may have consequential impacts on the health of populations residing in an area.

The discussion in the chapters that follow offers additional insights on the performance of the healthcare system that may be uniquely illuminated, as well as omitted, by a singular focus on any one point of view.

A Historical Overview of Policy-Related Health Services Research

Health services research is a relatively new field of inquiry, although its origins may be traced to the early 1900s in the United States. Selected historical contributions of health services research to the formulation of health policy are highlighted here. (For more detail, see Anderson 1991; Flook and Sanazaro 1973; Institute of Medicine 1995; and U. S. National Library of Medicine 1997.)

The Flexner report, based on a comprehensive study of medical schools in the United States and Canada, was published in 1910. This report led to a major reorganization of medical education in the United States.

The Committee on the Costs of Medical Care (CCMC) was established in 1927. That prestigious 42-member committee played a major role in the design and conduct of research on the utilization and costs of care and on the inequities of access that existed among income groups. The committee published 28 reports, including a series of reports and recommendations that affected and continue to affect how medical care is organized and delivered in the United States.

In 1935–36, the Public Health Service conducted a national health survey and a business census of hospitals to provide basic data on the health and healthcare needs of the population and on the financial structure of U.S. hospitals. An outgrowth of this early research was the development of the concept of health service areas for general hospitals and health centers. In 1944, the American Hospital Association (AHA) established its Commission on Hospital Care that provided the first complete inventory of the nation's hospitals. This and the earlier business census identified a need for more general hospital beds, especially in rural areas, that in 1946 resulted in the passage of the Hill-Burton Act, authorizing a massive nationwide hospital survey and construction program.

The Commission on Chronic Illness, established in 1949 under the auspices of the AHA, the American Medical Association (AMA), the American Public Health Association (APHA), and the American Public Welfare Association (APWA), carried out a number of studies dealing with the community prevalence and prevention of chronic illness, long-term care, and home care. The AHA Commission on Financing, established in 1951, attempted to address many of the issues related to the financing of hospital care (i.e., the factors affecting cost, prepayment, and financing care for non-wage and low-income groups) that had not been dealt with directly by the 1944 AHA Commission on Hospital Care. The research carried out by these national commissions contributed to early deliberations concerning the appropriate role of the federal government in healthcare (as in President Truman's Commission on the Health Care Needs of the Nation), as well as to the development of survey research methodologies and statistical and economic analysis methodologies that were to provide the foundation for contemporary health services research.

The U.S. Department of Health, Education, and Welfare (DHEW) was established in 1953. The National Health Survey Act, which provided authorization for the major data-gathering efforts of the National Center for Health Statistics, was passed in 1956. The research undertaken under the auspices of these agencies documented continuing inequities in health and healthcare for the poor and the elderly in particular—inequities identified over 20 years earlier by the Committee on the Costs of Medical Care. The evidence of these persistent disparities provided an empirical foundation for passage of the Medicaid and Medicare legislation in 1965 that extended federally subsidized coverage to these groups.

The lead federal agency for support of formal health services research activities, the National Center for Health Services Research and Development (NCHSRD), was established in 1968. During the intervening period, a number of other federal agencies (e.g., the Veterans Administration, Health Care Financing Administration, National Institute of Mental Health, and National Institute of Aging) as well as private foundations (e.g., the Robert Wood Johnson Foundation, the Commonwealth Fund, the Kaiser Family Foundation, and the Pew Foundation) assumed a greater role in supporting the design and conduct of health services research activities. The first national meeting of the Association for Health Services Research (AHSR) and the Foundation for Health Services Research (FHSR) was held in Chicago in June 1984. In 1989, the National Center for Health Services Research received a substantial boost in funding for research on patient outcomes and medical effectiveness as a result of major outcomes research bills introduced by Congress; the agency itself was subsequently renamed the Agency for Health Care Policy and Research (AHCPR) to reflect its more policy-oriented focus.

In the chapters that follow, the contributions of health services research in general as well as the contributions of specific studies in particular, such as the RAND Health Insurance Experiment and the Medical Outcomes Study, in clarifying and evaluating health policies in terms of effectiveness, efficiency, and equity will be examined.

Dimensions of Health Policy Analysis Framework

As indicated by the conceptual framework introduced earlier (Figure 1.4), health policy has been directed at a variety of factors that may ultimately determine the health of individuals and populations. The discussion that follows provides an overview of historical and current trends with respect to each of these dimensions and the role of health policy in influencing them.

Health Policy

The diversity and complexity of contemporary health policy has its roots historically in the evolution of the role played by different levels of government—federal, state, and local—in the policymaking process, as well as in the variant investments at these respective levels in public health– versus medical care–oriented programs and services.

The U.S. Constitution provided a broad foundation for the evolution of federal involvement in health through the assignment of governmental powers to promote and provide for the general welfare and to regulate commerce. This translated initially into public health–oriented interventions to prevent the importation of epidemics and to assist states and localities with their periodic needs for communicable disease control. The earliest federal health unit, the Marine Hospital Service, was established in 1798 to serve merchant seamen and to prevent the spread of epidemic diseases; it grew over time into what is now the U.S. Public Health Service (Turnock 1997).

The primary basis for the role of states in health and healthcare policy was lodged in their so-called "police powers" that permitted state and local governments to limit the actions of individuals in order to control and abate health nuisances or risks related to communicable diseases and environmental hazards from wastes, water, and food. State health departments were formed throughout the 1800s and early 1900s to carry out disease control activities and to run state mental institutions and state-owned university hospitals. From the 1930s to the 1960s states established a variety of medical indigency programs and also began supporting medical education (Altman and Morgan 1983).

With the passage of the 16th Amendment to the U.S. Constitution, which permitted the federal tax on income in the early twentieth century, the federal government was in an enhanced position to assume a larger role in both the regulation and provision of healthcare. Through federal grants-in-aids to the states, major investments in broader public health– and medical care–oriented programs and services evolved. The bulk of federal resources came to be devoted to the expansion of coverage for medical care, and to a lesser extent, public health–oriented programs and services.

The 1935 Social Security Act established a significant federal role in funding health programs with the creation of the social security "safety net" programs for the elderly, disabled, and families with dependent children. Federal grants to states were initiated in maternal and child health, public health, and healthcare for the aged and poor. The power and influence of the federal government grew rapidly from the 1930s to the 1960s with the support of biomedical research, a nationwide program of hospital planning and construction, and direct federal aid to professional schools of medical education. After 1965, the federal government's role was expanded as a major purchaser of healthcare with the creation of the Medicaid and Medicare programs (Lee and Benjamin 1993).

States, then, had served as the initial locus for programs and policies oriented to the health of the public until the federal government began to use its vast resource potential to meet changing public expectations after the Depression. State actions were soon driven by federal grant programs for public health, and eventually and centrally, for personal medical care service programs, especially during the 1960s. These developments then set the stage for what may now be seen as a burgeoning commitment of public, particularly federal, resources to medical care provision and coverage, and as a substantially lesser investment in population- or public health–oriented programs and services. The tides of political change at the federal level in the mid-1990s did, however, begin to shift more responsibility to the states for providing and paying for publicly supported medical care services, a shift that has catalyzed a corresponding reexamination of the importance and interface of public health and medical care service provision at both the federal and local levels.

A key assumption underlying the framework and the associated approaches to measuring effectiveness, efficiency, and equity presented here (Figure 1.4) is the importance of highlighting improvements in the health of individuals and communities as the essential and desired endpoint of health policy. The framework also assigns a greater importance to the "health" descriptor in "health policy," and to non-medical as well as medical factors in producing this valued policy outcome. In the chapters that follow, state healthcare reform in general and Medicaid managed care activities within states in particular will be examined in the light of this framework to illustrate the role of health services research and health policy analysis in assessing the impact of health policy on achieving the goals of effectiveness, efficiency, and equity, and ultimately, of improvements in the health of individuals and communities.

Environment

The physical, social, and economic environments in which individuals live and work significantly influence exposures to health-related risk factors. The physical environment directly affects the prevalence and distribution of health risks resulting from exposures to toxic hazards transmitted through the soil, water, and air (Goldfarb 1997; McKinney and Schoch 1996). Such risks, for example, have been variously blamed for the prevalence of childhood lead paint poisoning; rising rates of childhood asthma, particularly among minority children; the high incidence of birth defects among residents along the U.S.–Mexican border; and excessive cancer prevalence and death rates along the Mississippi River valley (i.e., "cancer alley"), in which there is a high concentration of pollution-producing industries. Further, research on environmental justice has documented that such risks, and associated adverse health consequences, are disproportionately inflicted on low socioeconomic and minority neighborhoods through the siting of high-risk industries or toxic waste sites in such areas (Brown 1995).

A large body of public health and health services research has substantiated the importance of socioeconomic factors in influencing the differential distribution of health and health risks (Aday 1993; Adler et al. 1994; Evans, Barer, and Marmor 1994; Feinstein 1993; Syme and Berkman 1976). Evans, Barer, and Marmor (1994) provide a compelling synthesis and argument regarding the impact of social and economic hierarchies (e.g., occupation, education, income, race, and gender), and of individuals' location within them, on health. Research based on animal models, as well as human populations, has consistently documented the poorer health status of those at lower, compared to higher, positions in such hierarchies. The dynamic that appears to be operating is that individuals in the lower ranks are more likely to be exposed to greater risks and associated stresses in their social and economic environment that can lead to both physiological and behavioral responses (e.g., biochemical changes and adoption of high-risk addictive practices). Ultimately, these responses give rise to health disparities by social position. Whiteis (1997) and others (Abraham 1993; Wilson 1980, 1987, 1989) have convincingly documented the role of public and corporate disinvestments in the poor and minority neighborhoods of large urban centers and the pervasive effect on the economic, social, and physical health and well-being of the people residing within them.

Detailed evidence on the impact of environmental risk factors, and particularly on the disproportionate distribution of health outcomes as a consequence, will be reviewed in Chapter 7.

Health and Health Risks

The Healthy People 2000 process, guided by the Office of Disease Prevention and Health Promotion, U.S. Department of Health and Human Services, involves people of the community in establishing health objectives at the local, state, and federal level. Healthy People 2000 set three broad public health goals for the 1990s:

1. Increase the span of healthy life for Americans
2. Reduce disparities of health among Americans
3. Achieve access to preventive services for all Americans

To help meet these goals, 300 more specific objectives have been established in 22 separate priority areas, and quantifiable targets have been set for improvements in health status, risk reduction, and service delivery. Organized under the broad approaches of health promotion, health protection, and preventive services, the national objectives have provided direction for a ten-year drive to improve health. Individuals, organizations, and communities have been challenged to change personal behaviors and their environments to promote good health. These goals and objectives are under continuous review (NCHS 1995b, 1996b, 1997).

The Healthy People 2000 goals and objectives are used here to provide a framework for reviewing, in terms of the descriptors in Figure 1.4, the health of the community and associated environmental and behavioral health risks. The health of the community is examined in terms of the three goals listed above that address specific diseases in the U.S. population. Environmental health risks are addressed by a series of health protection objectives, and the behavioral risks by the health promotion objectives. Out of the over 300 specific objectives, 47 sentinel objectives have been identified. Progress toward these sentinel objectives is summarized in Appendix 1.1 and is highlighted in the discussion that follows, based on the 1995 and 1996 mid-course reviews (NCHS 1995b, 1996b).

Health promotion

The health promotion objectives relate to physical activity, nutrition, tobacco use, alcohol and other drug use, family planning, mental health and mental disorders, violent and abusive behavior, and the development of educational and community-based programs. Progress on these objectives is mixed (see Appendix 1.1).

More people, 24 percent, were exercising regularly, but this rate still fell short of the objective of 30 percent. The proportion of people who reported never exercising, 24 percent, has not changed since the baseline measurement. The proportion overweight, 34 percent, actually increased and moved further from the goal of 20 percent, although the proportion of the U.S. population consuming lower-fat diets was reportedly moving in the desired direction.

The 26 percent of the U.S. population who reported smoking represented a decrease, but nonetheless still fell short of the objective of 15 percent, as did the proportion of youth who started smoking (30 percent versus a target of 15 percent). Alcohol use (21.6 percent versus the objective of 12.6 percent) and marijuana use (6 percent versus the objective of 3.2 percent) among youth remained higher than the desired objectives, but were moving in the right direction. The goal of reducing alcohol-related automobile deaths (5.5 per 100,000) is being approached (6.4 per 100,000).

Teen pregnancies, at 74.6 per 1,000 births, fetal losses, and abortions, were moving away from, rather than toward, the objective of 50.0. Suicides (11.6 per 100,000 persons versus the objective of 10.5) had decreased only slightly, but the rate of people reporting stress-related problems, 39.2 percent, had declined toward the objective of 35 percent. Both assault-related injuries (12.7 per 100,000 persons versus the objective of 8.7) and homicides (10.6 per 100,000 persons versus the objective of 7.2) increased rather than diminished.

Health protection

The principal health protection objectives relate to unintentional injuries, occupational safety and health, environmental health, food and drug safety, and oral health (see Appendix 1.1).

Unintentional injuries at 29.8 per 100,000 persons were essentially at the objective level of 29.3, but seatbelt use at 67 percent had not yet reached the desired level of 85 percent. In terms of occupational safety and health, work-related injuries (8.4 per 100,000 persons) were moving away from rather than toward the objective of 6.0. Work-related deaths (5 per 100,000 persons), on the other hand, were moving toward the objective of 4. Children with blood lead at levels of 15 µg/dL or higher numbered 503,000, still short of the objective of 300,000. Many more people, 75.1 percent, lived in communities with clean air, although this level was still short of the goal of 85 percent. Only 11 percent of people (versus the objective of 40 percent) lived in radon-tested homes. Salmonella outbreaks were down to 44 versus the objective of 25 per year. The prevalence of dental caries among children (54 percent) and edentulousness among the elderly (30 percent) diminished, but remained short of the desired goals of 35 percent and 20 percent, respectively.

Preventive services

The preventive services objectives encompass maternal and infant health, heart disease and stroke, cancer, diabetes, HIV infection, sexually transmitted diseases, immunization and infectious diseases, and clinical preventive services (see Appendix 1.1).

For maternal and infant health, the Healthy People 2000 goal was to achieve 90 percent of mothers having prenatal care in the first trimester, and a rate of only 5 percent of newborns with low birth weight. As of the 1995–96 review, although moving in the right direction, neither goal had been achieved, with 80.2 percent of mothers getting first trimester prenatal care and 7.3 percent of infants having low birth weights.

Both heart disease mortality rates and lower cholesterol levels were well on the way to being achieved with heart disease mortality at 114 per 100,000 people (versus the objective of 100), and average cholesterol levels at 205 mg/dl (versus the objective of 200). Stroke deaths were more slowly approaching the objective of 20 per 100,000 persons (versus 26.7), while the proportion of those with hypertension who had it controlled (29 percent) was just over half of the desired goal of 50 percent.

Cancer deaths overall at 132 per 100,000 persons were slowly being reduced to the objective of 130. Screening rates for breast cancer (56 percent versus the objective of 60 percent) and cervical cancer (94 percent, which was almost the same as the desired rate of 95 percent) were rapidly being achieved. Fecal occult blood testing screening for colo-rectal cancer, at 30 percent, still fell considerably short of the objective of 50 percent.

Diabetes-related deaths at 38 per 100,000 persons were not closer to the goal of 34 than they were at the baseline. The prevalence of chronic disabling conditions due to diabetes (10.3 percent) actually increased, thereby widening the gap in its relationship to the objective of 8 percent .

HIV infections were at 300 per 100,000 persons, which represented a decrease relative to both the baseline and the objective of 400. Both gonorrhea and syphilis infection rates had decreased substantially from the baseline. Gonorrhea infection rates were 168 per 100,000 persons versus the objective of 100, and syphilis rates were at 8.1 per 100,000 persons—moving toward the goal of 4.0.

In terms of other infectious diseases, the objective of no measles cases had not yet been achieved; there were 301 cases nationally as of the 1996 review. Childhood immunization rates, at 75 percent, also fell short of the objective of 90 percent. Pneumonia and influenza deaths at 15.7 per 100,000 persons, mostly in adults and preventable with vaccines, have met the objective of 15.9.

In summary, although progress has been made toward achieving a number of the health goals for the nation, most have not yet been accomplished. In addition, environmental and behavioral risks remain, and the attendant health impacts for some groups in particular are significant.

Population at Risk

The population at risk may be characterized in terms of predisposing (e.g., demographics, attitudes), enabling (e.g., personal and family resources), and need (e.g., perceived and evaluated health

status) characteristics. Health status differs according to characteristics such as race, gender, and socioeconomic status (Hertzman,
Frank, and Evans 1994; NCHS 1995a), and the differences are substantial (see Appendix 1.2). For example, in the United States the
age-adjusted mortality rate from all causes in 1990 varied from a
high of 1,061.3 deaths per 100,000 population for black males to
a low of 369.9 for white females. Specific relative risk ratios were
1.6 for black versus white males and 1.7 for white males versus
white females.

The racial and gender differences were found across most of the
major causes of death, and from 1980 to 1990 most of the racial differences widened (see Appendix 1.2). For deaths from heart disease,
accidents, and cirrhosis, the gender differences exceeded racial differences. For heart disease, cancer, stroke, homicide, unintentional
injuries, HIV, cirrhosis, and diabetes mellitus, the 1990 age-adjusted
mortality rates for both black males and black females exceeded
those for their white counterparts, ranging from a relative risk ratio
of 1.2 for black versus white females dying of cancer to highs of 7.7
for black versus white males dying of homicide and 9.0 for black
versus white females dying of HIV. Many of the relative risks by
race increased over the decade from 1980 to 1990.

In summary, although progress has been made in achieving
many of the goals set out by the Healthy People Year 2000 objectives,
most remain short of the desired level of achievement. Further,
health disparities between groups remain substantial and show
little evidence of narrowing. The discussion that follows describes
the dimensions and trends of health disparities with respect to the
U.S. healthcare delivery system, while subsequent chapters introduce approaches for evaluating system performance with respect
to effectiveness, efficiency, and equity criteria, and ultimately in
contributing to improvements in the health of the U.S. population.

Delivery System

The discussion that follows highlights the availability, organization,
and financing of the U.S. healthcare system, focusing in particular
on the major changes that have taken place over the past three
decades. Much of the information is based on an annual publication

of the National Center for Health Statistics, *Health: United States* (NCHS 1997).

Availability

In the 1960s, a worsening physician shortage was perceived to exist in the United States. In response, federal and state governments greatly expanded investment in medical schools, which resulted in a corresponding increase in the number of medical graduates. These trends raised subsequent concerns in the 1980s and 1990s about a burgeoning physician surplus (NCHS 1997, 232, 239; Reinhardt 1991).

The surplus was anticipated to be even greater due to the rapid growth in managed care organizations (Politzer et al. 1996; Weiner 1994). Group and staff model HMOs in particular use more generalists and fewer specialists than the fee-for-service sector. Forecasts suggest that unless more generalist physicians are produced, there may be a shortage in that area, with the surplus of specialists being commensurately higher. An even greater imbalance will ensue if managed care programs increase their use of non-physician providers for the delivery of primary care.

The hospital industry has also undergone tremendous changes during the past 30 years. These include the rapid advancement in medical technology; an expansion in outpatient services; a growth in multihospital systems; the emergence of increased competition among hospitals and between hospitals and other providers; increasing mergers and conversion of community nonprofit hospitals to for-profit status; and a fundamental change in the Medicare payment system that supplies about half of the hospital revenue in the United States. The shift, described in more detail later in this chapter, has been from a retrospective reimbursement system to a prospective payment system (PPS) based on diagnosis-related groups (DRGs) (NCHS 1997, 243, 245, 246).

Organization

Managed care systems. Managed care encompasses various forms of health maintenance organizations (HMOs), point-of-service plans (POSs), and preferred provider organizations (PPOs). HMOs are organizations that guarantee delivery of a comprehensive prepaid benefit package to a voluntarily enrolled population through an organized system of care. POSs represent HMOs that offer partial reimbursement for services that an enrollee chooses to obtain outside of the HMO network. PPOs contract to provide services at a discounted rate under conditions of utilization review that offer providers a wider network of enrolled populations, and enrolled populations a wider choice of providers, while restricting the scope or increasing the out-of-pocket costs of the benefits provided (Havlicek 1996; Reinhardt 1996).

HMO plans and enrollment have grown since the early 1970s. HMOs have also become vigorous competitors of traditional health insurance plans in several metropolitan areas, enrolling about 22.3 percent of the U.S. population (or 52.5 million persons) in 1996 (NCHS 1997, 271, 283). Trends also include growth in for-profit managed care plans, such as PPOs and nontraditional HMOs that allow enrollees to select a non-HMO provider in exchange for a financial penalty. In 1995, 73 percent of Americans who received health insurance through an employer were enrolled in managed care (Jensen et al. 1997). The most rapid growth in the early 1990s was in enrollment in PPOs and POSs. By 1994, the majority of HMO members (58 percent) were enrolled in for-profit plans (Gabel 1997).

As growth in the commercial market slowed in the early to mid-1990s, HMOs began to compete vigorously to enroll public beneficiaries. Medicare enrollment in HMOs was 4 million in 1996, 10 percent of beneficiaries. Strong growth is projected to continue into the next century, reaching one-third of beneficiaries by 2007 (Lamphere et al. 1997). The growth of Medicaid managed care arrangements will be discussed later in this chapter.

Physician organizations. Thirty-four percent of nonfederal physicians worked in group practice settings in 1995, compared to 10.6 percent in 1965. The mean size of physician groups increased from 6.6 to 10.5 physicians during the same period. Eighty-five percent of groups contracted with one or more HMOs, and 16 percent did business with HMOs on a referral basis. Eighty-four percent of groups contracted with one or more PPOs (Havlicek 1996).

Hospitals. About one percent of hospitals changed ownership status each year between 1980 and 1995, but most of the change was concentrated in California, Florida, Georgia, and Texas

(Needleman, Chollett, and Lamphere 1997). Among those converting, three out of four public hospitals converted to not-for-profit status, and 63 percent of not-for-profit hospitals converted to for-profit status. Another reaction to managed care and other cost-containment strategies has been the development of strategic alliances between hospitals. In the proprietary sector, large hospital corporations began purchasing hospitals in different markets and instituting centralized and standardized management practices to achieve greater efficiency and profits. Not-for-profit hospitals began affiliations with hospitals in their region of the country to establish referral patterns and share services, and possibly for protection against the expansion of the proprietary chains (Luke, Begun, and Pointer 1989). This move to horizontal integration has been followed by efforts to achieve vertical integration. Hospital systems and physician groups are increasingly forming organized systems of care (Shortell and Hull 1996).

Public health. In 1992–93 there were approximately 2,000 local public health departments in the United States, distributed among county (56 percent), city/county (13 percent), multi-county (11 percent), town/township (11 percent), city (7 percent), and other (2 percent) organizational entities. This number represents a decrease of about 10 percent from 1989. These departments were funded through a variety of sources: state government (40 percent of total department funds), local government (34 percent), fees (7 percent), Medicaid (7 percent), federal government (6 percent), Medicare (3 percent), and other sources (3 percent) (National Association of County and City Health Officials [NACCHO] 1995). The personnel who worked in these departments included environmental workers (36 percent of all personnel), public health nurses (23 percent), administrators (20 percent), health educators (10 percent), and others (11 percent) (U.S. Department of Health and Human Services [USDHHS] 1992).

The services they provided included immunizations (96 percent of departments), tuberculosis screening and treatment (86 percent), health education (84 percent), well-baby care (79 percent), Women, Infants and Children (WIC) Program services (78 percent), testing and counseling for sexually transmitted diseases (71 percent), treatment for sexually transmitted diseases (66 percent), family planning (68 percent), HIV testing and counseling (68 percent), dental health (45 percent), HIV treatment (33 percent), and primary care (30 percent) (NACCHO 1995).

A 1995 study of public health expenditures in nine states revealed that two of every three dollars spent on public health services ($6.1 billion of $8.8 billion) went for personal health services (Eilbert et al. 1996). Population-based health services spending was $2.7 billion ($43 per capita), and represented only one percent of the total healthcare expenditures ($3,342 per capita) in the participating states. The largest amount of this ($2.7 billion) went to enforcing laws and regulations that protect the health and ensure the safety of the public (26 percent), while training (4 percent) and research (2 percent) received the smallest investments.

Health departments face major new challenges today. One is the financial vulnerability of their primary care clinics in this time of movement to managed care. Another is concern about the provision of preventive services as clients traditionally served by these public health clinics are moved into private sector medical care (Pearson, Spencer, and Jenkins 1995). These challenges are calling upon health departments to reconsider their mission, and ways in which it can be accomplished. Among the responses have been renewed interest in public-private cooperative agreements, and a national medicine/public health initiative (Gabel 1997; The Medicine/Public Health Initiative 1997). At the same time, other organizations, such as community agencies, hospitals, clinics, and managed care organizations, have begun to provide some traditional public health services.

Financing

Payment arrangements. Until the 1980s, physicians in the United States controlled their means of payment and the amount they could charge through fee-for-service reimbursement. This led to high physician incomes relative to the average full-time employee as well as to other professionals (Organization for Economic Cooperation and Development [OECD] 1996), and to healthcare delivery practices that were both inefficient and inequitable. The fee-for-service system resulted in overpayments for procedural care at the expense of visits and consultations, physicians providing identical services yet receiving very different fees, and systems of charges and reimbursement that were both difficult to understand and complex to administer (Simon and Born 1996).

A new physician payment system under Medicare, the resource-based relative value scale (RBRVS), was developed in the early 1980s in response to these problems (Physician Payment Review Commission [PPRC] 1991). The relative value was the sum of physician work, practice expense, and malpractice costs, adjusted for geographic cost differences and converted to dollars using a conversion factor. The attempt was to develop a physician payment system that would (1) rationalize fee-for-service payments under Medicare, (2) reduce the rate of growth in physician expenditures, (3) protect access to care for Medicare enrollees, and (4) support quality care (Epstein and Blumenthal 1993).

The implementation of Medicare's prospective payment system in 1984 was the cornerstone for a corresponding movement to contain hospital costs. Under PPS, hospitals are paid a prospectively determined amount per discharge, rather than on a retrospective reasonable-cost basis. Payment varies by DRG category and is updated annually to reflect changes in a hospital input price index (Russell 1989).

Hospital payment also has been sharply affected by the growth in managed care and competition in the private sector. Resulting developments include hospitals increasingly engaging in cost cutting, mergers, forging closer relations with physicians and other providers, assumption of insurance functions, and contracting directly with employers. The result for most hospitals has been stable, rather than deteriorating, and in some cases improved, financial status (Duke 1996).

Expenditures and costs. National healthcare expenditures (NHE) for the complex and highly technological U.S. medical care enterprise were $988.5 billion in 1995 compared to $26.9 billion in 1960. For the same period, healthcare expenditures grew from $141 to $3,621 per capita and from 5.1 to 13.6 percent of the gross domestic product (GDP) (NCHS 1997, 249).

While all national healthcare expenditures have grown, the 30-year shifts in the distribution of spending for services has been mainly toward nursing home and home care. Hospitals still represent the largest sector, followed by expenditures for physician services. Although the absolute levels of expenditures increased, the relative share for drugs and other medical nondurables declined over this same period (NCHS 1997, 254).

The growth in personal healthcare expenditures (i.e., in spending for the direct provision of care) increased sharply after the passage of Medicare and Medicaid in 1965 and continued a strong upward trend in the 1970s, a period of high general inflation. Growth declined initially in the 1980s in response to cost-containment measures and the decline in general inflation. However, average annual cost increases continued between 9 to 10 percent during the late 1980s and early 1990s. Growth in personal healthcare expenditures slowed in the mid-1990s, however (Levit et al. 1996, 132; NCHS 1997, 254). The major factors affecting growth in personal health expenditures have been economy-wide inflation, medical price inflation in excess of general inflation, the increased use and intensity of services per capita, and more recently, slower growth in healthcare spending and increased growth in the gross domestic product (GDP) (Levit et al. 1991; 1996).

Government and private insurers have increased their roles in financing healthcare services in the United States. Government programs covered 44 percent (12 percent state and local and 32 percent federal) of the cost in 1994, almost double the proportion covered in 1960 (Levit et al. 1991, 50; Levit et al. 1996, 141). Around 18 percent of personal health expenditures were paid for out of pocket in 1994, compared to 56 percent in 1960. Private insurance, primarily including Blue Cross and Blue Shield plans, employer self-insurance, independent plans, and commercial insurance companies, covered 33 percent of the cost in 1994, compared to 21 percent in 1960. Despite the growth in government and private insurance, there were 40.6 million uninsured persons in 1995, and an equal or greater number without adequate insurance coverage (NCHS 1997, 284). (Additional evidence on the uninsured will be presented in Chapter 7.)

Realized Access

Health services research has documented substantial variations by geography in the levels of medical care resources, in the rates of administering various medical diagnostic procedures, and in the rates of performing surgical operations. These variations have, however, not been correspondingly associated with variations in health outcomes. The discussion that follows focuses on this variations evidence. Descriptive information on widely used indicators of the utilization of and satisfaction with healthcare will be highlighted in Chapter 7.

Glover (1938) is credited with first reporting the phenomenon of variations in the rate of surgical procedures, specifically for tonsillectomy rates in England. Since then a host of studies have reported findings of variations in rates for common surgical procedures within a state (Lewis 1969; Wennberg and Gittelsohn 1973) of the United States, within a Canadian province (Roos 1984), within a country (McPherson et al. 1981; Wennberg, Bunker, and Barnes 1980), and between countries (Bunker 1970; McPherson et al. 1981, 1982; Vayda 1973; Wennberg, Bunker, and Barnes 1980). All of these studies have found that the rates for common surgical procedures being done can vary as much as five- and sixfold from one geographic area of a state to another and as much as two and threefold between countries. In addition, the same has been found for the rates of various diagnostic and medical procedures within the United States (Chassin et al. 1986; Wennberg 1990). Wennberg (1990), using data from 16 university hospital or large community hospital market areas, found that the ratios of high to low varied from 2.0 for inguinal hernia repair to 3.6 for coronary artery bypass graft (CABG) surgery and 19.4 for carotid endarterectomy.

In summary, dramatic changes are under way in the U.S. healthcare system, as managed care comes to increasingly dominate the provision of and payment for medical care services. Trends in healthcare expenditures suggest that these changes may offer some promising constraints on the continued increases in healthcare costs. Nonetheless, wide variations in the patterns of providing medical care prevail across regions and delivery settings.

The discussion that follows reviews Medicaid managed care, a major healthcare reform initiative that is being developed and implemented in many states, as an attempt to address the array of quality, cost, and access issues identified here.

An Application: Medicaid Managed Care

Medicaid managed care, an important policy issue being addressed at the federal and state levels, offers a timely and relevant example to illustrate the application of the concepts of effectiveness, efficiency, and equity.

The economic problems faced by state Medicaid programs mirror those faced by other payors. The program was designed according to private insurance specifications prevailing in 1965. Key elements were fee-for-service payment of providers, free choice of provider by beneficiaries, and reimbursement from third party intermediaries. This combination, along with eligibility expansion, resulted in expenditure growth that was much greater than originally predicted. Total expenditures increased from $27 billion in 1981 to $151.3 billion in 1995 (Kaiser Commission on the Future of Medicaid 1997). State government was responsible for 43 percent of the bill in 1995. Without the ability to incur deficits, states soon faced difficult decisions regarding state resource allocation and control of Medicaid costs.

States have tried a number of separate unsuccessful policies to address Medicaid costs. They have limited benefits to enrollees and payments to providers; instituted utilization review, rate setting, and health planning; and curtailed other state spending priorities—such as public education.

The particular appeal of managed care arrangements for Medicaid programs lies in addressing the interlocking, mutually reinforcing problems endemic to the programs that have not been responsive to single-focus interventions (Freund and Hurley 1995; Hurley and Freund 1991). Concerns about escalating program costs contributed to disappointing payment levels and declining provider participation. Limited provider involvement resulted in corresponding diminished access to quality services, especially to mainstream primary care providers and to obstetricians and gynecologists. This diminished access led to reliance on inappropriate sites of care that are unnecessarily costly and lack the capacity to provide continuity and coordination of services (e.g., emergency rooms), or that are high-volume providers of questionable competence (e.g., the so-called Medicaid mills). This syndrome of related problems has demanded concerted efforts to attempt to deal with them. A variety of managed care models have been introduced in response.

Unlike the private sector, Medicaid initially relied on primary care case management (PCCM) and limited-risk prepaid health plans. Under PCCM, primary care providers are paid a monthly fee per patient to approve and monitor medical services for assigned beneficiaries, but do not assume financial risk. Limited-risk prepaid plans contract on a risk or non-risk basis to provide a limited range of services (e.g., ambulatory care). The number of Medicaid beneficiaries in managed care plans reached 12.8 million in 1996, and they were enrolled in 511 separate organizations, 349 of which were HMOs. HMOs enrolled 63 percent of the Medicaid managed care enrollees, with 31 percent in PCCM plans, 4 percent in health insuring organizations (HIOs), and 2 percent in prepaid health plans (PPRC 1997). This represented an increase of 12.5 million since 1981, when passage of the Omnibus Budget Reconciliation Act (OBRA) enabled substantial numbers of Medicaid beneficiaries to be enrolled in managed care plans. Managed care enrollment in 1996 represented 38.6 percent of all Medicaid beneficiaries and 50 percent of low-income adults and children covered by Medicaid.

The theoretical presumption underlying Medicaid managed care is that by enrolling individuals in managed care plans and restricting access to certain providers faced with financial incentives and utilization controls, one can simultaneously control cost, coordinate care, and ensure access to needed medical services for low-income populations. While these assumptions are appealing, analysts have difficulty documenting the effectiveness and efficiency of Medicaid managed care. Meaningful healthcare cost control would provide an opportunity, however, to allocate more state funds to education and social programs that, in the long run, may have a greater impact on the health of the population.

The shift of public beneficiaries to commercial HMOs nonetheless has financially threatened the community-based providers that have tended to serve the vulnerable population. HMOs enroll patients that have traditionally been served by teaching hospitals and thereby siphon away revenues and cases from medical education and provision of service to the uninsured. These changes are forcing academic health centers and other safety net providers to develop a variety of cost-cutting and strategic alliance strategies (Blumenthal and Meyer 1996; Lairson et al. 1997). Thus, Medicaid managed care raises important equity of access research questions and policy issues for state and federal decision makers.

Payors and policymakers are struggling to formulate policy to address these problems in the context of the uniquely pluralistic American healthcare system. Attention is focused on the medical care system due primarily to the nation's large and growing investment in the system. Ironically, medical care may draw resources and policy attention away from programs that address problems of the social and physical environment, which are the root causes of many health problems. The challenge, therefore, is to achieve a better balance between the corporate- and community-level efforts to address simultaneously the demand to cure and care for current health problems and the need to mitigate those environmental and behavioral health risks that give rise to them.

The chapters that follow examine the conceptual, methodological, and empirical underpinnings of the effectiveness, efficiency, and equity objectives of the U.S. healthcare system. Health services research regarding Medicaid managed care is reviewed to illustrate the application of health services research to health policy in the light of these objectives.

In the final chapter the relationship of health services research and policy analysis is described and illustrated by comparing alternative state healthcare reform options using criteria derived from effectiveness, efficiency, and equity research.

Note

1. More generally, we are concerned about allocating resources among all possible goods and services to achieve maximum social welfare (or well-being).

References

Abraham, L. K. 1993. *Mama Might Be Better Off Dead: The Failure of Health Care in Urban America*. Chicago: University of Chicago Press.

Aday, L. A. 1993. *At Risk in America: The Health and Health Care Needs of Vulnerable Populations in The United States*. San Francisco: Jossey-Bass.

Aday, L. A., C. E. Begley, D. R. Lairson, and C. H. Slater. 1993. *Evaluating the Medical Care System: Effectiveness, Efficiency, and Equity*, 1st ed. Chicago: Health Administration Press.

Adler, N. E., T. Boyce, M. A. Chesney, S. Cohen, S. Folkman, R. L. Kahn, and S. L. Syme. 1994. "Socioeconomic Status and Health: The Challenge of the Gradient." *American Psychologist* 49: 15–24.

Altman, D. E., and D. H. Morgan. 1983. "The Role of State and Local Government In Health." *Health Affairs* 2 (4): 7–31.

Altman, S. H., and U. E. Reinhardt, eds. 1996. *Strategic Choices for a Changing Health Care System.* Chicago: Health Administration Press.

Anderson, O. W. 1991. *The Evolution of Health Services Research: Personal Reflections on Applied Social Science.* San Francisco: Jossey-Bass.

Blumenthal, D., and G. S. Meyer. 1996. "Academic Health Centers in a Changing Environment." *Health Affairs* 15 (2): 200–215.

Brown, L. D. 1991. "Knowledge and Power: Health Services Research as a Political Resource." In *Health Services Research: Key to Health Policy.* Edited by E. Ginzberg, 20–45. Cambridge, MA: Harvard University Press.

Brown, P. 1995. "Race, Class, and Environmental Health: A Review and Systematization of the Literature." *Environmental Research* 69: 15–30.

Bunker, J. P. 1970. "Surgical Manpower: A Comparison of Operations and Surgeons in the United States and in England and Wales." *The New England Journal of Medicine* 282: 135–44.

Chassin, M. R., R. H. Brook, R. E. Park, J. Keesey, A. Fink, J. Kosecoff, K. Kahn, N. Merrick, and D. H. Solomon. 1986. "Variations in the Use of Medical and Surgical Services by the Medicare Population." *The New England Journal of Medicine* 314: 285–90.

Choi, T., and J. N. Greenberg. 1982. *Social Science Approaches to Health Services Research.* Chicago: Health Administration Press.

DeFriese, G. H., T. C. Ricketts III, and J. S. Stein, eds. 1989. *Methodological Advances in Health Services Research.* Chicago: Health Administration Press.

Duke, K. S. 1996. "Hospitals in a Changing Health Care System." *Health Affairs* 15 (2): 49–61.

Dunn, W. N. 1994. *Public Policy Analysis: An Introduction.* 2nd ed. Englewood Cliffs, NJ: Prentice Hall.

Eilbert, K. W., M. Barry, R. Bialek, and M. Garufi. 1996. *Measuring Expenditures for Essential Public Health Services.* Washington, D.C.: Public Health Foundation.

Epstein, A. M., and D. Blumenthal. 1993. Physician Payment Reform: Past and Future. *Milbank Quarterly* 71: 193–215.

Evans, R. G., M. L. Barer, and T. R. Marmor, eds. 1994. *Why Are Some People Healthy and Others Not? The Determinants of Health of Populations.* New York: Aldine De Gruyter.

Feinstein, J. S. 1993. "The Relationship Between Socioeconomic Status and Health: A Review of The Literature." *Milbank Quarterly* 71: 279–322.

Flook, E. E., and P. J. Sanazaro, eds. 1973. *Health Services Research and R & D in Perspective*. Chicago: Health Administration Press.

Freund, D. A., and R. E. Hurley. 1995. "Medicaid Managed Care: Contribution to Issues of Health Reform." *Annual Review of Public Health* 16: 473–95.

Gabel, J. 1997. "Ten Ways HMOs Have Changed During the 1990s." *Health Affairs* 16 (3): 134–45.

Ginzberg, E., ed. 1991. *Health Services Research: Key to Health Policy*. Cambridge, MA: Harvard University Press.

Glover, J. A. 1938. "The Incidence of Tonsillectomy in School Children." *Proceedings of the Royal Society of Medicine* 31: 1219–36.

Goldfarb, T., ed. 1997. *Taking Sides. Clashing Views on Controversial Environmental Issues*. 7th ed. Guilford, CT: Dushkin/McGraw-Hill.

Havlicek, P. L. 1996. *Medical Groups in the U.S.: A Survey of Practice Characteristics*. Chicago: American Medical Association.

Hertzman, C., J. Frank, and R. G. Evans. 1994. "Heterogeneities in Health Status and the Determinants of Population Health." In *Why Are Some People Healthy and Others Not? The Determinants of Health of Populations*. Edited by R. G. Evans, M. L. Barer, and T. R. Marmor, 67–92. New York: Aldine De Gruyter.

Hurley, R. E., and D. A. Freund. 1991. "Rollover Effects in Gatekeeper Programs: Cushioning the Impact of Restricted Choice." *Inquiry* 28: 375–84.

Institute of Medicine. 1979. *Report on Health Services Research*. Washington, D.C.: National Academy of Sciences.

———. 1991. *Improving Information Services for Health Services Researchers: A Report to the National Library of Medicine*. Washington, D.C.: National Academy of Sciences.

———. 1995. *Health Services Research: Work Force and Educational Issues*. Washington, D.C.: National Academy of Sciences.

Jensen, G. A., M. A. Morrisey, S. Gaffney, and D. K. Liston. 1997. "The New Dominance of Managed Care: Insurance Trends in the 1990s." *Health Affairs* 16 (1): 125–36.

Kaiser Commission on the Future of Medicaid. 1997. *Medicaid Facts: Medicaid and Managed Care*. Washington, D.C.: Kaiser Commission on Managed Care.

Lairson, D. R., G. Schulmeier, C. E. Begley, L. A. Aday, Y. Coyle, and C. H. Slater. 1997. "Managed Care and Community-Oriented Care: Conflict or Complement." *Journal of Health Care for the Poor and Underserved* 8: 36–55.

Lamphere, J. A., P. Neuman, K. M. Langwell, and S. Sherman. 1997. "The Surge in Medicare Managed Care: An Update." *Health Affairs* 16 (3): 127–33.

Lee, P. R., and A. E. Benjamin. 1993. "Health Policy and the Politics of Health Care." In *Introduction to Health Services*, 4th ed. Edited by S. J. Williams and P. R. Torrens, 399–420. New York: Delmar Publishers Inc.

Levit, K. R., H. C. Lazenby, C. A. Cowan, and S. W. Letsch. 1991. "National Health Expenditures 1990." *Health Care Financing Review* 13 (1): 29–54.

Levit, K. R., H. C. Lazenby, and L. Sivarajan. 1996. "Health Care Spending in 1994: Slowest in Decades." *Health Affairs* 15 (2): 130–144.

Lewis, C. E. 1969. "Variations in the Incidence of Surgery." *The New England Journal of Medicine* 281: 880–884.

Longest, B. B. Jr. 1994. *Health Policymaking in the United States*. Chicago: AUPHA Press/Health Administration Press.

Luke, R. D., J. W. Begun, and D. D. Pointer. 1989. "Quasi Firms: Strategic Interorganizational Forms in the Health Care Industry." *Academy of Management Review* 14: 9–19.

McKinney, M. L., and R. M. Schoch. 1996. *Environmental Science: Systems and Solutions*. Minneapolis: West Publishing Company.

McPherson, K., P. M. Strong, A. Epstein, and L. Jones. 1981. "Regional Variations in the Use of Common Surgical Procedures: Within and Between England and Wales, Canada, and the United States of America." *Social Science and Medicine* 15 (Part A): 273–88.

McPherson, K., J. E. Wennberg, O. B. Hovind, and P. Clifford. 1982. "Small-Area Variations in the Use of Common Surgical Procedures: An International Comparison of New England, England, and Norway." *The New England Journal of Medicine* 307: 1310–14.

National Association of County and City Health Officials. 1995. *1992–1993 National Profile of Local Health Departments*. Washington, D.C.: The National Association of County and City Health Officials.

National Center for Health Statistics. 1983. *Health, United States, 1983 and Injury Profile*, DHHS Pub. No. (PHS) 84-1232. Hyattsville, MD: Public Health Service.

———. 1995a. *Health, United States, 1994*, DHHS Pub. No. (PHS) 95-1232. Hyattsville, MD: Public Health Service.

———. 1995b. *Healthy People 2000—Midcourse Review and 1995 Revisions*, Hyattsville, MD: Public Health Service.

———. 1996a. *Health, United States, 1995*, DHHS Pub. No. (PHS) 96-1232. Hyattsville, MD: Public Health Service.

———. 1996b. *Healthy People 2000 Review, 1995–96*, Hyattsville, MD: Public Health Service.

————. 1997. *Health, United States, 1996–97 and Injury Chartbook*. Hyattsville, MD: Public Health Service.

Needleman, J., D. Chollet, and J. A. Lamphere. 1997. "Hospital Conversion Trends." *Health Affairs* 16 (2): 187–95.

Organization for Economic Cooperation and Development. 1996. *OECD Health Data 1996*. Paris, France: OECD.

Pearson, T. A., M. Spencer, and P. Jenkins. 1995. "Who Will Provide Preventive Services? The Changing Relationships Between Medical Care Systems and Public Health Agencies in Health Care Reform." *Journal of Public Health Management and Practice* 1 (1): 16–27.

Peterson, M. A. 1995. "How Health Policy Information Is Used in Congress." In *Intensive Care: How Congress Shapes Health Policy*. Edited by T. E. Mann and N. J. Ornstein, 79–125. Washington, D.C.: American Enterprise Institute, The Brookings Institution.

Physician Payment Review Commission. 1991. *Annual Report to Congress, 1991*. Washington, D.C.: Physician Payment Review Commission.

————. 1997. *Annual Report to Congress, 1997*. Washington, D.C.: Physician Payment Review Commission.

Politzer, R. M., S. R. Gamliel, J. M. Cultice, C. M. Bazell, M. L. Rivo, and F. Mullan. 1996. "Matching Physician Supply and Requirements: Testing Policy Recommendations." *Inquiry* 33: 181–94.

Reinhardt, U. E. 1991. "Health Manpower Forecasting: The Case of Physician Supply." In *Health Services Research: Key to Health Policy*. Edited by E. Ginzberg, 234–83. Cambridge, MA: Harvard University Press.

————. 1996. "A Social Contract for the 21st Century Health Care: Three-Tier Health Care with Bounty Hunting." *Health Economics* 5: 479–99.

Roos, N. P. 1984. "Hysterectomy: Variations in Rates Across Small Areas and Across Physicians' Practices." *American Journal of Public Health* 74: 327–35.

Roos, N. P., C. Black, N. Frohlich, C. DeCoster, M. Cohen, D. J. Tataryn, C. A. Mustard, L. L. Roos, F. Toll, K. C. Carrière, C. A. Burchill, L. MacWilliam, and B. Bogdanovic. 1996. "Population Health and Health Care Use: An Information System for Policy Makers." *Milbank Memorial Fund Quarterly* 74: 3–31.

Russell, L. B. 1989. *Medicare's New Hospital Payment System: Is It Working?* Washington, D.C.: The Brookings Institution.

Shi, L. 1997. *Health Services Research Methods*. Albany, NY: Delmar Publishers Inc.

Shortell, S. M., and K. E. Hull. 1996. "The New Organization of the Health Care Delivery System." In *Strategic Choices for a Changing Health Care System*. Edited by S. H. Altman, and U. E. Reinhardt, 101–48. Chicago: Health Administration Press.

Shortell, S. M., and U. E. Reinhardt, eds. 1992. *Improving Health Policy and Management: Nine Critical Research Issues for the 1990s.* Chicago: Health Administration Press.

Shortell, S. M., and W. C. Richardson. 1978. *Health Program Evaluation.* St. Louis: C. V. Mosby.

Simon, C. J., and P. H. Born. 1996. "Physician Earnings in a Changing Managed Care Environment." *Health Affairs* 15 (3): 124–33.

Syme, S. L., and L. F. Berkman. 1976. "Social Class, Susceptibility And Sickness." *American Journal of Epidemiology* 104: 1–8.

The Medicine/Public Health Initiative. 1997. The Medicine/Public Health Initiative [Online]. Available: http://www.sph.uth.tmc.edu/mph/ [09/17/97].

Turnock, B. J. 1997. *Public Health: What It Is and How It Works.* Gaithersburg, MD: Aspen Publishers.

U.S. Department of Health and Human Services. 1992. *Health Personnel in the United States, Eighth Report to Congress 1991.*Washington, D.C.: Health Resources and Services Agency and Public Health Service.

U.S. National Library of Medicine. 1997. NICHSR Introduction to HSR: Class Manual. Brief History: Issues of Health Services in the United States [Online]. Available: http://www.nlm.nih.gov/nichsr/ihcm/ hsrchist.html [07/17/97].

Vayda, E. 1973. "A Comparison of Surgical Rates in Canada and in England and Wales." *The New England Journal of Medicine* 289: 1224–29.

Weiner, J. P. 1994. "Forecasting the Effects of Health Reform on U.S. Physician Workforce Requirement: Evidence From HMO Staffing Patterns." *Journal of the American Medical Association* 272: 222–30.

Wennberg, J. E. 1990. "Small Area Analysis and the Medical Care Outcome Problem." *Research Methodology: Strengthening Causal Interpretations of Nonexperimental Data.* Edited by L. Sechrest, E. Perrin, and J. Bunker. Pub. No. PHS 90-3454. Rockville, MD: Agency for Health Care Policy and Research.

Wennberg, J. E., J. P. Bunker, and B. Barnes. 1980. "The Need for Assessing the Outcome of Common Medical Practices." *Annual Review of Public Health* 1: 277–95.

Wennberg, J. E., and A. Gittelsohn. 1973. "Small Area Variations in Health Care Delivery." *Science* 182: 1102–8.

White, K. L. 1992. *Health Services Research: An Anthology*, Scientific Publication No. 534. Washington D.C.: Pan American Health Organization, Pan American Sanitary Bureau, Regional Office of the World Health Organization.

Whiteis, D. G. 1997. "Unhealthy Cities: Corporate Medicine, Community

Economic Underdevelopment, and Public Health." *International Journal of Health Services* 27: 227–42.

Wilson, W. J. 1980. *The Declining Significance of Race: Blacks and Changing American Institutions*, 2nd ed. Chicago: The University of Chicago Press.

———. 1987. *The Truly Disadvantaged: The Inner City, the Underclass, and Public Policy*. Chicago: The University of Chicago Press.

———. 1989. "The Ghetto Underclass: Social Science Perspectives." *The Annals of the American Academy of Political and Social Science* 501 (Entire Volume).

World Health Organization. 1994. *WHO Progress Towards Health For All: Statistics of Member States 1994*. Albany, NY: WHO Publications Office.

Objective	Baseline	1995–96 Update	Year 2000 Targets
HEALTH PROMOTION			
1. Physical Activity			
1.3 more people exercising regularly	22%	24%	30%
1.5 fewer people never exercising	24%	24%	15%
2. Nutrition			
2.3 fewer people overweight	26%	34%	20%
2.5 lower fat diets	36%	34%	30%
3. Tobacco			
3.4 fewer people smoking cigarettes	29%	26%	15%
3.5 fewer youth beginning to smoke	30%	30%	15%
4. Alcohol and other drugs			
4.1 fewer alcohol-related automobile deaths (per 100,000)	9.8	6.4	5.5
4.6 less alcohol use among youth ages 12–17 years	25.2%	21.6%	12.6%
4.6 less marijuana use among youth ages 12–17 years	6.4%	6.0%	3.2%
5. Family planning			
5.1 fewer teen pregnancies (per 1,000)	71.1	74.6	50.0
5.2 fewer unintended pregnancies	56%	NA	30%
6. Mental health and mental disorders			
6.1 fewer suicides (per 100,000)	11.7	11.6	10.5
6.5 fewer people reporting stress-related problems	44.2%	39.2%	35%
7. Violent and abusive behavior			
7.1 fewer homicides (per 100,000)	8.5	10.6	7.2
7.6 fewer assault injuries (per 100,000)	9.7	12.7	8.7
8. Educational and community-based programs			
8.4 more schools with comprehensive school health education	2.3%	NA	75%
8.6 more workplaces with health promotion programs	65%	81%	85%
HEALTH PROTECTION			
9. Unintentional injuries			
9.1 fewer unintentional injury deaths (per 100,000)	34.7	29.8	29.3
9.2 more people using automobile safety restraints	42%	67%	85%
10. Occupational safety and health			
10.1 fewer work-related deaths (per 100,000)	6	5	4
10.2 fewer work-related injuries (per 100,000)	7.7	8.4	6.0
11. Environmental health			
11.4 no children with blood lead 15 $\mu g/dL$	3 million	503,000	300,000
11.5 more people with clear air in their communities	49.7%	75.1%	85%
11.6 more people in radon-tested houses	5%	11.0%	40%

Appendix 1.1   (*continued*)

Objective	Baseline	1995–96 Update	Year 2000 Targets
12. Food and drug safety			
12.3 fewer salmonella outbreaks	77	44	25
13. Oral health			
13.1 fewer children with dental caries	54%	54%	35%
13.4 fewer older people without teeth	36%	30%	20%
PREVENTIVE SERVICES			
14. Maternal and infant health			
14.5 fewer newborns with low weight	6.9%	7.3%	5%
14.11 more mothers with first trimester care	76.0%	80.2%	90%
15. Heart disease and stroke			
15.1 fewer coronary heart disease deaths (per 100,000)	135	114	100
15.2 fewer stroke deaths (per 100,000)	30.4	26.7	20.0
15.4 better control of high blood pressure	11%	29%	50%
15.6 lower cholesterol levels	213 mg/dL	205 mg/dL	200 mg/dL
16. Cancer			
16.1 decrease cancer deaths (per 100,000)	134	132	130
16.11 increase screening for breast cancer (age >50)	25%	56%	60%
16.12 increase screening for cervical cancer (age >18)	88%	94%	95%
16.13 increase fecal occult blood testing (age >50)	27%	30%	50%
17. Diabetes and chronic disabling conditions			
17.2 fewer people disabled by chronic conditions	9.4%	10.3%	8%
17.9 fewer diabetes-related deaths (per 100,000)	38	38	34
18. HIV infection			
18.2 slower increase in HIV infection (per 100,000)	400	300	400
19. Sexually transmitted diseases			
19.1 fewer gonorrhea infections (per 100,000)	300	168	100
19.3 fewer syphilis infections (per 100,000)	18.1	8.1	4.0
20. Immunization and infectious diseases			
20.1 no measles cases	3058	301	0
20.2 fewer pneumonia and influenza deaths (per 100,000)	19.9	15.7	15.9
20.11 higher immunization levels (ages 19–35 months)	54–64%	75%	90%
21. Clinical preventive services			
21.4 no financial barrier to recommended preventive services	16%	17.8%	0
SURVEILLANCE AND DATA SYSTEMS			
22.1 common and comparable health status indicators in use across States	0 states	51 states	40 states

Appendix 1.2   Age-Adjusted Death Rates by Selected Cause, Race, and Sex, United States, 1990 and 1980   (Rate per 100,000 Population)   Italic = 1980   Plain = 1990

	Black Male	White Male	Black Female	White Female	Relative Risk Race/Male	Relative Risk Race/Female	Relative Risk Gender/Black	Relative Risk Gender/White
Total Deaths (All Causes)	1061.3 *1112.8*	644.3 *745.3*	581.6 *631.1*	369.9 *411.1*	1.5 *1.5*	1.6 *1.5*	1.8 *1.8*	1.7 *1.8*
Heart Disease	275.9 *327.3*	202 *277.5*	168.1 *201.1*	103.1 *134.6*	1.4 *1.2*	1.6 *1.5*	1.6 *1.6*	2.0 *2.1*
Cancer	248.1 *229.9*	160.3 *160.5*	137.2 *129.7*	111.2 *107.7*	1.5 *1.4*	1.2 *1.2*	1.8 *1.8*	1.4 *1.5*
Stroke	56.1 *77.5*	27.7 *41.9*	42.7 *61.7*	23.8 *35.2*	2 *1.9*	1.8 *1.8*	1.3 *1.3*	1.2 *1.2*
Homicide	68.7 *71.9*	8.9 *10.9*	13 *13.7*	2.8 *3.2*	7.7 *6.5*	4.6 *4.3*	5.3 *5.2*	3.2 *3.4*
Accidents	62.4 *82*	46.4 *62.3*	20.4 *25.1*	17.6 *21.4*	1.3 *1.3*	1.2 *1.2*	3.1 *3.3*	2.6 *2.9*
HIV	44.2 *NA*	15 *NA*	9.9 *NA*	1.1 *NA*	2.9 *NA*	9 *NA*	4.5 *NA*	13.6 *NA*
Cirrhosis	20 *30.6*	11.5 *15.7*	8.7 *14.4*	4.8 *7*	1.7 *2*	1.8 *2.1*	2.3 *2.1*	2.4 *2.2*
Diabetes	23.6 *17.7*	11.3 *9.5*	25.4 *22.1*	9.5 *8.7*	2.1 *1.9*	2.7 *2.5*	0.9 *0.8*	1.2 *1.1*

Sources: *Health, United States, 1995*, Tables 30 and 36 (NCHS 1996a); *Health, United States, 1983*, Tables 9 and 15 (NCHS 1983).

Chapter 2

Effectiveness: Concepts and Methods

Overview

The fundamental questions posed in this chapter are (1) What is effectiveness? and (2) How should the effectiveness of healthcare be assessed? Chapter 3 considers (3) To what extent has effectiveness been achieved? and (4) What policy strategies contribute to enhancing effectiveness?

Questions of effectiveness have assumed great importance in the last decade because of the continually escalating costs of medical care; evidence of wide and unexplained variations in the rates of utilization of medical care across states and regions; community-level evidence suggesting the limited effectiveness of medical care as contrasted to non-medical factors in improving the health of populations; clinical evidence of the potential for improvement in the provision of medical care; and healthcare reform, originally attempted at the federal level and now taking place at the state level in the United States.

While the health of the population overall in the United States has improved substantially over the past century, as judged by the mortality and life expectancy figures cited in Chapter 1, the health of certain vulnerable groups has declined. Specifically, over the last century, trends make evident the near elimination of acute infectious disease mortality, sharp reductions in mortality from major chronic diseases, and resulting increases in life expectancy. But, as pointed out in Chapter 1, health status continues to differ by race as well as by other demographic variables; the differences are substantial, and from the early 1980s into the late 1990s, many disparities have widened. In addition, substantial geographic variations exist in the levels of medical care resources as well as in the rates for various medical and surgical procedures. These findings raise the questions of whether health improvements are in fact attributable to medical care or to some other factor or set of factors; whether the continuing disparities for selected groups are a result of failures in medical care; and whether geographic variations are associated with varying outcomes for patients across areas. These and related questions are addressed by effectiveness research.

This chapter presents and discusses a conceptual framework for effectiveness research. Key methods of effectiveness research from both the clinical and population perspectives are presented and illustrated. Chapter 3 categorizes the various policy strategies for enhancing population health, reviews the evidence on the effectiveness of each strategy, develops a set of criteria for assessing policy alternatives in terms of effectiveness, and presents an evaluation of Medicaid managed care as a current application of effectiveness research.

Conceptual Framework and Definitions

Two Perspectives

Effectiveness research reflects two seemingly competing, but complementary, definitions of effectiveness (see Figure 2.1). One represents a population perspective, or macrolevel view, that considers the role of physical, social, and economic environments on the health of the population. This macrodefinition is represented in the earlier conceptual work of Milio (1983) and the later work of Evans, Barer, and Marmor (1994). It can be characterized as the *epidemiology of health*. It includes in its purview both patients who have received medical care, as well as individuals in the population as a whole who have not.

The second is a clinical perspective that represents the microlevel view and focuses on the interactions of patients and providers in the medical care system and institutions and the resulting clinical improvement or health benefits achieved by patients. Research conducted from this point of view examines the impact of the

Figure 2.1   Factors Contributing to Population Health

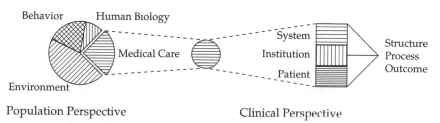

Levels of Analysis of Medical Care

Population Perspective   Clinical Perspective

Sources: Blum 1976; Lalonde 1975; and Milio 1983.

structures and processes associated with delivering medical care in achieving improvements in the health of patients. It is represented in the work of Donabedian (1966, 1980, 1982); Wennberg (1990), who has labeled this area "clinical evaluation science"; and Brook and Lohr (1985), who have called for an *epidemiology of medical care.*

Figure 2.1 displays the difference in these two views. The population perspective attends to the health of the population as a whole and to all of the factors contributing to it. The clinical perspective tends to treat the magnitude of the problem as being related only to that segment of the population utilizing medical care, and it assumes that medical care is the primary means of improving health.

Health services research related to each of these views mirrors their differing perspectives. The epidemiology of health focuses on the benefits from both medical and non-medical determinants of the health of the population, including environment, behavior, human biology, and medical care. The epidemiology of medical care, or clinical evaluation science, delineates the benefits from medical care for patients. The following example illustrates these differing views.

The National Health and Nutrition Examination Survey (NHANES) conducted by the National Center for Health Statistics periodically collects both interview and physical examination data on a representative sample of the U.S. population. Based on the 1991 survey, Burt et al. (1995) determined that of 1,000 people in the population, 204 had elevated blood pressure, that is, hypertension.

Of these 204 people, 112 were under medical care for their hypertension, and 62 had their blood pressure effectively controlled by this treatment. Translating this into the perspectives discussed, from a *clinical perspective* 62 of 112, or 55 percent, of hypertensive *patients* had their blood pressure effectively controlled, but from a *population perspective* 62 of 204, or 30 percent, of the hypertensive *individuals* in the population had their hypertension effectively controlled. The difference between the two views leads to widely varying empirical estimates of primary care effectiveness: 55 percent versus 30 percent.

The differing perspectives also explore different factors to account for the respective rates: biological or clinical factors, or patient compliance, versus social or behavioral factors, or medical care access. A point worth noting, however, is that while this description of two perspectives is instructive, a middle ground may exist between the two perspectives involving health promotion and disease prevention services that encompasses both medical and nonmedical interventions. This middle ground might be labeled *health-* (in contrast to *medical*) care, and represents the transition to a broader set of policy alternatives for improving the health of the population (see Figure 1.1).

Conceptual Frameworks

The major conceptual frameworks that guide effectiveness research derive in the population perspective from Evans, Barer, and Marmor (1994), and in the clinical perspective from the work of White, Williams, and Greenberg (1961) and Donabedian (1966). The Evans, Barer, and Marmor framework, represented in the population perspective displayed in Figure 2.1, defines the determinants of health as the physicial and social environment, human biology, individual behavior, and medical care services. White and his colleagues (1961) are responsible for describing what they termed the ecology of medical care, represented within the clinical perspective displayed in Figure 2.1 at the system, institution, and patient levels, but also including the community level as represented by the medical care component of the population perspective displayed in this figure. From the clinical perspective, Donabedian (1966) first offered the categorization of medical care in terms of structure, process, and outcomes for the purpose of determining those aspects that might be indicators of quality. This is shown in Figure 2.1 as the components that can be examined at the patient, institution, and system levels.

The four levels of effectiveness research include the *community* level, associated with the population perspective, and the *system*, *institution*, and *patient* levels, associated with the clinical perspective. *Community* includes the population as a whole and the environments in which its members reside. *System* refers to the health-care system, " . . . the resources (money, people, physical infrastructure, and technology) and the organizational configurations used to transform these resources into health care services" (Longest 1994, 2). It includes all of the elements within the system nationally or in a specific region. *Institution* refers to a specific organizational entity such as a hospital, clinic, or managed care organization. *Patient* refers to the recipient of services at the clinical level where the focus is on prevention, treatment, or follow-up, and includes an encounter between a patient and a provider. As illustrated in Figure 2.1, each of the three levels within the clinical perspective, as well as the medical care system as a component of the population perspective, can be further elaborated in terms of *structure, process,* and *outcome.*

Structure refers to "the settings in which it [narrowly, medical care, or broadly, health services] takes place and the instrumentalities of which it is the product" (Donabedian 1966, 169), where instrumentalities include the diagnostic and therapeutic procedures and interventions used in the delivery of medical care. Delivery system characteristics include the organization, specialty mix, workload, and access and convenience of care; provider characteristics of specialty training, preferences, and job satisfaction; and patient characteristics of diagnosis and condition, severity, comorbidity, and health habits (Tarlov et al. 1989). The population perspective would view this component relative to the denominator of a community's population as a whole, while the clinical perspective would lodge it in relationship to the enrollees or patients to be served by a given system or institution.

Process refers to the "set of activities that go on within and between practitioners and patients" (Donabedian 1980, 79). Examples of process variables within the clinical perspective include technical aspects such as visits, medications, referrals, test ordering, and hospitalizations; and interpersonal characteristics such as interpersonal manner, counseling, and communication level on the part of patients or enrollees (Tarlov et al. 1989). A population perspective would consider utilization rates or *de facto* (realized) access for the target population in an area.

Outcomes are defined as the "consequences to the health and welfare of individuals and of society" (Donabedian 1980, 80). Examples of clinical outcomes include endpoints such as symptoms and signs of problems, laboratory values, disability, and death; and health-related quality of life including the physical, mental, social, and role dimensions (Tarlov et al. 1989). The population perspective would focus on overall population mortality, morbidity rates, or health status.

Structure, process, and outcome are linked conceptually in a research paradigm that assumes structural elements of healthcare as having an influence on what is and is not done in the process as well as how well it is done; this process in turn influences the health outcome people experience as a result of their encounters with the process. This categorization and the implied linkage among these components has become the basic conceptualization in studying the effectiveness of medical care and its determinants. These relationships are captured in the summary framework shown in Table 2.1.

Definitions

Table 2.1 provides several illustrative definitions for the major components of the structure, process, and outcomes of care; the discussion that follows summarizes the key idea of each. *Quantity* refers to the number of physicians, nurses, and other providers as well as the quantity of monetary resources. *Efficacy* is concerned with the benefits achievable from a therapy or an intervention under ideal conditions, such as those found in a randomized clinical trial (Brook and Lohr 1985; Cochrane 1971; Sackett 1980; Williamson 1978). *Variations in use* relate to the quantity, or what is more commonly referred to as utilization, of healthcare services and procedures (Brook and Lohr 1985). It also includes the frequency or volume of procedures done.

Quality is an attribute of the healthcare process having to do both with whether the right thing is done and whether it is done well (Brook and Lohr 1985; Donabedian 1980). Quality assessment thus

Table 2.1 Dimensions of Effectiveness

STRUCTURE	PROCESS	OUTCOMES
Quantity Efficacy	Variations in Use • Quantity • Quality • Appropriateness	Effectiveness • Mortality • Morbidity • Health status
QUANTITY Refers to the number of physicians, nurses, and other providers as well as the quantity of monetary resources	VARIATIONS IN USE "different observed levels of per capita consumption of a service, especially hospital care, office visits, drugs, and specific procedures" (Brook and Lohr 1985)	EFFECTIVENESS "achieved benefit" (Williamson 1978) "Does it work?" "Does the maneuver, procedure, or service do more good than harm to those people to whom it is offered?" (Sackett 1980)
EFFICACY "maximum achievable benefit" (Williamson 1978) "Can it work?" "Does the health maneuver, procedure, or service do more good than harm to people who fully comply with the associated recommendations or treatment?" (Sackett 1980) Refers to the ability of "a particular medical action in altering the natural history of a particular disease for the better," under ideal conditions (Cochrane 1971)	QUALITY "a judgment concerning the process of care, based on the extent to which that care contributes to valued outcomes" (Donabedian 1982) "quality of medical care is that component of the difference between efficacy and effectiveness that can be attributed to care providers, taking account of the environment in which they work" (Brook and Lohr 1985) APPROPRIATENESS "refers to the extent to which available knowledge and techniques are used or misused in the management of illness and health" (Donabedian 1973)	Refers to the ability of "a particular medical action in altering the natural history of a particular disease for the better," under actual conditions of practice and use (Cochrane 1971)

deals with evaluating this aspect of the process of healthcare. *Appropriateness* is the subset of quality that concerns determining whether the right thing was done for the patient. *Effectiveness* concerns the results achieved in the actual practice of healthcare with typical patients and providers, in contrast to efficacy, which is assessed by the benefits achieved under ideal conditions (Brook and Lohr 1985; Cochrane 1971; Sackett 1980; Williamson 1978). Quality is that part of the gap between efficacy, or what is achievable, and effectiveness, or what is achieved, that can reasonably be attributed to healthcare itself.

In conclusion, the argument has been made that both the population and clinical perspectives are important in examining the effectiveness of healthcare. The population perspective argues that non-medical, as well as medical, investments are required to improve the health of individuals and communities, while the clinical perspective illuminates how enhancing the precision of medical care can contribute to this improvement.

Key Methods of Assessing Effectiveness

Two basic questions related to effectiveness were presented at the beginning of this chapter: (1) what is effectiveness, and (2) how should the effectiveness of healthcare be assessed? Table 2.2 introduces a framework for effectiveness research that attempts to integrate the two perspectives, population and clinical, and the four levels, community, system, institution, and patient, in empirically addressing these questions. The population perspective focuses on addressing these questions in the context of a community-level analysis, while the clinical perspective can seek to address them at the system, institution, or patient level of analysis, or at a combination of these levels.

The outcome measures, risk-adjustment procedures, study designs, and data sources that might be drawn upon at each level, as well as examples that illustrate the application of these methods at each of the levels, are highlighted in Table 2.2 and are discussed in the sections that follow.

| | Level of Analysis | | | |
| | Population Perspective → | Clinical Perspective → | | Patient |
	Community	System	Institution	

Outcome Measures	Mortality
	  Population death rates
	Morbidity
	  Population morbidity rates
	  Disability rates
	  Health status
	  Disease incidence & prevalence rates
	  Perceived health status
		Mortality
		  Case fatality rates
		Morbidity
		  Complication rates
		  Disability rates
		  Health status
		  Diagnosis rates
			Mortality
			  Case fatality rates
			Morbidity
			  Complication rates
			  Disability rates
			  Health status
			  Diagnosis rates
				Mortality
				  Individual deaths
				Morbidity
				  Adverse events
				  Disability limitation
				  Health status
				  Clinical endpoints

Risk Adjustment	Demographic characteristics	Averaged HRQOL Demographic characteristics Comorbidity rates Risk-adjustment systems	Averaged HRQOL Demographic characteristics Comorbidity rates Risk-adjustment systems	Health-related QOL Patient profiles Comorbidities Diagnoses

Study Designs	Observational-
	Epidemiological
		Observational-
		Interorganizational
			Observational-
			Intraorganizational
				Observational-
				Case reports/series
				Experimental – RCT
				Synthetic
				  Meta-analysis
				  Decision analysis

Data Sources	Records
	  Population health information system
	  Vital Statistics
	  Disease surveillance
	Surveys
		Records
		  Medical records
		  Discharge data
		  Claims data
		Surveys
			Records
			  Medical records
			  Discharge data
			  Claims data
			Surveys
				Records
				  Medical records
				  Discharge data
				  Claims data
				Surveys

Example *(references)*	Boston-New Haven (Wennberg et al. 1989)	Medical Outcomes Study (Tarlov et al. 1989)	Hospital Quality & Mortality (Park et al. 1990)	PORT (e.g., BPH) (Wennberg et al. 1988)

TYPICAL EFFECTIVENESS RESEARCH QUESTIONS BY LEVEL OF ANALYSIS

Community	What is the contribution of medical care to the health of the population?
System	What is the impact of system level variables (e.g., provider specialty mix, organizational form, payment mechanism) on the processes and outcomes of medical care?
Institution	What is the impact of the quality of care on the outcomes of medical care?
Patient	What patient treatment options result in the best outcomes for patients with a specific condition?

Outcome Measures

Outcome measures fit into the general categories of mortality, morbidity, and health status, although specific indicators of each of these broad outcome measures may be used at different levels. The usefulness of a measure depends, in part, on the degree to which it meets the criteria of reliability, validity, feasibility, and sensitivity (McDowell and Newell 1996). Reliability concerns the reproducibility of the measure under various conditions of administration. Validity relates to the accuracy of the measure, in the sense that it measures what it is intended to measure. Feasibility refers to the ease with which the scale can be used in various populations. Sensitivity refers to the ability of the measure to detect changes—improvement or deterioration—in the condition of the person as a result of healthcare. Sensitivity to healthcare variation is particularly important for outcome measures being used to assess the effectiveness of care.

Community-level outcome measures include population death, morbidity, and disability rates, as well as disease prevalence and incidence rates and perceived health status. One problem with these measures is how to combine them into a positive index of the community's or population's health, as opposed to negative indexes such as death rates, to yield a representation of health-adjusted life expectancy (Kindig 1997). The disability-adjusted life year (DALY) represents one attempt to combine these community-level measures in a way that reflects the burden of disease upon a population (Murray and Lopez 1996). Specifically, the DALY "expresses years of life lost to premature death and years lived with a disability of specified severity and duration. One DALY is thus one lost year of healthy life" (Murray and Lopez 1996, 7). Another attempt to index a population's health is based on the years of healthy life, derived from a combination of the responses to the activity limitation and self-perceived health status questions from the National Health Interview Survey (Erickson, Wilson, and Shannon 1995).

Population-based data, as exemplified by mortality rates, while relatively high in reliability, validity, and feasibility, have been shown repeatedly to be insensitive to medical care variation. This suggests that these data are useful for addressing the question of medical care's contribution to the health of the population, but they have limited applicability in assessing the clinical effectiveness of medical care.

For examining mortality, morbidity, and health status outcomes across institution and system levels, outcomes may be aggregated from the patient level within these categories. Patient-level outcome measures focus on individual deaths, on morbidity as reflected both in adverse outcomes and disability limitations, and on the health status outcomes of clinical endpoints, such as blood sugar and blood pressure, and subjective health status measures. At the institution and system levels, these patient-level measures are aggregated to produce case fatality, complication, disability, and diagnosis rates as well as averaged subjective health status for groups of patients.

Subjective health status measures

Subjective health status (SHS) measures, based on individuals' self-reports, are singled out here for a more detailed discussion because they have undergone extensive development and have achieved widespread use in the past decade (Leplege and Hunt 1997). They may be of a generic type, applicable across all disease conditions, or of a disease-specific type. Both types are needed in the assessment of the medical care outcomes—the generic indicators for comparisons across disease conditions, and the disease-specific ones to more sensitively identify the effects of diseases on people and the effects of treatments on particular disease conditions. A range of possible SHS measures has been collected in *Measuring Health—A Guide to Rating Scales and Questionnaires* (McDowell and Newell 1996). For each of over 100 instruments, this book presents a description, copies of the actual questionnaire, information on the reliability and validity of the instrument, and a complete listing of references. Ware (1995) has also provided a brief summary and review of the ten most widely used SHS measures.

One example of generic SHS measures is the Medical Outcomes Study Short Form (SF-36), with its simpler companion, the SF-12. This questionnaire contains an array of questions related to the effect of disease on physical health, mental health, and social health, as well as on health perceptions. The scores on each of eight dimensions were originally kept separate and presented as a profile.

They have subsequently been grouped into two categories to yield summary scores for physical and mental health, respectively (Ware, Kosinski, and Keller 1994).

In addition to the generic measures are disease-specific subjective health status measures, such as the Arthritis Impact Measurement Scale (AIMS) questionnaire (Meenan, Gertman, and Mason 1980). Such questionnaires focus on unique aspects of the disease for which they were developed. They are, as illustrated by the AIMS questionnaire, reliable, valid, feasible, and above all sensitive to the changes following medical treatment.

The optimum strategy for outcomes assessment, given the different levels of sensitivity, may be to use a generic instrument, such as the SF-36 or the SF-12, supplemented with disease-specific questions or a disease-specific questionnaire (Patrick and Deyo 1989). The generic instrument would allow comparisons to be made across diseases, while the disease-specific instrument would be more likely to provide sufficient sensitivity to detect small changes in patients' conditions.

Risk Adjustment

Ultimately the value of all effectiveness research depends on the ability to validly adjust for differences in risks associated with final outcomes. Risk adjustment of patient outcomes is necessary in effectiveness research to account for the differing risks patients bring to the clinical setting. Clearly, patients who differ at admission to a hospital in their risks, and who receive similarly effective treatments, will experience different outcomes. When randomized clinical trials are possible, these differences can be minimized by the random allocation of subjects to experimental and control groups. But under nonexperimental conditions, under which most effectiveness research is done, these differences and their potential confounding should be adjusted for in the analysis. These differing risks that require adjustments include differences in patient demographic characteristics such as age, gender and race; comorbidities, or conditions unrelated to the primary illness that can negatively affect treatment outcomes; and diagnoses that may differ in the initial severity of illness.

At the patient level, two general approaches may be taken in this adjustment. A subjective approach, relying on the informed judgments of experienced clinicians in rating the severity of the patient's illness at entry, may provide a valid assessment of a patient's status (Charlson et al. 1986), but such an expensive procedure, in terms of the physician's time, is rarely possible. In its place, an objective approach, utilizing clearly identified data related to the patient's risk, clinical state, and probable outcome, are used in an algorithm or formula to generate a score characterizing the patient's risk. These data may include characteristics of patients, their comorbid conditions, and their diagnoses, which at the institution and system levels may be incorporated into risk-adjustment systems, such as the Acute Physiological and Chronic Health Evaluation (APACHE) scale or the Medical Illness Severity Grouping System (MedisGroups) described later. Also at the institution and system levels, where some of the detailed patient data such as discharge and claims data may be lacking, demographic characteristics or comorbidity rates may be used as proxies for actual severity measures. At the community level, demographic characteristics such as age and gender are used to adjust for differing risk of illness.

The risk-adjustment methods in common use assume the objective approach described above; 14 of them, all at the patient level, are described and thoroughly analyzed in *Risk Adjustment for Measuring Health Care Outcomes* (Iezzoni 1997). This resource also provides information on the dimensions of risk, data sources, and performance of these measures. Iezzoni specifies several issues important to the assessment and measurement of risk: level of analysis, time frame for observation, timing of data collection, feasibility, reliability, and validity. The level or unit of analysis determines both the data that are available and the dimensions important to consider. Health-related quality of life (HRQOL), for example, is not likely to be found when entire systems are being analyzed, because HRQOL is not routinely collected on all patients in all settings. The time frame for observation of outcomes—for example, whether consideration is to be given only to hospital inpatient events or to things occurring within six months post-discharge—determines which dimensions are important. The timing of data collection is also important; if the severity of illness at admission is to be the basis for the risk adjustment, it is not appropriate to use risk data gathered from the entire stay in the hospital because the results may be confounded by the treatments subsequent to admission.

Iezzoni (1997) catalogs describes 14 different systems for risk adjustment. They represent a mix of dimensions as well as disease-specific and generic measures. All are proprietary to some extent, and are therefore less available for the kind of critical analyses done of outcome measures. Two, APACHE and MedisGroups, will be described now in greater detail. Both are grounded in the clinical perspective on effectiveness. APACHE, one of the first risk-adjustment systems developed, continues to be updated and widely applied. MedisGroups has been mandated in several states as the system to be used by hospitals.

The APACHE scale was developed for the evaluation of patients in hospital critical care units and uses a dozen physiologic values generated from physical findings and laboratory data in the first 24 hours after admission (Knaus, Draper, and Wagner 1985). Scale scores for each of these values are added, and are combined with adjustments for age and chronic health conditions, to yield an overall score. The APACHE score is generic in that it can be applied across diseases for comparisons of severity.

MedisGroups has assumed great importance because several states have now mandated it as the risk-adjustment measure to be used by hospitals in reporting data to state agencies. The Medis-Groups system produces a generic set of severity categories across illnesses, using medical record data processed by a proprietary program (Brewster et al. 1985). It uses what are called "key clinical findings," including laboratory, radiology, pathology, and physical examination data. This information can be input into the system's coding scheme to permit the severity of patients' conditions at admission, as well as their progress over the course of the hospitalization, to be monitored.

These risk-adjustment methods and severity-of-illness measures can and should be evaluated by the same criteria as health status measures—namely, reliability, validity, feasibility, and sensitivity. Several reviews have summarized the information from studies comparing measures of these attributes (Geehr 1989; Hornbrook 1982; Iezzoni 1990, 1997; Thomas and Ashcraft 1991). Because the objective methods use factual data and are computerized, they are both basically reliable and feasible. Their validity continues to be a question, and they vary in sensitivity. Risk adjustment is less well developed than outcome measurement, and is impeded by the fact that much of the work is in the proprietary domain. Iezzoni, however, has contributed greatly to removing the veil from these systems.

Study Designs

Study designs for effectiveness research cover a range of possibilities (see Table 2.2). The design principles are the same as those for any study: maximize experimental variance, control extraneous variance, and minimize error variance. On one hand, applying these principles results in outcomes research designs that follow true experimental design principles of random allocation, control groups, blinding, and homogeneity, and lead to efficacy studies. On the other hand are nonexperimental observational designs, in which investigators do not directly intervene but instead develop methods for describing events that occur naturally and their effect on study subjects. These types of studies characterize much of effectiveness research, and are represented by examples of effectiveness studies presented later in this chapter. Alternatives include meta-analysis and decision analysis, sometimes called synthetic designs (Fineberg 1990). All of these methods, as they apply to effectiveness research, were reviewed in a conference sponsored by the AHCPR (Sechrest, Perrin, and Bunker 1990) and in a report prepared for Congress (U.S. Office of Technology Assessment [OTA] 1994). The following discussion reflects the content of the conference and the report.

The assessment of efficacy—the determination of the benefits of a particular medical therapy, health service activity, or public health intervention under ideal conditions—involves the randomized clinical trial (RCT) as the primary method of analysis. The hallmark of the RCT is random assignment of patients to experimental and control groups, and hence, control of much of the extraneous variation and sources of error. Good examples of RCTs concerning medical therapies include trials of pravastatin in the treatment of patients with acute myocardial infarctions (Sacks et al. 1996), and drug therapy to prevent future obstruction of coronary artery bypass grafts (The Post Coronary Artery Bypass Graft Trial Investigators 1997). To extend the range of RCTs to situations where treatment effects are modest in size, large, simple trials have been used (Peto, Collins, and Gray 1995).

RCT designs have also been used to assess the benefits of ways in which medical care is delivered, for instance, in the evaluation of inpatient versus outpatient cardiac catheterization (Block et al. 1988), and of day hospital versus inpatient care for cancer patients (Mor et al. 1988). This design was also used to assess the effects of different medical care payment plans on use and outcomes in the RAND Health Insurance Experiment (Brook et al. 1983). RCTs have been used less frequently, unfortunately, to evaluate public health interventions (Orleans 1995); the polio vaccine trials conducted in the 1950s are, however, an outstanding exception and a good example of large public health trials.

RCTs are a powerful method, but are not often feasible because of the expense necessitated by the large sample sizes and the length of time required to conduct them. Ethical issues involved in depriving patients of treatment may also preclude their use. Another problem with RCTs is that many are done on a small local scale and therefore the results often are not highly significant nor widely disseminated. Because of the difficulties and expense inherent in RCTs, they must be used selectively. As a result, many important treatment questions cannot be answered by such designs.

An alternative to RCTs is the use of synthetic methods such as meta-analysis and decision analysis. Meta-analysis involves quantitatively and statistically combining the results of several RCTs to estimate the results of therapy when no single trial may be sufficient in number of patients to yield a statistically significant result (Goldschmidt 1986; Mullen and Ramirez 1987). Meta-analyses have been used, for example, to obtain estimates of the effectiveness of respiratory rehabilitation in chronic obstructive pulmonary disease (Lacasse et al. 1996), the effects of Hypericum extracts in the treatment of depression (Linde et al. 1996), and health outcomes associated with antihypertensive therapies used as first-line agents (Psaty et al. 1997). Meta-analyses are also being used in the Cochrane Collaboration (1997), which is a major international effort that "aims to ensure that all areas of healthcare which have been evaluated using RCTs will be covered." Collaborators in this process prepare and maintain systematic reviews of RCTs as well as other evidence where appropriate. These reviews are then maintained in a database and disseminated for use.

Decision analyses synthesize information about effectiveness to determine the value of one approach versus another for policy analysis and ultimately for clinical decisions. A decision analysis requires information on the actual treatment of patients with disease, the outcomes, and the value of those outcomes to patients. Information from large databases and other sources is used to estimate the probabilities of different outcomes from therapy for patients. Patient surveys provide information on patients' symptoms as well as their preferences for different outcomes. The advantage of a decision analysis is that it synthesizes a large amount of information relevant to effectiveness. The disadvantage is that necessary data on patient values or preferences are often not available. An example of a decision analysis using national-level Medicare data concerning the most effective treatment for benign prostatic hypertrophy (Wennberg et al. 1988) is presented later in this chapter in discussing examples of effectiveness research.

Observational nonexperimental designs, chiefly cross-sectional studies, are another design type, and characterize the bulk of the literature on effectiveness. Community-level epidemiological studies use existing registries or databases such as the Medicare database. System- and institution-level studies use databases appropriate to these levels, such as hospital discharge and claims data, to address issues within the organization (intraorganizational) and between organizations (interorganizational). At the patient level, when RCTs are not possible, reports of individual cases and series of them are reported. One problem with these observational studies is that the databases used may have significant biases due to missing values, lack of validating evidence, or the unrepresentativeness of the database, and that these biases may limit the generalizability of study results. Another problem is that random allocation has not been possible, and that therefore statistical adjustments are applied to account for the differences in mix of patients that may result from possible selection biases. Despite these limitations, however, observational studies are more feasible than experimental studies and draw upon large volumes of data reflecting actual experience. Most of the studies of effectiveness, and thus much of the evidence about effectiveness to be presented and reviewed in the next section of this chapter, derive from these observational designs.

Data Sources

Where clinical trials and true experiments are not possible, effectiveness research relies on a variety of data sources for the cross-sectional studies (as shown in Table 2.2). Surveys of institutions, providers, and patients, as well as records of medical care, discharges, and claims, provide information for effectiveness research at the patient, institution, and system levels, dependent on the level of aggregation of the data. At the community level, public health surveillance systems and vital statistics data that may be used to construct population health information systems provide the data for effectiveness studies.

Community-level outcome measures, such as population mortality rates, can be obtained from state and U.S. Vital Statistics data, as well as from WHO and OECD data for international comparisons. Morbidity rates can be acquired from the NCHS National Health Interview Surveys (NHIS). These surveys are conducted annually on a sample of the U.S. population and yield, among other data, information on limited activity days and restricted activity days. Disease prevalence and incidence data can also be obtained from NHIS data, as well as from other federal sources such as the *Mortality and Morbidity Weekly Report* of the Centers for Disease Control and Prevention.

The surveys conducted by the NCHS provide a rich source of information for effectiveness research. Information is gathered, for example, by the NHIS on respondents' use of medical care. Provider surveys, such as the National Ambulatory Medical Care Survey, the National Hospital Discharge Survey, and the National Long-Term Care Survey, provide aggregate information on patients and their use of healthcare services. Diseases are also recorded in national registries, some maintained by the government and some by private sources. An example of the former is the National Cancer Institute's Surveillance Epidemiology and End Results (SEER) system (SEER 1997).

The majority of effectiveness research studies, however, rely on medical records and related sources such as claims data collected for billing purposes and hospital discharge abstract data collected principally for quality assurance purposes. The largest single source of claims data is the Health Care Financing Administration (HCFA) Medicare database, of which the Medicare Provider Analysis and Review (MEDPAR) file is the most utilized. In addition, HCFA, through state-level peer review organizations, gathers medical record–level information about the quality of care. Private insurers, such as Blue Cross and Blue Shield, also maintain large claims databases, but their usefulness is limited by the fact that there are over 1,500 private insurers in this country. In addition, these sources gather information only on patients who have health insurance.

An increasing number of states have mandated that hospitals and health plans contribute to state-level databases on hospital-level activities (Iezzoni, Schwartz, and Restuccia 1991). In addition, these states have required hospitals to adopt uniform risk-adjustment methods to accompany their data. While a majority of states have mandated these data activities, as of 1997 only about half of the states in the United States had actually implemented such systems (Epstein 1997).

Finally, the Joint Commission on Accreditation of Healthcare Organizations (JCAHO) has also created a national hospital database derived from its new clinical indicators, and the National Committee for Quality Assurance (NCQA) has done the same for managed care organizations through its Health Plan Employer Data and Information Set (HEDIS). For a common set of indicators, all participating institutions provide information on their experience to these monitoring organizations. These data are used for accreditation decisions as well as for external comparisons of organizational performance (JCAHO 1997; NCQA 1997).

Reviews of claims and discharge data reveal that they have both strengths and weaknesses (Blumberg 1991; Jencks 1990). The strengths include the possible linking of large databases, the large numbers of patients included, the reliability of the factual information, and the usefulness of the data for documenting variations in practices as well as a range of outcomes. Their weaknesses are that important research variables may be missing, there is usually little information for risk adjustment, and post-discharge data generally are missing.

Examples

Several studies are presented as prototypical examples illustrating each level of effectiveness research—community, system, institution, and patient (see Table 2.2). They also demonstrate the use of the various effectiveness research methods discussed earlier (i.e., outcomes measured, risk adjustment used, basic study design, and data sources). The prototypical examples that will be reviewed include a comparison of Boston and New Haven mortality outcomes for Medicare patients as the community-level example, the Medical Outcomes Study as the system-level example, a study of the relationship between quality and hospital mortality rates as the institution-level example, and a decision analysis of the survival and quality-of-life outcomes for men with benign prostatic hypertrophy as the patient-level example.

Community-level example: Boston–New Haven

A study by Wennberg and his colleagues (Wennberg et al. 1989) compared Boston and New Haven in terms of their utilization of medical care and the mortality outcomes for Medicare beneficiaries. For outcomes they used mortality rates, both inpatient and within 30 days of admission, and as denominators used both hospital discharges and Medicare beneficiaries in the population. Risk adjustment was done using the demographic variables of age, race, and gender. The study design was observational, using only cross-sectional data to compare Boston and New Haven. For data sources, the authors used Medicare hospital claims (Medicare Part A) and enrollment files. They found that even though Boston Medicare patients used up to twice as many medical care resources, no difference in mortality rates between the two cities was found when the denominator used was total Medicare beneficiaries in each city.

System-level example: Medical Outcomes Study

The Medical Outcomes Study was designed to observe, over a period of time, the effects of different combinations of system-level variables on the health outcomes of patients with various chronic health conditions (Tarlov et al. 1989). Analyses based on variant conditions, patient groups, and outcomes will be highlighted here: clinical outcomes of patients with hypertension and diabetes (Greenfield et al. 1995), and general health status outcomes for older and poorer patients (Ware et al. 1996) in fee-for-service as compared to prepaid medical care. The outcomes selected in the first study included physiological measures such as blood pressure and glycosolated hemoglobin, and the second study included functional health status as determined by the SF-36. Risk adjustment was done using initial health status as well as the demographic variables of age and poverty status. The study design was observational but longitudinal, following the selected patients for up to seven years. The data sources used were the medical records of the selected patients and self-report questionnaires.

In the study of the outcomes of patients with hypertension and diabetes, clinical and functional outcomes were examined two and four years after the beginning of the study. Greenfield et al. (1995, 1436) reported, "No meaningful differences were found in the mean health outcomes for patients with hypertension or [non-insulin dependent diabetes mellitus] NIDDM, whether they were treated by different care systems or by different physician specialists." In the study of the outcomes for older and poorer patients in fee-for-service as compared to prepaid medical care, physical health for those who were both poor and elderly decreased more under the prepaid than under the fee-for-service arrangements, when mean scores on the SF-36 were used. For mental health, as measured by mean scores on the SF-36, there was no difference in changes over time for the poor and elderly between prepaid and fee-for-service arrangements (Ware et al. 1996).

Institution-level example: quality and hospital deaths

A RAND study of quality and hospital deaths (Park et al. 1990) was undertaken to answer the question of whether hospital-level mortality rates were indicators of problems with the quality of medical care in these hospitals. The outcome measure was probability of death, both in-hospital and within 30 days. Risk adjustment was done using the APACHE II, a severity rating system using data abstracted from the medical records. The study design was observational and used only cross-sectional data. The data sources included both Medicare hospital claims files and information abstracted from the medical records of patients with either acute myocardial infarctions or congestive heart failure. At the institutional level of analysis, these researchers found no relationship between the quality of medical care in the hospitals and their mortality rates for these two selected medical conditions. They did, however, find that the quality of medical care that individual patients received was related to their probability of death.

Patient-level example: benign prostatic hypertrophy

An example comparing the treatment outcomes of watchful waiting versus immediate surgery for benign prostatic hypertrophy (BPH) in older men is presented as the prototype for the effectiveness research at the patient level (Wennberg et al. 1988). For outcomes, the researchers examined complications, long-term mortality results, and quality of life related to symptoms. Risk adjustment was done in terms of both patient demographics and quality of life. The study designs employed were both observational, using longitudinal data, and synthetic, using decision analysis to assemble the various data for answering the fundamental question of differences in survival and quality of life. In various parts of this study, the authors used as data sources claims databases, medical records, and quality-of-life questionnaires. What they found was a slight advantage in terms of survival only for watchful waiting, but that adjustment for quality of life slightly favored immediate surgery.

Summary and Conclusions

In this chapter, effectiveness has been defined in terms of two complementary views—that is, a population perspective and a clinical perspective. The population view asks what contributions medical care makes to the health of the population. The clinical view, by contrast, asks how medical care improves the health of patients who enter the system for care. The key methods of effectiveness research that help provide answers to these questions have been described, discussed in terms of their strengths and weaknesses, and illustrated in a set of example studies. The next chapter illustrates the useful application of these methods in a broad range of outcomes research answering the basic effectiveness questions.

References

Block, P. C., I. Ockene, R. J. Goldberg, J. Butterly, E. H. Block, C. Degon, A. Beiser, and T. Colton. 1988. "A Prospective Randomized Trial of Outpatient Versus Inpatient Cardiac Catheterization." *The New England Journal of Medicine* 319: 1251–55.

Blum, H. I.. 1976. "From a Concept of Health to a National Health Policy." *American Journal of Health Planning* 1 (1): 3–22.

Blumberg, M. S. 1991. "Potentials and Limitations of Database Research Illustrated by the QMMP AMI Medicare Mortality Study." *Statistics in Medicine* 10: 637–46.

Brewster, A., B. Karlin, L. Hyde, C. Jacobs, R. Bradbury, and Y. Chae. 1985. "MEDISGRPS: A Clinically Based Approach to Classifying Hospital Patients at Admission." *Inquiry* 22: 377–87.

Brook, R., and K. Lohr. 1985. "Efficacy, Effectiveness, Variations, and Quality: Boundary-Crossing Research." *Medical Care* 23 (Supplement): 710–22.

Brook, R., J. Ware, W. Rogers, E. Keeler, A. Davies, C. Donald, G. Goldberg, K. Lohr, P. Masthay, and J. Newhouse. 1983. "Does Free Care Improve Adults' Health? Results from a Randomized Controlled Trial." *The New England Journal of Medicine* 309: 1426–34.

Burt, V. L., J. A. Cutler, M. Higgins, M. J. Horan, D. Labarthe, P. Whelton, C. Brown, and E. J. Roccella. 1995. "Trends in the Prevalence, Awareness, Treatment, and Control of Hypertension in the Adult U.S. Population: Data from the Health Examination Surveys, 1960 to 1991." *Hypertension* 26: 60–69.

Charlson, M. E., F. L. Sax, C. R. MacKenzie, S. D. Fields, R. L. Braham, and R. G. Douglas. 1986. "Assessing Illness Severity: Does Clinical Judgement Work?" *Journal of Chronic Diseases* 39: 439–52.

Cochrane, A. L. 1971. *Effectiveness and Efficiency*. London: The Nuffield Provincial Hospitals Trust.

Cochrane Collaboration. 1997. The Cochrane Collaboration [Online]. Available: http://hiru.mcmaster.ca/COCHRANE/DEFAULT.HTM [9/26/97].

Donabedian, A. 1966. "Evaluating the Quality of Medical Care." *Milbank Memorial Fund Quarterly* 44 (Part 2): 166–206.

————. 1973. *Aspects of Medical Care Administration: Specifying Requirements for Health Care.* Cambridge, MA: Harvard University Press.

————. 1980. *Explorations in Quality Assessment and Monitoring. Volume I— The Definition of Quality and Approaches to Its Assessment.* Chicago: Health Administration Press.

————. 1982. *Explorations in Quality Assessment and Monitoring. Volume II— The Criteria and Standards of Quality.* Chicago: Health Administration Press.

Epstein, M. 1997. Personal Communication. National Association of Health Data Organizations.

Erickson, P., R. Wilson, and I. Shannon. 1995. *Years of Healthy Life.* Hyattsville, MD: National Center for Health Statistics.

Evans, R. G., M. L. Barer, and T. R. Marmor, eds. 1994. *Why Are Some People Healthy and Others Not? The Determinants of Health of Populations.* New York: Aldine De Gruyter.

Fineberg, H. V. 1990. "The Quest for Causality in Health Services Research." In *Research Methodology: Strengthening Causal Interpretations of Nonexperimental Data.* Edited by L. Sechrest, E. Perrin, and J. Bunker. PHS 90-3454. Rockville, MD: Agency for Health Care Policy and Research.

Geehr, E. D. 1989. *Selecting a Proprietary Severity-of-Illness System.* Tampa, FL: American College of Physician Executives.

Goldschmidt, P. G. 1986. "Information Synthesis: A Practical Guide." *Health Services Research* 21: 215–37.

Greenfield, S., W. Rogers, M. Mangotich, M. F. Carney, and A. R. Tarlov. 1995. "Outcomes of Patients with Hypertension and Non-Insulin Dependent Diabetes Mellitus Treated by Different Systems and Specialties." *Journal of the American Medical Association* 274: 1436–44.

Hornbrook, M. C. 1982. "Hospital Case Mix: Its Definition, Measurement, and Use: Part I. The Conceptual Framework. Part II. Review of Alternative Measures." *Medical Care Review* 39: 1–43, 73–123.

Iezzoni, L. I. 1990. "Severity of Illness Measures—Comments and Caveats." *Medical Care* 28: 757–61.

————. 1997. *Risk Adjustment for Measuring Health Care Outcomes,* 2nd ed. Chicago: Health Administration Press.

Iezzoni, L. I., M. Schwartz, and J. Restuccia. 1991. "The Role of Severity Information in Health Policy Debates: A Survey of State and Regional Concerns." *Inquiry* 28: 117–28.

Jencks, S. 1990. "Issues in the Use of Large Data Bases for Effectiveness Research." In *Effectiveness and Outcomes in Health Care.* Edited by K. A. Heithoff, and K. Lohr, 94–104. Washington, D.C.: National Academy Press.

Joint Commission on Accreditation of Healthcare Organizations. 1997.

JCAHO Home Page [Online]. Available: http://www.jcaho.org/ [9/12/97].

Kindig, D. A. 1997. *Purchasing Population Health: Paying for Results.* Ann Arbor, MI: The University of Michigan Press.

Knaus, W. A., E. A. Draper, and D. P. Wagner. 1985. "APACHE II: A Severity of Disease Classification System." *Critical Care Medicine* 13: 818–29.

Lacasse, Y., E. Wong, G. H. Guyatt, D. King, D. J. Cook, and R. S. Goldstein. 1996. "Meta-Analysis of Respiratory Rehabilitation in Chronic Obstructive Pulmonary Disease." *The Lancet* 348: 1115–19.

Lalonde, M. 1975. *A New Perspective on the Health of Canadians: A Working Document.* Ottawa: Information Canada.

Leplege, A., and S. Hunt. 1997. "The Problem of Quality of Life in Medicine." *Journal of the American Medical Association* 278: 47–50.

Linde, K., G. Ramirez, C. D. Mulrow, A. Pauls, W. Weidenhammer, and D. Melchart. 1996. "St. John's Wort for Depression—Overview and Meta-Analysis of Randomised Clinical Trials." *British Medical Journal* 313: 253–58.

Longest, B. B. Jr. 1994. *Health Policymaking in the United States.* Chicago: AUPHA Press/Health Administration Press.

McDowell, I., and C. Newell. 1996. *Measuring Health: A Guide to Rating Scales and Questionnaires,* 2nd ed. New York: Oxford University Press.

Meenan, R., P. Gertman, and J. Mason. 1980. "Measuring Health Status in Arthritis: The Arthritis Impact Measurement Scales." *Arthritis and Rheumatism* 23: 146–52.

Milio, N. 1983. *Primary Care and the Public's Health.* Lexington, MA: Lexington Books.

Mor, V., M. Z. Stalker, R. Gralla, H. I. Scher, C. Cimma, D. Park, A. M. Flaherty, M. Kiss, P Nelson, L. Laliberte, R. Schwartz, P. A. Marks, and H. F. Oettgen. 1988. "Day Hospital as an Alternative to Inpatient Care for Cancer Patients: A Random Assignment Trial." *Journal of Clinical Epidemiology* 41: 771–85.

Mullen, P. D., and G. Ramirez. 1987. "Information Synthesis and Meta-Analysis." In *Advances in Health Education and Promotion.* Edited by W. Ward, M. Becker, P. D. Mullen, and S. Simonds, 201–39 . Greenwich, CN: JAI Press.

Murray, C. J. L., and A. D. Lopez, eds. 1996. *The Global Burden of Disease: A Comprehensive Assessment of Mortality and Disability from Diseases, Injuries, and Risk Factors in 1990 and Projected to 2020.* Cambridge, MA: Harvard School of Public Health on behalf of the World Health Organization and the World Bank.

National Committee for Quality Assurance. 1997. NCQA Home Page [Online.] Available: http://www.ncqa.org/index.htm [9/12/97].

Orleans, M. 1995. "The Cochrane Collaboration: Lessons for Public Health Practice and Evaluation?" *Public Health Reports* 110: 633–34.

Park, R. E., R. H. Brook, J. Kosecoff, J. Keesey, L. Rubenstein, E. Keeler, K. L. Kahn, W. H. Rogers, and M. R. Chassin. 1990. "Explaining Variations in Hospital Death Rates: Randomness, Severity of Illness, Quality of Care." *Journal of the American Medical Association* 264: 484–90.

Patrick, D. L., and R. A. Deyo. 1989. "Generic and Disease-Specific Measures in Assessing Health Status and Quality of Life." *Medical Care* 27(Supplement): S217-S232.

Peto, R., R. Collins, and R. Gray. 1995. "Large-Scale Randomized Evidence: Large, Simple Trials and Overviews of Trials." *Journal of Clinical Epidemiology* 48: 23–40.

Psaty, B. M., N. L. Smith, D. S. Siscovick, T. D. Koepsell, N. S. Weiss, S. R. Heckbert, R. N. Lemaitre, E. H. Wagner, and C. D. Furberg. 1997. "Health Outcomes Associated with Antihypertensive Therapies Used as First-Line Agents." *Journal of the American Medical Association* 277: 739–45.

Sackett, D. L. 1980. "Evaluation of Health Services." In *Maxcy-Rosenau Public Health and Preventive Medicine.* Edited by J. Last, 1800–23. Norwalk, CT: Appleton-Century-Crofts.

Sacks, F. M., M. A. Pferrer, L. A. Moyé, J. L. Rouleau, J. D. Rutherford, T. G. Cole, L. Brown, J. W. Warnica, J. M. Arnold, C. C. Wun, B. R. Davis, and E. Braunwald. 1996. "The Effect of Pravastatin on Coronary Events after Myocardial Infarction in Patients with Average Cholesterol Levels." *The New England Journal of Medicine* 335: 1001–9.

Sechrest, L., E. Perrin, and J. Bunker, eds. 1990. *Research Methodology: Strengthening Causal Interpretations of Nonexperimental Data,* PHS 90-3454. Rockville, MD: Agency for Health Care Policy and Research.

Surveillance, Epidemiology, and End Results. 1997. Surveillance, Epidemiology, and End Results [Online]. Available: http://www-seer.ims.nci. nih.gov/index.html [9/26/97].

Tarlov, A., J. E. Ware, S. Greenfield, E. C. Nelson, E. Perrin, and M. Zubkoff. 1989. "The Medical Outcomes Study: An Application of Methods for Monitoring the Results of Medical Care." *Journal of the American Medical Association* 262: 925–30.

The Post Coronary Artery Bypass Graft Trial Investigators. 1997. "The Effect of Aggressive Lowering of Low-Density Lipoprotien Cholesterol Levels and Low-Dose Anticoagulation on Obstructive Changes in Saphenous-Vein Coronary-Artery Bypass Grafts." *The New England Journal of Medicine* 336: 153–62.

Thomas, J. W., and M. L. Ashcraft. 1991. "Measuring Severity of Illness:

Six Severity Systems and Their Ability to Explain Cost Variations." *Inquiry* 28: 39–55.

U.S. Congress Office of Technology Assessment. 1994. *Identifying Health Technologies That Work: Searching for Evidence*, OTA-H-608. Washington D.C.: U.S. Government Printing Office.

Ware, J. E. 1995. "The Status of Health Assessment 1994." In *Annual Review of Public Health*. Edited by G. S. Omenn, J. E. Fielding, and L. B. Lave, 327–54. Palo Alto, CA: Annual Reviews Inc.

Ware, J. E., M. S. Bayliss, W. H. Rogers, M. Kosinski, and A. R. Tarlov. 1996. "Differences in 4-Year Health Outcomes for Elderly and Poor, Chronically Ill Patients Treated in HMO and Fee-For-Service Systems." *Journal of the American Medical Association* 276: 1039–47.

Ware, J. E., M. Kosinski, and S. D. Keller. 1994. *SF-36 Physical and Mental Health Summary Scales: A User's Manual*. Boston: The Health Institute, New England Medical Center.

Wennberg, J. E. 1990. "Small Area Analysis and the Medical Care Outcome Problem." *Research Methodology: Strengthening Causal Interpretations of Nonexperimental Data*. Edited by L. Sechrest, E. Perrin, and J. Bunker. PHS 90-3454. Rockville, MD: Agency for Health Care Policy and Research.

Wennberg, J. E., J. L. Freeman, R. M. Shelton, and T. A. Bubolz. 1989. "Hospital Use and Mortality among Medicare Beneficiaries in Boston and New Haven." *The New England Journal of Medicine* 321: 1168–73.

Wennberg, J. E., A. Mulley, D. Hanley, R. Timothy, F. Fowler, N. P. Roos, M. Barry, K. McPherson, E. R. Greenberg, D. Soule, T. Bubolz, E. Fisher, and D. Malenka. 1988. "An Assessment of Prostatectomy for Benign Urinary Tract Obstruction: Geographic Variations and the Evaluation of Medical Care Outcomes." *Journal of the American Medical Association* 259: 3027–30.

White, K. L., T. F. Williams, and B. G. Greenberg. 1961. "The Ecology of Medical Care." *The New England Journal of Medicine* 265: 885–92.

Williamson, J. W. 1978. "The Estimation of Achievable Health Care Benefit." In *Assessing and Improving Health Care Outcomes*. Edited by J. W. Williamson, 51–69. Cambridge, MA: Ballinger Publishers.

Chapter 3

Effectiveness: Policy Strategies, Evidence, Criteria, and an Application

The basic health policy question, from an effectiveness viewpoint, is: What policy strategies contribute most to improving the health of the population? The answer to this question clearly depends upon the perspective—population versus clinical—taken. In metaphoric terms, the answer relies on whether the role of Hygeia, reflecting the population perspective, or Panakeia, reflecting the clinical perspective, is adopted:

> In ancient times, Asklepios was the god of health . . . Asklepios had two daughters, Hygeia and Panakeia. Panakeia was a true healing goddess, learned in the use of drugs derived from either plants or from the earth: her cult is alive and well today in the universal search for a panacea. In contrast, her sister Hygeia was the goddess for whom health was the natural order of things. We still honor her memory through the use of the word hygiene. (Renaud 1994)

The answer offered and the policies adopted depend on whether the focus is on public health, in the tradition of Hygeia, or on medical care solutions, in the tradition of Panakeia.

This chapter begins with a review of the health policy strategies available and implemented in improving the health of the population, from both a population perspective and a clinical perspective. It then proceeds to a review of health status indicators at the population level on the assumption that ultimately the question is whether the strategies and interventions derived from either the population or the clinical perspective contribute to improvements in the health of the population. The evidence bearing on each of the broad policy strategies just discussed is then reviewed and translated into a set of effectiveness criteria for evaluating various policy strategies. The chapter concludes with an evaluation, from the effectiveness viewpoint, of a specific policy option—Medicaid managed care.

Policy Strategies Relating to Effectiveness

Health policy strategies can be related to the overall conceptual framework of factors contributing to population health discussed in Chapter 2 (see Figure 2.1). A population perspective considers strategies aimed at environment, behavior, human biology, and medical care as major contributors to population health, while a clinical perspective considers strategies related to structures, processes, and outcomes of medical care and is directed at improving patient-, institution-, and system-level performance. Grounded in these respective determinants, an overview of broad policy strategies that have been applied is presented in Table 3.1. The population perspective yields strategies such as investing in overall population health information monitoring systems, health protection, health promotion, and preventive services; and for medical care, strategies such as biomedical research, investment in resources, health planning and regionalization of services, organized delivery systems, and enhanced access. The clinical perspective yields regulation of professional performance, and outcomes assessment and management with its attention to practice guidelines and performance monitoring.

Population Perspective

One set of policy strategies relates to the population perspective, or to what in Renaud's words Hygeia represents—that is, a focus on health rather than illness. While the contribution of non-medical factors to health improvement has not had a significant influence on the formulation of health policy in general, it is broadly reflected in public health strategies. An example of a population health strategy comes from Canada, where the Lalonde (1975) report set

Table 3.1 Health Policy Strategies Related to Factors
Contributing to Population Health

CONTRIBUTING FACTOR	POLICY STRATEGY
Population Perspective	Population Health Information Systems
Environment	Health Protection
Behavior	Health Promotion
Human Biology	Biomedical Research
	Preventive Services
Medical Care	
Structure	
Efficacy	Biomedical Research
Quantity	Investment in Resources
Distribution and	Health Planning and Regionalization of
Organization	Services
Process	Organized/Integrated Delivery Systems
Utilization	Enhanced Access
Clinical Perspective	
Medical Care	
Process	
Quality	Regulation of Professional Performance
Outcomes	Outcomes Assessment and Management
	Practice Guidelines
	Performance Monitoring Systems

forth an agenda for improving the population's health based on the recognition that health is determined as much by environment, lifestyle, and human biology as by healthcare services. The pursuit of this population health strategy led to a Canadian policy of equal access to *health*, as opposed to equal access to health*care* (Mhatre and Deber 1992); to a focus on the full range of health determinants in formulating health policy (Evans et al. 1994); and, finally, to the adoption of a population health information system (Roos et al. 1996) in British Columbia, Canada, to guide the development of a comprehensive health policy.

In the United States the growing knowledge about health determinants was responsible in part for the development of an explicit policy strategy of health promotion and disease prevention, beginning with the adoption of the Healthy People Report (U.S. DHEW 1979) and the establishment of the Office of Health Promotion and

Disease Prevention. This effort began with a set of specific objectives, the Healthy People 1990 Objectives, and moved on to Healthy People 2000 Objectives; efforts have begun to formulate Healthy People 2010 Objectives. This initiative has addressed a range of health determinants and has identified health promotion, health protection, and preventive services objectives, but has not explicitly identified strategies for achieving each of these objectives.

An overall population-based strategy calls for the establishment of population health information systems to monitor the health of the population and all of its determinants. One example of such a system is the Population Information System (POPULIS) in British Columbia, Canada (Roos et al. 1996). In the United States, the Healthy People 2000 Objectives, described in detail in Chapter 1, serve as the national-level performance monitoring system for population health, and Objective 22 of the Healthy People 2000 framework specifies the elements for state-level population health monitoring (see Appendix 1.1). An Institute of Medicine report (1997) provides a set of 25 specific indicators for population health monitoring at the community level.

Specific policy strategies relate to the various determinants of health, with the non-medical ones being covered by health protection and health promotion. Health policy strategies directed at the environment are referred to as Health Protection in the Healthy People 2000 Objectives and include such things as regulation of auto emissions. Health policy strategies directed at individual behavior are termed Health Promotion in the Healthy People 2000 Objectives and include lifestyle-oriented strategies such as cigarette-smoking cessation programs. Health policy strategies directed at human biology include biomedical research and the part of what in the Healthy People 2000 Objectives are encompassed within the Preventive Services goals, including, for example, childhood immunizations.

These various strategies are included in one way or another in the core functions of public health. Hence, the establishment of public health itself represents a commitment to a major population health policy strategy. Public health in the United States can trace its origins to the establishment of the Marine Hospital Service in 1798, but it might be said that 1912, the year of its renaming as the United States Public Health Service, marks the beginning of federal policy in this direction. The next major step in this direction came with the

Social Security Act of 1935, which included, among other things, a provision calling for the federal government to assist states " . . . in establishing and maintaining public health services . . ." (Institute of Medicine 1988, 68). Since that time, as described in Chapter 1, public health has become a significant enterprise at the state, county, and city levels, but may be viewed as now facing a crisis of identity in the medical, and increasingly managed, care–dominated healthcare and health policy environment.

Another large set of policy strategies has focused on medical care services as the means of improving population health. These strategies relate to the elements of both the structure and process of care delivery. The predominant strategy for most of this half-century has been investment in the structure of healthcare delivery, related to the efficacy, quantity, distribution, and organization of medical care resources through such programs as the NIH, Hill-Burton, Health Professions Educational Assistance, and Comprehensive Health Planning.

Early federal policy in this direction was reflected in the establishment of the NIH with their mandate to fund biomedical research as the means of developing the knowledge base for understanding the causes and treatment of diseases—for example, for addressing the improvement of the efficacy of medical care. This effort began with the establishment of the NIH from the Marine Hospital Service Hygienic Laboratory in 1930, and expanded to a broader biomedical research focus with the establishment of the National Cancer Institute in 1937, which was integrated into the NIH along with a second institute, the National Heart Institute, established in 1948 (Harden 1986). In an example of one of those great ironies of public policy, it was out of the public health service, a policy strategy clearly anchored in the population perspective, that the NIH arose and became such a dominant force for the clinical perspective.

Such a successful research policy was ultimately challenged to become more practical and accountable. Accordingly, it went a step further in disseminating the results of this research into practice through the establishment of the Regional Medical Program and later, the Consensus Development Program. The Regional Medical Program, also known as A National Program to Conquer Heart Disease, Cancer and Stroke, was established in 1965 to bring, among other things, the results of the biomedical research to the practice of medicine through such vehicles as continuing medical education (Komaroff 1971). The Consensus Development Program, beginning in the mid-1970s, represented an additional effort to translate the research findings into medical practice. One of the problems a practitioner faces is distilling the enormous amount of research into specific medical practices. To assist in this process, NIH began a process of convening consensus development conferences to bring about this synthesis and to provide medical practitioners with more specific guidelines based on the research (Burtram 1994).

A second major structural policy strategy sought to improve the health of the population through increasing the quantity of medical care resources. The Hill-Burton legislation enhanced the number as well as the distribution of hospitals, while the Health Professions Educational Assistance Act increased the numbers of doctors, nurses, and other health professionals.

A third major structural policy thrust, embodied in the Comprehensive Health Planning and Regional Medical Programs, addressed the distribution and organization of medical care through regionalization (Bodenheimer 1969) and the intentional building of comprehensive healthcare systems (Kissick 1970) or organized/ integrated delivery systems (Shortell et al. 1993). The Comprehensive Health Planning legislation provided grants for both state- and areawide health planning, while the Regional Medical Program legislation fostered the development of a technical infrastructure for integrated delivery systems (Kissick 1970). These programs and subsequent private-sector efforts attempted to put together healthcare services across the continuum of need to improve both the effectiveness and the efficiency of services. Organized delivery systems have been defined as "a network of organizations that provides or arranges to provide a coordinated continuum of services to a defined population and is willing to be held clinically and fiscally accountable for the outcomes and the health status of the population served" (Shortell et al. 1996, 7).

A number of efforts in the direction of increasing the distribution and organization of services were also targeted at special populations, thus increasing access to medical care; Maternal and Child Health Programs, State and Local Health Departments, Medicare, Medicaid, and the Office of Economic Opportunity Neighborhood Health Centers are examples. Some of these examples will be discussed in Chapters 6 and 7 in the context of achieving equity.

Clinical Perspective

An alternative set of health policy strategies has focused on improving clinical effectiveness and includes both regulation of professional performance, a principally process-oriented strategy, and outcomes assessment and management, an outcome-oriented strategy. A burst of activity following the establishment of Medicare in 1965 sought to improve professional performance through monitoring the quality of medical care. The first federal effort in this direction was the Professional Standards Review Organization (PSRO) in 1972. This effort of the federal government mandated professional review of medical care, but allowed the review to be delegated to the local institutional level. When this proved unsatisfactory over time, the Health Care Financing Administration mandated state-level professional review organizations (PROs).

The establishment of AHCPR in 1989 as the flagship agency for outcomes research, and its subsequent development and dissemination of practice guidelines, represents a recent thrust in this direction and is focused on the outcomes rather than just the process of care. Besides practice guidelines as an operational strategy at the patient level, outcomes assessment and management has also been responsible for the development of performance monitoring at the institution and system levels.[1]

Practice guidelines are "systematically developed statements to assist practitioner and patient decisions about appropriate health care for specific clinical circumstances" (Institute of Medicine 1992, 27), that are expected to reduce inappropriate care, control geographic variations, and improve efficiency (Woolf 1990). They are known by a variety of names: clinical guidelines (AHCPR), practice standards (Brook 1989), clinical practice guidelines (American Academy of Medical Directors [AAMD]), practice policies (Eddy 1990), practice parameters (AMA), medical necessity guidelines (American College of Physicians [ACP]), clinical indicators (JCAHO), and consensus statement guidelines (NIH). Lomas (1993) estimated that there may be as many as 1,200 different practice guidelines, developed by as many as 50 different organizations, including professional societies, public agencies, and private groups. One of the most systematic efforts has been the development of practice guidelines by the AHCPR, which has developed and widely disseminated clinical guidelines for the treatment of acute pain management, urinary incontinence in adults, pressure ulcers in adults, cataracts in adults, depression in primary care, sickle cell disease, early HIV infection, benign prostatic hyperplasia, management of cancer pain, unstable angina, heart failure, otitis media with effusion, quality mammography, acute low back problems, post-stroke rehabilitation, cardiac rehabilitation, and smoking cessation. Patient, provider, and researcher versions for each of these practice guidelines can be found at the Agency's web site (AHCPR 1997). AHCPR has also launched the Evidence-Based Practice Initiative to assist other organizations in developing guidelines.

The outcomes assessment and management effort has also fostered the development of performance monitoring systems. The JCAHO has defined a performance monitoring system as "an inter-related set of process measures, outcome measures, or both, that facilitates internal comparisons over time and external comparisons of an organization's performance" (JCAHO 1997). Performance monitoring systems are being sponsored by state, employer, federal government, professional, and provider organizations. One of the most prominent of these systems is the HEDIS developed by the NCQA. "HEDIS is . . . a set of standardized performance measures to assure that purchasers and consumers have the information they need to reliably compare the performance of managed health care plans . . ." (NCQA 1997). The eight performance domains of HEDIS include effectiveness of care, accessibility and availability of care, satisfaction with the experience of care, cost of care, stability of the health plan, informed healthcare choices, use of services, and plan descriptive information. Besides providing for accreditation and performance measurement, HEDIS produces Quality Compass, a national database of comparative information on 226 health plans. From this information, NCQA has selected a group of 17 measures for reporting national averages that are updated regularly and posted on the NCQA web site (NCQA 1997).

Evidence Relating to Effectiveness

This section will address the evidence related to effectiveness first, by asking what the current health status of the population of the United States is, and how it compares to other developed nations;

second, by asking what general evidence there is supporting the importance of non-medical determinants of health; and third, by asking what evidence exists on the effectiveness of the various health policy strategies outlined earlier.

Population Health Indicators

Through its Healthy People 2000 Objectives, and in an effort to develop a consensus set of indicators to be used by each state in monitoring its progress, the U.S. Public Health Service has developed a set of 18 indicators of population health status (Centers for Disease Control and Prevention 1991). These include measures of mortality, disease incidence, low birth weight, prenatal care outcomes, childhood poverty, and air quality standards (see Table 3.2). While progress is being made on most of these 18 indicators, as of the 1995–96 Healthy People Review, for only four of them—work-related injuries, lung cancer deaths, AIDS incidence, and syphilis incidence—had the target been reached or exceeded. In comparison with most other developed nations, most of whom spend far less on healthcare, the United States ranked at the bottom on many of these indicators, specifically for infant mortality, total mortality, and work-related injury deaths (OECD 1995). Chapter 5 will provide specific evidence comparing the United States with other countries.

There is a mixed picture of progress for racial and ethnic population groups; significant health disparities between these groups and the white population continue to exist. Hispanics appeared to be faring better than blacks. For blacks, only the rates for work-related injury deaths and suicide had reached the target objectives. For Hispanics, the rates for work-related injuries, suicides, lung cancer, female breast cancer, heart disease, and stroke, as well as syphilis incidence, had met the desired target levels.

Major Determinants of Health

At the population level, many other important determinants of health besides medical care exist. The body of literature reviewed by Evans, Barer, and Marmor (1994) points to these predictors, and over the past two decades has resulted in a redefinition of the importance

Table 3.2 Health Status Indicators, United States, 1993

	Objective	Total	White	Black	Hispanic
1. Race/ethnicity-specific infant mortality as measured by the rate (per 1,000 live births) of deaths among infants under 1 year of age	7.0	8.4	6.8	16.5	7.1
2. Total deaths per 100,000 population	none	513.3	485.1	785.2	385.2
3. Motor vehicle crash deaths per 100,000 population	14.2	16.0	16.1	16.3	16.8
4. Work-related injury deaths per 100,000 population	4.0	3.3	3.2	3.1	3.5
5. Suicides per 100,000 population	10.5	11.3	12.0	7.2	7.3
6. Homicides per 100,000 population	7.2	10.7	6.0	40.9	11.0
7. Lung cancer deaths per 100,000 population	42.0	39.3	38.9	48.9	14.5
8. Female breast cancer deaths per 100,000 women	20.6	21.5	21.2	27.1	12.4
9. Cardiovascular disease deaths per 100,000 population	none	181.8	173.9	269.6	120.4
Heart disease deaths per 100,000 population	100.0	145.3	139.9	208.9	94.8
Stroke deaths per 100,000 population	20.0	26.5	24.5	45.0	19.5
10. Reported incidence (per 100,000 population) of AIDS	43.0	26.9	14.8	93.3	44.9
11. Reported incidence (per 100,000 population) of measles	0.0	0.4	—	—	—
12. Reported incidence (per 100,000 population) of tuberculosis	3.5	9.4	3.4	26.8	19.5
13. Reported incidence (per 100,000 population) of syphilis	10.0	8.1	1.0	59.5	3.5
14. Prevalence of low birthweight as measured by the percentage of live-born infants weighing under 2,500 grams at birth	5.0	7.3	6.1	13.2	6.2
15. Births to adolescents (ages 10–17 years) as a percentage of total live births	5.0	5.3	4.2	10.8	7.6
16. Prenatal care as measured by the percentage of mothers delivering live infants who did not receive care during the first trimester of pregnancy	10.0	19.8	17.2	31.7	31.1
17. Childhood poverty, as measured by the proportion of children under 15 years of age living in families at or below the poverty level					
Under 18 years	none	21.8	16.9	43.8	41.5
Under 15 years	none	22.5	—	—	—
5–17 years	none	20.1	—	—	—
18. Proportion of persons living in counties exceeding U.S. Environmental Protection Agency standards for air quality during the previous year	15.0	24.9	23.6	29.6	45.2

Source: Healthy People 2000 Review, 1995–96, Appendix A and Table V (NCHS 1996, 206).

of factors other than medical care as the determinants of health. Reconceptualizing the determinants of health as a means of altering health policy, Lalonde (1975), Blum (1976), and Evans, Barer, and Marmor (1994) identified the physical environment, social environment, individual behavior, genetic endowment, and medical care all as contributors to the health of the population. Also, over the past two decades a great deal of evidence has accumulated documenting the importance of both the physical and the social environment as determinants of the health of populations.

It has been estimated that 60 to 90 percent of cancers are environmentally caused (Blumenthal 1985) with as much as one-third of cancer deaths being attributed to diet (Scheuplein 1992). Specifically, the causes of cancer have been estimated epidemiologically (Doll and Peto 1981) as diet (35 percent), tobacco (30 percent), infection (10 percent), occupational exposures (4 percent), and geophysical factors (3 percent) such as radiation. Environmental risks as a group include food contamination, food additives, water pollution, air pollution, indoor chemicals, occupational exposure, toxic wastes, carcinogens, radiation, and physical agents such as trauma, accidents, and noise (Beasley and Swift 1989; Blumenthal 1985; Wilson and Crouch 1987). Besides cancer mortality, environmental factors cause nervous system, endocrine system, and immune system problems as well as acute poisoning and birth defects (Misch 1994).

The social environment, reflecting social class and status hierarchies, income, social ties, and cultural change, has also been demonstrated to be powerfully influential in determining the health of population groups (Cassel 1976; Syme 1996; Syme and Berkman 1976). Status hierarchy in work has been shown to be a major determinant of the mortality of individuals in England (Marmot, Kogevinas, and Elston 1987; Marmot et al. 1997). In addition, it has been demonstrated that income in both the United States (Hadley 1982; Stockwell 1961) and internationally (Wilkinson 1992) relates positively to mortality. Social ties and cultural change are also clearly related to mortality. The existence and strength of social ties have been shown to relate to decreased mortality from all causes (House, Robbins, and Metzner 1982), and acculturation of Japanese immigrants to the U.S. culture has been demonstrated to relate to increased heart disease mortality (Marmot et al. 1975).

Evidence About the Various Policy Strategies

The above evidence on the health of the U.S. population, as well as the general evidence concerning non-medical determinants of health, suggests the need for a careful examination of evidence on the effectiveness of the various policy strategies that have been proposed or tried as means of improving the health of the population. These findings raise questions about possible ways to improve effectiveness, but the answers proposed depend on the perspective, population or clinical, assumed. These perspectives lead to quite different proposals regarding the problems to be addressed and the solutions for doing so.

Population perspective: health protection, health promotion, and preventive services

The population perspective focuses on evidence regarding the effectiveness of public health services in general and health protection, health promotion, and preventive services in particular in improving the health of the population. Turnock (1997) cites evidence that community and public health have contributed to an increase in life expectancy in the United States from 47 to 75 years over the period from 1900 to the 1990s. He also claims that 67 percent of the reduction in stroke mortality, 49 percent of the reduction for cardiovascular mortality, and 28 percent of the reduction in motor vehicle crash mortality from 1960 to 1993 can be attributed to community and public health services. McKeown (1976), using a historical approach similar to that of McKinlay and McKinlay (1977) but based on data from the nineteenth century, argues that the major declines in population mortality preceded the introduction of public health services and were in fact more directly attributable to broader health-related changes in the society, including improved nutrition.

The effectiveness of health promotion and preventive services in general is somewhat mixed. The effectiveness of various prevention strategies was reviewed by Fielding (1978) who concluded that population-focused strategies, such as mass fluoridation of community water supplies, proved far more effective than individually focused strategies, such as anti-smoking campaigns. Glanz, Lewis, and Rimer (1997), in a review of cardiovascular disease interventions in communities, noted that each of these interventions showed only modest, and in some cases nonsignificant, reductions in risk factors and mortality that were obscured by the strong downward trends in the risk factors in control communities. Thacker et al. (1994) of the Centers for Disease Control and Prevention, in a review of methods for assessing the effectiveness of preventive services, presented evidence substantiating the 95–98 percent effectiveness of vaccinations in preventing measles, the 20–70 percent effectiveness of mammography in preventing breast cancer deaths, and the 50 percent effectiveness of retinal screening and treatment in preventing blindness in patients with diabetes. Finally, Bunker, Frazier, and Mosteller (1994), using statistical estimation techniques based on clinical preventive services of demonstrated efficacy, concluded that hypertension and cervical cancer screening as well as childhood immunizations have contributed significantly to the increase in life expectancy over this century in the United States.

Population perspective: medical care

Increasing investments in medical care has long been the strategy of choice for improving the health of the population, but the evidence of its effectiveness in achieving this goal is mixed. A major conclusion of the effectiveness evidence that follows is that variations in medical care resources and utilization have modest relationships to quality and effectiveness, especially at the population level. The evidence is presented in terms of the strategies listed in Table 3.1 under medical care from the population perspective.

Biomedical research as a policy strategy is ultimately directed at improving the efficacy of medical care. While the RCT is the principal method for determining the efficacy of medical care interventions, the example that follows illustrates the creative use of a cross-sectional study design—in this case, observations over time—to assess the effectiveness of medical care given efficacious therapies for the conditions under consideration.

As mentioned in Chapter 2, between the early and late 1900s in the United States there was a dramatic shift in mortality from deaths due to acute infectious diseases to deaths due to chronic disease such as heart disease, cancer, and strokes. This shift was assumed to be due to the introduction of antibiotics to cure the acute infectious diseases and vaccines to prevent the occurrence of them. Using mortality data over this time period, available from U.S. Vital Statistics sources, McKinlay and McKinlay (1977) set out to test this hypothesis. They examined the data for ten common infectious diseases: tuberculosis, scarlet fever, influenza, pneumonia, diphtheria, whooping cough, measles, smallpox, typhoid fever, and poliomyelitis. They demonstrated that for every condition examined except smallpox, most of the decline in mortality from the disease had occurred before the introduction of the antibiotic or the vaccine specific for that disease. For the ten diseases examined, the average net reduction after the introduction of the disease-specific intervention was 25 percent, although the range was from 0.29 percent for typhoid fever to 100 percent for smallpox. Even for poliomyelitis, the decline following the 1955 introduction of the Salk and Sabin vaccines was a modest 25 percent. In other words, specific medical interventions appear to have made only small contributions to the decline in mortality from the acute infectious diseases in this country. This study, its sequel (McKinlay, McKinlay, and Beaglehole 1989), and others similar to it (Charlton and Velez 1986) have revealed only marginal benefits from efficacious medical care.

Investment in resources is the second major policy strategy related to the structure of medical care. This strategy has taken, for example, the form of investment in increasing the quantity of hospitals and doctors. The relationship between the quantity of resources and outcomes at the population level has been explored in studies with nonexperimental designs using cross-sectional observational data. Cochrane, St. Leger, and Moore (1978), using various mortality rates from 18 developed nations as the outcomes and resource-to-population rates as the structural variables, found no consistent relationship of mortality to the levels of medical care resources. Martini et al. (1977), drawing on data from the various regions of the National Health Service in England, showed mortality to be more highly correlated with environmental and sociodemographic variables than with medical care. Newhouse and Friedlander (1979) found that disease prevalence rates from the U.S. Health and Nutrition Examination Survey were unrelated to the levels of medical care resources across census regions. Each of these studies confirmed the suggestion that medical care makes only a modest contribution to the health of the population, whether the outcome measure is mortality or disease prevalence and whether the comparison is across countries or within a single country.

Health planning and regionalization of services is a third medical care policy strategy within the population perspective. It has been suggested that it is not merely the quantity of medical care resources, but their distribution and organization as well, that is important to the health of the population, and this has been the premise for policy strategies aimed at health planning and regionalization of medical care. Using city health department data in an analytic study design, Gordis (1973) determined the effect of the presence of comprehensive community health centers on the incidence of rheumatic fever in Baltimore. He found a lower incidence of rheumatic fever among children in the geographic areas of the city that had introduced comprehensive community health centers, the assumption being that these children had better access to definitive treatment of streptococcal infections.

Once the efficacy of procedures has been established, the effects of greater quantities of procedures on outcomes can also be examined, and such studies have been used as an argument for regionalization of surgical services. An example of such a study is one that examined the relationship between the number of surgical procedures done in hospitals and each hospital's mortality experience for those operations. Using adjusted case fatality rates by hospital as the outcome and frequency of the surgical procedure as the process variable, the researchers (Luft, Bunker, and Enthoven 1979) showed that greater frequency of procedures is associated with better outcomes—that is, lower mortality rates. For example, for coronary bypass surgery they showed that hospitals doing more than 200 procedures per year had lower mortality rates. The same threshold level of 200 held for vascular and prostate surgery. For other surgeries, the threshold volume level was much lower: 50 for bowel surgery and total hip replacement, and 10 for gallbladder surgery. A later review of the several studies of this type confirmed the basic findings (U.S. Congress, Office of Technology Assessment 1988). The implication of such studies is that the effectiveness of medical care, in the case of surgical procedures, can be improved. One policy alternative for doing so is to regionalize surgery services for the procedures that require a high volume to maximize effectiveness.

An observational study done using longitudinal data from England investigated the impact of improving the distribution of healthcare resources on population mortality rates (Hollingsworth 1981). The author used data from before and after the introduction of the National Health Service to determine the effect of changing the distribution of medical care resources on population mortality rates by social class. He found that despite the achievement of equity in distribution of healthcare resources by geographic health region, increased use of services by lower social class patients, and improvements in mortality rates, differences in health status between those at opposite ends of the socioeconomic scale persisted after nearly 40 years of experience in the British National Health Service. For example, the data show that while overall neonatal mortality rates declined over 50 percent during this period of time, the difference in neonatal mortality by social class increased by 25 percent for the lowest social class relative to the highest by 1972. Substantial social class variations in health status have persisted, although access to basic medical care services has historically been more universally assured in that country than in the United States (Gray 1982).

Shortell and his colleagues examined structural and process variables related to functional integration, physician integration, clinical integration, and governance and management in a selected sample of integrated healthcare systems (Shortell et al. 1996). Their study, however, did not encompass health outcomes at either the system or the population level. Lacking this direct evidence, perhaps a brief consideration of performance evaluations of HMOs, which were early forms of integrated health systems, will provide some insights. Luft in his early review of health maintenance organization performance did examine the then few outcomes studies and concluded that "HMO outcomes are not very different from those of conventional practice" (Luft 1981, 250). In later updates, it was found that while there were many more studies, the conclusion was still equivocal, meaning the outcomes were in general no better nor worse on average (Miller and Luft 1994, 1997). The primary exception was negative outcomes for Medicare enrollees with chronic conditions noted in several studies.

Enhanced access is one of the policy strategies related to the process of care involving attempts to increase healthcare utilization for certain groups. Evidence relating to process and outcomes includes studies examining the relationships between the process variables of utilization, quantity of procedures and quality of care, and various outcome variables as the measures of effectiveness. Even though a host of studies (briefly reviewed in Chapter 1) have documented great variation in the geographic distribution of medical care resources and procedure rates, these variations have not been consistently linked to differences in outcomes. This is the clear conclusion from the Boston–New Haven comparison (Wennberg et al. 1989), in which twice the level of utilization of medical care resources in Boston showed no clear mortality advantage for Medicare beneficiaries in the population.

A similar conclusion, that differences in utilization have a modest relationship, if any, to outcomes, can be drawn from studies focused on the clinical perspective. The RAND Health Insurance Experiment (Brook et al. 1983) provides an example of the examination of the effects of varying utilization rates on health outcomes. The study was undertaken to determine what influence various levels of copayment in a national health insurance scheme might have, primarily on utilization and secondarily on health status. The utilization examined included both outpatient treatment and hospitalization for both adults and children. The clinical outcomes assessed were blood pressure and vision for adults; and anemia, hay fever, hearing, fluid in the middle ear, and vision for children. The utilization differences were 33 percent greater for adults and 22 percent greater for children in the free care versus the 95 percent copay plan (Valdez et al. 1985). These utilization differences were accompanied by only slight differences in blood pressure and vision correction in the adults and no differences in clinical outcomes in the children.

An important caveat, however, is that it may not be valid to extrapolate these results to all population groups, because there is substantial heterogeneity in health outcomes across different socioeconomic and racial groups as well as differences by gender and geography. This was pointed out in the data on disparities in population health outcomes for blacks versus whites presented in Chapter 1. It was also confirmed in the RAND (Brook et al. 1983) and the Medical Outcomes studies (Ware et al. 1996), which showed that restrictions, limitations, and managing care did not negatively affect average patients, but that the poor and the elderly were adversely affected.

The importance of this caveat is emphasized by studies of what are called avoidable or preventable hospitalizations. The premise of these studies is that there are identifiable hospital diagnoses that indicate an advanced stage of disease that could have been prevented by accessible primary medical care. By studying the occurrence of these preventable hospitalizations, several studies have shown that poorer populations without access to adequate primary medical care do more often become hospitalized for preventable conditions (Begley et al. 1994; Billings et al. 1993; Parchman and Culler 1994; Weissman, Gatsonis, and Epstein 1992).

Clinical perspective

Regulation of professional performance has only modest evidence to support its effectiveness. As of the time of implementation of the first public regulation of professional performance, the PSRO program, no consistent evaluation evidence existed to support the effectiveness of such a strategy (Slater and Bryant 1975). A decade later, a comprehensive review of the literature by the OTA (1988) found only modest support for the effectiveness of most quality assessment methods, whether process or outcome based. And more recently, Blumenthal (1996), McGlynn (1997), and Lohr (1997) argue that there are still many challenges left in trying to make quality monitoring effective.

One example of the relationship of quality to outcomes from the clinical perspective is an investigation of quality and variation in hospital mortality rates. Using a cross-sectional design and a hospital database, investigators (Dubois et al. 1987) examined the relationship between hospital mortality rates for three specific conditions—heart attack, pneumonia, and stroke—and two different measures of quality of care. They found that 64 percent of the variation in outcomes was explained by the severity of illness in patients admitted to these hospitals, but that there was an association between poorer quality and mortality for one quality assessment method based on a subjective judgment of preventability of death. A subsequent study (Park et al. 1990) confirmed the finding of a modest association between the quality of medical care given and the subsequent death of individual patients.

Outcomes assessment and management suggests that practice guidelines and performance monitoring systems, such as HEDIS, can improve the outcomes of medical care. Evidence for the effectiveness of clinical practice guidelines has been slowly developing. The Consensus Development Program, an example of practice guidelines, was assessed and found lacking by Kosecoff and her colleagues (1987), who investigated the effectiveness of this process for 12 consensus recommendations. They found little impact from any of the recommendations although physicians were aware of them. More importantly, they observed that with regard to several of the guidelines, physician behaviors were changing even before the consensus statements were disseminated. Lomas et al. (1989), investigating the effectiveness of Canadian national guidelines for cesarean-section rates, found that while the majority of obstetricians had knowledge of and agreed with the guidelines and reported reducing their cesarean-section rates, actual practice had in fact changed little. In reviewing a number of studies, Woolf (1990) found similar results, as did Grimshaw and Russell (1993, 1317), who undertook an information synthesis of 59 evaluations of clinical practice guidelines, concluding that "explicit guidelines do improve clinical practice" when the focus is on the process of care, but that less than 20 percent of these studies had looked at the impact on outcomes.

No systematic evaluations of performance reporting systems have been undertaken to assess their usefulness. However, selected examples of evaluations of single-focus programs (Blumenthal and Epstein 1996; Epstein 1995) have been examined, demonstrating mixed results. Outcomes have not regularly been shown to alter, but reporting behavior, in the form of increased severity of illness for patients, has changed. It is perhaps too early to find thorough evaluations of performance monitoring systems, but health services research can contribute to their design and implementation, and hence to determining whether such systems most directly contribute to improved outcomes for patients.

Summary

From the population perspective, variations in population health by race and other characteristics (described in Chapter 1) on the one hand, and geographic variations in care resources and procedures on the other hand, have only modest relationships to one another at the population level. Research in England (Gray 1982; Hollingsworth 1981) illustrates this point: improvements in the distribution of healthcare resources and evidence of better access by the poor did not contribute over time to reducing the disparities in health between members of different social classes. The reasons are complex but can be reduced in part to the assertions that the determinants of population health include more than medical care, and medical care is not a precise science. One implication of these findings about the effectiveness of medical care is that increasing the quantity of medical care resources and improving their distribution and access do not produce substantial improvements in population mortality or morbidity, and appear unable to reduce the sociodemographic disparities in population health. Healthcare in the United States appears to have reached a point of diminishing returns in improving the health of the population. This evidence will be reviewed in greater detail in Chapters 4 and 5.

In summary, while it may be true that further investments in medical care will not improve the health of the population, it does not follow that the same is the case for particularly vulnerable populations, such as the poor and the elderly (Brook et al. 1983; Ware et al. 1996). An important point, however, is that if health policy is intended to improve the health of the population as a whole, it may be better directed at non-medical contributors to population health, such as public health–oriented health protection and health promotion strategies.

From the clinical perspective, despite massive and expensive efforts to improve medical care effectiveness through professional performance regulation and outcomes assessment and management, there is little evidence to date of the success of these efforts. Of the various policy strategies for improving effectiveness, including enhancing public health services, health promotion and disease prevention, biomedical research and its dissemination, increasing the investments in medical care resources, improving the distribution and organization of medical care, regulation of professional performance through quality assessment, enhanced system integration, and outcomes assessment and management, the last has become the dominant focus of federal policy on effectiveness, reflected in the research and policy agenda of AHCPR.

Criteria for Assessing Policy Alternatives in Terms of Effectiveness

The conceptualization by Shortell et al. of the Community Health Care Management System (Shortell, Gillies, and Devers 1995), reflecting both population and clinical perspectives as well as community, system, and institution levels of healthcare, provides the conceptual grounding for a set of criteria for judging effectiveness. Such a system, they suggest, begins with the assessment of needs on a community level, proceeds to the development of resources and services across the continuum of care to meet those needs, develops guidelines and protocols to guide the care, and then suggests a monitoring system to assure that the needs are met. This framework leads to the following criteria for evaluating a health policy reform from a population perspective:

1. The health policy option should be based on the results of a community health needs assessment. This assumption implies that there should be a community health needs assessment from which information on policy options are derived, and that a population-based, community-level health information system should be in place to guide health policy development for the population. The Evans et al. (1994) model provides a framework for such population information and POPULIS (Roos et al. 1996) serves as a concrete example of such a system.

2. The health policy option selected should reflect an appropriate relationship to the continuum of healthcare services. The resources and services for maintaining and improving health need to be integrated across the entire continuum of care, including health promotion and disease prevention, and any specific policy option needs to be clearly related to this full continuum. The continuum of services displayed in Figure 1.1 in Chapter 1 illustrates the range of health services that needs to be considered.

Shortell's framework also leads to a set of criteria for evaluating, from a clinical perspective, health policy reform options:

1. Precision of medical care will be fostered by the specification in advance of guidelines for clinical performance. Such practice guidelines, protocols, or practice parameters can reduce the uncertainty in medical care, and can contribute not only to improved effectiveness, but also to enhanced efficiency.

2. Performance of medical care can also be improved through the monitoring of process and outcomes indicators for selected clinical conditions. JCAHO- and HEDIS-type process and outcome indicators would appear to be the measures of choice. These include such items as low birth weight, senior's health status, and satisfaction with care.

These criteria, along with indicators of their presence and adequacy, are summarized in Table 3.3. The presence of a population health information system is taken as an indicator of the possibility of population needs–based assessment. The existence of the full continuum of services indicates comprehensiveness. Practice guidelines indicate attention to precision, while a performance monitoring system indicates a focus on performance.

An Application of Effectiveness Criteria: Medicaid Managed Care

Medicaid managed care was introduced in Chapter 1 as an example of an important health policy issue, illustrating the application of the concepts of effectiveness, efficiency, and equity. The evidence regarding its effectiveness will be examined here.

A number of evaluations of the Medicaid managed care program have been undertaken to assess the impact on outcomes for enrollees compared to those in fee-for-service arrangements. In other words, these evaluations have examined professional performance in terms of outcomes from the clinical perspective. Three groups of Medicaid beneficiaries have been the subjects of these evaluations:

Table 3.3   Criteria for Assessing Health Policies in Terms of
            Effectiveness

Issue	Criteria	Indicators
Population Effectiveness		
Need-based	• Based on the results of a community health needs assessment	• Population health information system
Comprehensiveness	• Reflect an appropriate relationship to the continuum of healthcare services	• Full continuum of services
Clinical Effectiveness		
Precision	• Specify in advance expected guidelines for structure and process	• Practice guidelines
Performance	• Monitor process and outcome indicators for selected conditions	• Performance monitoring system

pregnant women, chronically mentally ill patients, and elderly patients. In general these studies have found no significant improvements for any of these groups under managed care arrangements,
but in most cases they have found no significant declines.

The majority of the studies have examined the impacts on
pregnant women, looking at their prenatal care and at the outcomes
of pregnancy in terms of complications, cesarean-section rates, gestational age, and low birth weight. Risk adjustments, when done
at all, have used mother's race and age as well as time of program
eligibility. Each of these is typical of a study with system-level independent variables—Medicaid managed care versus fee-for-service
care—and patient-level outcome variables aggregated to the system level. Study designs have been cross-sectional, retrospective
case control, or longitudinal. Data sources have included Medicaid
claims and enrollment files, birth certificates, and medical records.

The original Medicaid Managed Care Competition Demonstration Project (Freund et al. 1989) in the 1980s looked at birth weight
in comparing pregnancy outcomes in six states: California, Florida,
Minnesota, Missouri, New Jersey, and New York. Researchers found
no differences in mean birth weights and proportion of newborns
of low birth weight when the managed care demonstrations were

compared to fee-for-service in Medicaid programs in these states. They did discover, however, that prenatal care in the first trimester of pregnancy, a process variable, fell far short of desired standards; while the national average at the time was 76.4 percent, none of the demonstration projects rates exceeded 36 percent and some ranged as low as 32 percent.

Mean birth weights were shown to be greater in the prepaid program in California but lower in the Missouri prepaid program, although the latter result was not statistically significant (Carey, Weis, and Homer 1991). The proportion of children of low birth weight was shown to be less in both the California and Missouri prepaid programs as compared to fee-for-service, but neither of these differences was statistically significant. After adjustment for mother's race and age, time of eligibility, and prenatal care, the results remained the same. In a similar evaluation in Washington, Medicaid recipients in the managed care plans had equal or slightly better birthweight outcomes than those seen in the fee-for-service system (Krieger, Connell, and LoGerfo 1992).

A longitudinal evaluation of Iowa Medicaid recipients in managed care versus fee-for-service showed no significant differences in mean gestational age, but mixed results for birth weight (Schulman, Sheriff, and Momany 1997). These authors, however, subcategorized low birth weight into low (1500–2499 g) and very low (< 1500 g), and found contrasting results. Over the period from 1989–1992, the proportion of low-birthweight infants decreased in the FFS programs while the proportion of very low-birthweight infants increased in the same FFS programs. They also noted that the diagnosis "normal newborn" was significantly lower in the managed care programs.

A study undertaken to evaluate the impact of Medicaid managed care on the outcomes for patients with chronic mental illness was based on a RCT with Medicaid clients in the Medicaid Demonstration Project in Hennepin County, Minnesota (Lurie et al. 1992). About 700 patients were interviewed both at baseline and about one year later. Neither general health status nor psychiatric symptoms were significantly different between the managed care and the fee-for-service groups.

The same research team also conducted a study of the outcomes for elderly patients enrolled in Medicaid in Hennepin County, Minnesota (Lurie et al. 1994). In this RCT, 800 Medicaid beneficiaries 65 years of age or older were assessed both at baseline and a year later. There were no differences between the managed care and the fee-for-service groups in the number of deaths, the proportion of fair or poor health, physical functioning, activities of daily living, visual acuity, and blood pressure or diabetic control.

Given the preceding review of effectiveness evidence, these are not surprising findings. As shown previously, substantial changes in the utilization of medical care result in modest if any differences in outcomes. The change brought about by Medicaid managed care may have been an improvement, but it could hardly be called major or substantial. In fact, the Medicaid managed care intervention, especially the PCCM model in many states, was very weak and did not differ substantially from the fee-for-service system. In addition to being organizationally weak, the early history of performance was mixed. Given these limitations, a significant and positive impact of Medicaid managed care has yet to be unambiguously documented.

In addition, when changes in the average health of whole groups of clients is assessed, medical care makes only a small contribution to these changes. In other words, given significant health problems, many of which are rooted in environmental and behavioral determinants, a modest change in the form of delivering medical care is not likely to be reflected in altered health status for many particularly at-risk populations. The efficiency and equity evidence on the results of the Medicaid managed care program will provide further insight into the usefulness of this program. If effectiveness does not decline, then achieving the same result for less cost provides evidence of gains in efficiency. Data bearing on this issue will be presented in Chapter 5. Gains in efficiency pose the question of whether they have been translated into greater access in terms of more people getting care or the same number of people getting greater amounts of needed care. Evidence related to this question will be reviewed in Chapter 7.

Summary and Conclusions

This chapter has focused on the question: What policy strategies contribute most to improving the health of the population? The evidence reviewed from the population perspective suggests that while the point of diminishing returns from further investments in medical care with regard to improving the health of the population may have been reached, a case should still be made for investments in medical care for improving the health of vulnerable population groups. The health of populations in general, as well as at-risk groups in particular, is most likely to be enhanced, however, by focusing more resources on non-medical determinants of health, such as the physical, social, and economic environments in which individuals live and work. Chapters 4 and 5 provide arguments and evidence that economic, as well as health, benefits may be yielded as a consequence.

Note

1. It is interesting that it was a report written by Lemuel Shattuck in 1850 that early documented the need for services to improve the health of the public, a population perspective strategy—and that it was at the Shattuck Lecture (named in his honor) in 1988 that Paul Ellwood proclaimed the ascendancy of outcomes assessment, a policy strategy clearly situated in the clinical perspective.

References

Agency for Health Care Policy and Research. 1997. Guidelines and Medical Outcomes [Online]. Available: http://www.ahcpr.gov:80/clinic/ [12/17/97].

Beasley, J. D., and J. Swift. 1989. *The Kellogg Report: The Impact of Nutrition, Environment & Lifestyle on the Health of Americans.* Annandale-On-Hudson, NY: Institute of Health Policy and Practice, The Bard College Center.

Begley, C. E., C. H. Slater, M. J. Engel, and T. F. Reynolds. 1994. "Avoidable Hospitalizations and Socio-Economic Status in Galveston County, Texas." *The Journal of Community Health* 19: 377–87.

Billings, J., L. Zeitel, J. Lukomnik, T. S. Carey, A. E. Blank, and L. Newman. 1993. "Impact of Socioeconomic Status on Hospital Use in New York City." *Health Affairs* 12 (1): 162–73.

Blum, H. L. 1976. "From a Concept of Health to a National Health Policy." *American Journal of Health Planning* 1 (1): 3–22.

Blumenthal, D. 1996. "Quality of Health Care. Part 1: Quality of Care— What Is It?" *The New England Journal of Medicine* 335: 891–94.

Blumenthal, D. S. 1985. *Introduction to Environmental Health*. New York: Springer Publishing Company.

Blumenthal, D., and A. M. Epstein. 1996. "Quality of Health Care. Part 6: The Role of Physicians in the Future of Quality Management." *The New England Journal of Medicine* 335: 1328–31.

Bodenheimer, T. S. 1969. "Regional Medical Programs: No Road to Regionalization." *Medical Care Review* 26: 1125–66.

Brook, R. 1989. "Practice Guidelines and Practicing Medicine: Are They Compatible?" *Journal of the American Medical Association* 262: 3027–30.

Brook, R., J. Ware, W. Rogers, E. Keeler, A. Davies, C. Donald, G. Goldberg, K. Lohr, P. Masthay, and J. Newhouse. 1983. "Does Free Care Improve Adults' Health? Results from a Randomized Controlled Trial." *The New England Journal of Medicine* 309: 1426–34.

Bunker, J. P., H. S. Frazier, and F. Mosteller. 1994. "Improving Health: Measuring Effects of Medical Care." *The Milbank Quarterly* 72: 225–58.

Burtram, S. G. 1994. "A Critical Assessment of the National Institutes of Health Consensus Development Program Against the Eras Which Shaped It." Ph.D. Dissertation, University of Texas School of Public Health.

Carey, T. S., K. Weis, and C. Homer. 1991. "Prepaid Versus Traditional Medicaid Plans: Lack of Effect on Pregnancy Outcomes and Prenatal Care." *Health Services Research* 26: 165–81.

Cassel, J. C. 1976. "The Contribution of the Social Environment to Host Resistance." *American Journal of Epidemiology* 104: 107–23.

Centers for Disease Control and Prevention. 1991. "Consensus Set of Health Status Indicators for the General Assessment of Community Health Status–United States." *Morbidity and Mortality Weekly Report* 40: 449–51.

Charlton, J. H. R., and R. Velez. 1986. "Some International Comparisons of Mortality Amenable to Medical Intervention." *British Medical Journal* 292: 295–301.

Cochrane, A. L., A. S. St. Leger, and F. Moore. 1978. "Health Service 'Input' and Mortality 'Output' in Developed Countries." *Journal of Epidemiology and Community Health* 32: 200–205.

Doll, R., and R. Peto. 1981. *The Causes of Cancer: Quantitative Estimates of Avoidable Risks of Cancer in the United States Today*. New York: Oxford University Press.

Dubois, R. W., W. H. Rogers, J. H. Moxley, D. Draper, and R. H. Brook. 1987. "Hospital Inpatient Mortality: Is It a Predictor of Quality?" *The New England Journal of Medicine* 317: 1674–80.

Eddy, D. M. 1990. "Clinical Decision Making: From Theory to Practice—

Practice Policies—What Are They?" *Journal of the American Medical Association* 263: 877–78,880.

Epstein, A. M. 1995. "Performance Reports on Quality—Prototypes, Problems, and Prospects." *The New England Journal of Medicine* 333: 57–61.

Evans, R. G., M. L. Barer, and T. R. Marmor, eds. 1994. *Why Are Some People Healthy and Others Not? The Determinants of Health of Populations.* New York: Aldine De Gruyter.

Fielding, J. E. 1978. "Successes of Prevention." *Milbank Memorial Fund Quarterly* 56: 274–302.

Freund, D. A., L. F. Rossiter, P. D. Fox, J. A. Meyer, R. E. Hurley, T. S. Carey, and J. E. Paul. 1989. "Evaluation of the Medicaid Competition Demonstrations." *Health Care Financing Review* 11 (2): 81–97.

Glanz, K., F. M. Lewis, and B. Rimer, eds. 1997. *Health Behavior and Health Education: Theory, Research, and Practice.* 2nd ed. San Francisco: Jossey-Bass Publishers.

Gordis, L. 1973. "Effectiveness of Comprehensive-Care Programs in Preventing Rheumatic Fever." *The New England Journal of Medicine* 289: 331–35.

Gray, A. 1982. "Inequalities in Health: The Black Report. A Summary and Comment." *International Journal of Health Services* 12: 349–80.

Grimshaw, J. M., and I. T. Russell. 1993. "Effect of Clinical Guidelines on Medical Practice: A Systematic Review of Rigorous Evaluations." *The Lancet* 342: 1317–22.

Hadley, J. 1982. *More Medical Care, Better Health? An Economic Analysis of Mortality Rates.* Washington, D.C.: The Urban Institute Press.

Harden, V. A. 1986. *Inventing the NIH: Federal Biomedical Research Policy, 1887–1937.* Baltimore, MD: Johns Hopkins University Press.

Hollingsworth, J. R. 1981. "Inequality in Levels of Health in England and Wales, 1891–1971." *Journal of Health and Social Behavior* 22: 268–83.

House, J. S., C. Robbins, and H. L. Metzner. 1982. "The Association of Social Relationships and Activities With Mortality: Prospective Evidence From the Tecumseh Community Health Study." *American Journal of Epidemiology* 116: 123–40.

Institute of Medicine. 1988. *The Future of Public Health.* Washington, D.C.: National Academy Press.

———. 1992. *Guidelines for Clinical Practice.* Washington, D.C.: Institute of Medicine.

———. 1997. *Improving Health in the Community: A Role for Performance Monitoring.* Washington, D.C.: National Academy Press.

Joint Commission on Accreditation of Healthcare Organizations. 1997. JCAHO Home Page [Online]. Available: http://www.jcaho.org/ [9/12/97].

Kissick, W. L. 1970. "Health-Policy Directions for the 1970s." *The New England Journal of Medicine* 282: 1343–50.

Komaroff, A. L. 1971. "Regional Medical Programs in Search of a Mission." *The New England Journal of Medicine* 284: 758–64.

Kosecoff, J., D. Kanouse, W. Rogers, L. McCloskey, C. M. Winsolow, and R. H. Brook. 1987. "Effects of the National Institutes of Health Consensus Development Program on Physician Practice." *Journal of the American Medical Association* 258: 2708–13.

Krieger, J. W., F. A. Connell, and J. P. LoGerfo. 1992. "Medicaid Prenatal Care: A Comparison of Use and Outcomes in Fee-For-Service and Managed Care." *American Journal of Public Health* 82: 185–90.

Lalonde, M. 1975. *A New Perspective on the Health of Canadians: A Working Document.* Ottawa, Canada: Information Canada.

Lohr, K. N. 1997. "How Do We Measure Quality?" *Health Affairs* 16 (3): 22–25.

Lomas, J. 1993. "Making Clinical Policy Explicit." *International Journal of Technology Assessment in Health Care* 9: 11–25.

Lomas, J., G. M. Anderson, K. Domnick-Pierre, E. Vayda, M. W. Enkin, and W. J. Hannah. 1989. "Do Practice Guidelines Guide Practice? The Effect of a Consensus Statement on the Practice of Physicians." *The New England Journal of Medicine* 321: 1306–11.

Luft, H. S. 1981. *Health Maintenance Organizations: Dimensions of Performance.* New York: John Wiley & Sons.

Luft, H. S., J. P. Bunker, and A. C. Enthoven. 1979. "Should Operations Be Regionalized? The Empirical Relation Between Surgical Volume and Mortality." *The New England Journal of Medicine* 301: 1364–69.

Lurie, N., J. B. Christianson, M. Finch, and I. S. Moscovice. 1994. "The Effects of Capitation on Health and Functional Status of the Medicaid Elderly: A Randomized Trial." *Annals of Internal Medicine* 120: 506-11.

Lurie, N., I. S. Moscovice, M. Finch, J. B. Christianson, and M. K. Poplin. 1992. "Does Capitation Affect the Health of the Chronically Mentally Ill? Results From a Randomized Trial." *Journal of the American Medical Association* 276: 3300–04.

Marmot, M. G., H. Bosma, H. Hemingway, E. Brunner, and S. Stansfeld. 1997. "Contribution of Job Control and Other Risk Factors to Social Variations in Coronary Heart Disease Incidence." *The Lancet* 350: 235–39.

Marmot, M. G., M. Kogevinas, and M. Elston. 1987. "Social/Economic Status and Disease." *Annual Review of Public Health* 8: 111–35.

Marmot, M. G., S. L. Syme, A. Kagan, H. Kato, J. B. Cohen, and J. Belsky. 1975. "Epidemiological Studies of Coronary Heart Disease and Stroke in Japanese Men Living in Japan, Hawaii, and California: Prevalence of Coronary and Hypertensive Disease and Associated Risk Factors." *American Journal of Epidemiology* 102: 514–25.

Martini, C. J. M., G. J. B. Allan, J. Davison, and E. M. Backett. 1977. "Health Indexes Sensitive to Medical Care Variation." *International Journal of Health Services* 7: 293–309.

McGlynn, E. A. 1997. "Six Challenges in Measuring the Quality of Health Care." *Health Affairs* 16 (3): 7–21.

McKeown, T. 1976. *The Role of Medicine: Dream, Mirage, Or Nemesis?* London: Nuffield Provincial Hospitals Trust.

McKinlay, J. B., and S. M. McKinlay. 1977. "The Questionable Contribution of Medical Measures to the Decline of Mortality in the United States in the Twentieth Century." *Milbank Memorial Fund Quarterly* 55: 405–28.

McKinlay, J. B., S. M. McKinlay, and R. Beaglehole. 1989. "A Review of the Evidence Concerning the Impact of Medical Measures on Recent Mortality and Morbidity in the United States." *International Journal of Health Services* 19: 181–208.

Mhatre, S. L., and R. B. Deber. 1992. "From Equal Access to Health Care to Equitable Access to Health: A Review of Canadian Provincial Health Commissions and Reports." *International Journal of Health Services* 22: 645–68.

Miller, R. H., and H. S. Luft. 1994. "Managed Care Plan Performance Since 1980: A Literature Analysis." *Journal of the American Medical Association* 271: 1512–19.

———. 1997. "Does Managed Care Lead to Better Or Worse Quality of Care?" *Health Affairs* 16 (5): 7–25.

Misch, A. 1994. "Assessing Environmental Health Risks." In *State of the World 1994.* Edited by L. Starke, 117–36. New York: Norton & Co.

National Center for Health Statistics. 1996. *Healthy People 2000 Review, 1995–96.* Hyattsville, MD: Public Health Service.

National Committee for Quality Assurance. 1997. NCQA Home Page. [Online.] Available: http://www.ncqa.org/index.htm [9/12/97].

Newhouse, J. P., and L. J. Friedlander. 1979. "The Relationship Between Medical Resources and Measures of Health: Some Additional Evidence." *Journal of Human Resources* 15: 201–18.

Organization for Economic Cooperation and Development. 1995. *New Directions in Health Care Policy*, Health Policy Series No. 7. Paris, France: OECD.

Parchman, M. L., and S. Culler. 1994. "Primary Care Physicians and Avoidable Hospitalizations." *The Journal of Family Practice* 39: 123–28.

Park, R. E., R. H. Brook, J. Kosecoff, J. Keesey, L. Rubenstein, E. Keeler, K. L. Kahn, W. H. Rogers, and M. R. Chassin. 1990. "Explaining Variations in Hospital Death Rates: Randomness, Severity of Illness, Quality of Care." *Journal of the American Medical Association* 264: 484–90.

Renaud, M. 1994. "The Future: Hygeia Versus Panakeia?" In *Why Are Some People Healthy and Others Not: The Determinants of Health of Populations.* Edited by R. G. Evans, M. L. Barer, and T. R. Marmor, 317–34. New York: Aldine De Gruyter.

Roos, N. P., C. Black, N. Frohlich, C. DeCoster, M. Cohen, D. J. Tataryn, C. A. Mustard, L. L. Roos, F. Toll, K. C. Carrière, C. A. Burchill, L. MacWilliam, and B. Bogdanovic. 1996. "Population Health and Health Care Use: An Information System for Policy Makers." *Milbank Memorial Fund Quarterly* 74: 3–31.

Scheuplein, R. J. 1992. "Perspectives in Toxicological Risk—An Example: Foodborne Carcinogenic Risk." *Critical Reviews in Food Science & Nutrition* 32: 105–21.

Schulman, E. D., D. J. Sheriff, and E. T. Momany. 1997. "Primary Care Case Management and Birth Outcomes in the Iowa Medicaid Program." *American Journal of Public Health* 87: 80–84.

Shortell, S. M., R. R. Gillies, D. A. Anderson, K. M. Erickson, and J. B. Mitchell. 1996. *Remaking Health Care in America: Building Organized Delivery Systems.* San Francisco: Jossey-Bass.

Shortell, S. M., R. R. Gillies, D. A. Anderson, J. B. Mitchell, and K. L. Morgan. 1993. "Creating Organized Delivery Systems: The Barriers and Facilitators." *Hospital & Health Services Administration* 38: 447–66.

Shortell, S. M., R. R. Gillies, and K. J. Devers. 1995. "Reinventing the American Hospital." *Milbank Quarterly* 73 (2): 131–60.

Slater, C. H., and A. Bryant. 1975. *Regulation of Professional Performance: Background Discussion and Annotated Bibliography.* Denver, CO: Policy Center, Inc.

Stockwell, E. G. 1961. "Socioeconomic Status and Mortality in the United States." *Public Health Reports* 76: 1081–86.

Syme, S. L. 1996. "Rethinking Disease: Where Do We Go From Here?" *Annals of Epidemiology* 6: 463–68.

Syme, S. L., and L. F. Berkman. 1976. "Social Class, Susceptibility and Sickness." *American Journal of Epidemiology* 104: 1–8.

Thacker, S. B., J. P. Koplan, W. R. Taylor, A. R. Hinman, M. F. Katz, and W. L. Roper. 1994. "Assessing Prevention Effectiveness Using Data to Drive Program Decisions." *Public Health Reports* 109: 187–94.

Turnock, B. J. 1997. *Public Health: What It Is and How It Works.* Gaithersburg, MD: Aspen Publishers.

U.S. Congress Office of Technology Assessment. 1988. *The Quality of Medical Care: Information for Consumers*, OTA-H-386. Washington, D.C.: Government Printing Office.

U.S. Department of Health, Education, and Welfare (USDHEW). 1979. *Healthy People: The Surgeon General's Report on Health Promotion and Disease Prevention*, DHEW(PHS) Publication No. 79-55071. Washington, D.C.: USDHEW.

Valdez, R. B., R. H. Brook, W. H. Rogers, E. B. Keeler, C. A. Sherbourne, K. N. Lohr, G. A. Goldberg, P. Camp, and J. P. Newhouse. 1985. "Consequences of Cost-Sharing for Children's Health." *Pediatrics* 75: 952–61.

Ware, J. E., M. S. Bayliss, W. H. Rogers, M. Kosinski, and A. R. Tarlov. 1996. "Differences in 4-Year Health Outcomes for Elderly and Poor, Chronically Ill Patients Treated in HMO and Fee-For-Service Systems." *Journal of the American Medical Association* 276: 1039–47.

Weissman, J. S., C. Gatsonis, and A. M. Epstein. 1992. "Rates of Avoidable Hospitalization By Insurance Status in Massachusetts and Maryland." *Journal of the American Medical Association* 268: 2388–94.

Wennberg, J. E., J. L. Freeman, R. M. Shelton, and T. A. Bubolz. 1989. "Hospital Use and Mortality Among Medicare Beneficiaries in Boston and New Haven." *The New England Journal of Medicine* 321: 1168–73.

Wilkinson, R. G. 1992. "Income Distribution and Life Expectancy." *British Medical Journal* 304: 165–68.

Wilson, R., and E. A. C. Crouch. 1987. "Risk Assessment and Comparisons: An Introduction." *Science* 236: 267–70.

Woolf, S. H. 1990. "Practice Guidelines: A New Reality in Medicine. I. Recent Developments." *Archives of Internal Medicine* 150: 1811–18.

Chapter 4

Efficiency: Concepts and Methods

Overview

The fundamental questions in this chapter related to assessing the efficiency of healthcare are (1) What is efficiency? and (2) How might efficiency be measured?

The concepts and methods of efficiency research provide guidance for societal decision making regarding the combination of healthcare goods and services to be produced with society's limited resources, and the ways in which these goods and services are to be produced, as well as whether the maximum value is being achieved in terms of improving the health of the population relative to the costs required to produce these goods and services.

All modern societies allocate a large portion of their wealth to the provision of healthcare services. The United States leads the world both in the level of healthcare spending and in efforts to study the problems of access, quality, and cost of healthcare. In 1960, 5.3 percent of the U.S. GDP was spent on healthcare. By 1995 it had increased to 13.6 percent (NCHS 1997). Large variations in medical practice; evidence on the possible lack of effectiveness of many medical procedures; and the renewed interest in disease prevention, health promotion, and non-medical determinants of health suggest that the current allocation of healthcare resources is not efficient (OECD 1995).

In aggregate terms, both the efficiency and equity of the U.S. healthcare system compare unfavorably to Canada and several western European countries. Analysts in the United States have examined those countries both to obtain points of reference for U.S.

problems and to gain insight into possible solutions. Despite their relatively low expenditures and broad coverage, other countries also perceive severe problems with their healthcare systems and look to the United States for innovative healthcare delivery and financing systems. These countries look in particular to the extensive U.S. health services research base on the effectiveness, efficiency, and equity of alternative healthcare systems.

Because of the concern about past and projected public and private payor budgets for healthcare, macroeconomic cost control—assuring that the healthcare system consumes an "appropriate" share of GDP—is a major goal of developed countries (OECD 1995). Although it is not necessary to restrain the percentage of GDP spent on health simply because it is high or growing rapidly, such limits are desirable when government policies or private market failure lead to excess supply of, or to excess demand for, health services. Ideally, cost containment would first be achieved by eliminating spending on services that were detrimental to, or had no effect on, patient health status. If further reductions were required, services would be ranked and funded according to their yield in health improvement per dollar. While the state of Oregon in the United States has struggled to implement a system for efficiently rationing healthcare, policymakers to date have no fully satisfactory mechanism for these technically and ethically difficult decisions (Eddy 1991; Hadorn 1991; Tengs 1996). Research on the efficiency of health services delivery does provide some guidance, however, in making these decisions.

Evans and Stoddart (1990) have suggested that healthcare spending has risen to the point where it may actually cause a decline in the health of the population because it draws resources from areas, such as education, housing, and the environment, that provide a positive contribution to health, and applies them to medical services that have low, no, or even negative impacts on the health of the population as a whole (Evans, Barer, and Marmor 1994).

Thus, the questions of how much to spend on healthcare, what healthcare services to provide, and how to provide them have become important policy issues. Because of the nature of health and healthcare, the status of healthcare as a good that many feel should be available regardless of one's ability to pay, the impingement of healthcare costs on public budgets, the lack of information, and other healthcare market imperfections, the solution cannot simply be left to the operation of the private market. There is a constant search for a better understanding of these problems and of the operation of the healthcare system, and for policies that will improve the access, cost, and quality of healthcare.

The tools of efficiency analysis can assist in formulating these policies. This chapter introduces these tools and the theoretical underpinnings for each in the context of addressing the first question posed at the beginning of the chapter: What is efficiency? In particular, the concepts of allocative and production efficiency will be presented and defined, and the theoretical basis for need and market demand criteria for making resource allocation and production decisions will be discussed. The role of production functions; cost-effectiveness, cost-benefit, and cost-utility analysis; and international comparisons will be examined in addressing the second question: How might efficiency be measured? Chapter 5 (1) describes the broad approaches and specific means by which various countries have attempted to achieve efficiency goals; (2) reviews selected evidence on the performance of those policies with respect to efficiency; and (3) delineates and applies efficiency criteria to the evaluation of the Medicaid managed care policy in the United States.

Conceptual Framework and Definitions

For society as a whole, efficiency requires that the combination of goods and services with the highest attainable total value, given limited resources and technology, be produced (Byrns and Stone 1987). This requires attainment of both allocative and production efficiency. *Allocative efficiency* depends on attainment of the "right," or most valued, mix of outputs (Davis et al. 1990). *Production efficiency* refers to producing a given level of output at minimum cost. As implied in the conceptual framework introduced in Chapter 1 (Figure 1.4), improving the health of communities and individuals is the desired and valued endpoint, or output, of societal investments in health programs and policies. Culyer (1992) suggests that these decisions have important implications for the equity of healthcare provision as well, based on both the fairness and the effectiveness of the allocation of resources to achieve desired health outcomes.

Allocative Efficiency

Where healthcare is viewed as an input in the production of health improvements, the focus is on allocative efficiency (i.e., maximizing health given constrained resources). Allocative inefficiency may occur even in a production-efficient health system if the system produces too many or too few of some services relative to health improvements. Allocative efficiency problems arise in healthcare delivery, for example, when substantial resources are allocated to treatments of questionable effectiveness while proven prenatal screening and other preventive services are neglected. Primary health policy areas that reflect concerns with allocative efficiency include decision making regarding investments in (1) medical versus non-medical policy alternatives; (2) coverage of preventive services; and (3) mix or types of treatment, in relationship to health improvements.

Medical versus non-medical alternatives

In a broader context of health-oriented social policy, a society may achieve much greater health benefits by diverting resources from healthcare to activities that improve the physical and social environment, for example, air and water quality, education, job training, and community development (Evans, Barer, and Marmor 1994). Studies have documented that the marginal product of healthcare in the United States is small for the population as a whole, but may be higher for selected population groups such as the elderly (Folland, Goodman, and Stano 1997). Lifestyle factors, on the other hand, have been found to be major and significant predictors of population health status, as has education. One theory (Grossman 1972) has proposed that schooling improves the efficiency with which one produces one's own health; better-educated people know what is needed to stay healthy, and know how to use medical and other inputs, as well as their time, to produce better health (Behrman and Wolfe 1989; Berger and Lee 1989; Wolfe and Behrman 1987). These findings present interesting challenges to state policymakers in particular, who may be confronting significant trade-offs in deciding the relative allocation of state tax dollars to Medicaid versus public education.

Preventive services

There is concern within the healthcare sector that too much is spent on the treatment of cases for whom health improvements or survival are remote, and that too little is spent on preventive services (Lubitz and Prihoda 1984; Scitovsky 1988; Waldo and Lazenby 1984; Webster and Berdes 1990). Studies of effectiveness and cost-effectiveness (Eddy 1980) have been used in selecting preventive services to be covered by public and private insurance (Gold et al. 1996; Pear 1997; U.S. Preventive Services Task Force 1989). The U.S. Department of Health and Human Services (1990) reported an allocation of $5.2 billion to preventive activities in 1988, that represented about one percent of national health expenditures.[1] Recently, there has been a shift toward greater reimbursement and provision of preventive services. The continuing growth of health maintenance organizations, which typically provide a broad range of preventive care, is a major contributor to this shift (NCHS 1997).

Luft and Greenlick (1996) note that HMOs tend to cover preventive services without significant copayments. Staff and group model HMOs with lower disenrollment rates have a further incentive to encourage preventive services with potential for long-term benefits. While HMOs may offer increased preventive services, however, studies also recognize the existence of appointment delay, busy schedules, and other barriers to implementation of both primary and secondary prevention services (Kottke, Brekke, and Solberg 1993; Thompson 1996).

Mix or types of treatment

There is also policy concern about the appropriate and efficient mix or types of services delivered in treating patients. One area of concern is the misallocation of resources to technical procedures and away from services that improve patients' understanding of their health problems and of ways they can ameliorate and possibly avoid health problems in the future. Due to the malpractice and fee-for-service reimbursement systems, physicians have been induced to perform procedures such as surgery and diagnostic tests and to spend less time taking histories and providing congnitive services to patients (e.g., health education or motivational counseling).

Extensive testing provides documentation to use in the case of a medical liability lawsuit. Tests and other procedures also provide much higher remuneration per unit of time compared to cognitive services (Hsaio et al. 1988). This problem is exacerbated by physician ownership of diagnostic equipment and laboratories (Hillman et al. 1990). Given that most diseases have a strong behavioral component, one of the most important and potentially effective aspects of patient care is being neglected due to this concentration on procedures as opposed to patient education and counseling.

Production Efficiency

Health is viewed as the final output and health services the intermediate output of the healthcare system. Production efficiency (i.e., producing output at the least cost) is of concern for both intermediate and final outputs. Production efficiency addresses whether resources are organized and managed in a manner that minimizes the cost of production, as well as whether personnel, supplies, and equipment are paid for at rates that represent their cost in their next-best alternative use. Inefficiency occurs when care is not managed in a way that maximizes potential productivity. For example, inefficiency occurs when physicians provide services that could be provided just as well by nurses or other less expensive health personnel, and when practice does not take advantage of economies of scale, as in the production of laboratory services. These concepts of efficiency are relevant at the level of the individual patient and practitioner, and at institution, system, and community levels (see Table 1.1).

Figure 4.1 displays combinations of goods and services that could be produced with society's resources during a given period of time. Within the figure, the curve AB represents the production possibility frontier. Points on the curve represent the maximum possible output of all goods and services, given current technology and the most efficient production methods. If actual production is inside the curve, as at point C, production efficiency is not being achieved. Within the shaded area, improvements in production efficiency could expand healthcare without reducing output of other goods and services, and vice versa. From any point on the frontier, however, expansion of one commodity is at the expense of the other.

Thus, allocative decisions must be made in terms of the trade-off between healthcare and other goods and services.

The production possibility frontier only illustrates that alternative combinations are possible. It does not identify the allocatively efficient combination. Resource allocation is a complex, dynamic process that depends on a combination of private spending decisions and government tax and spending decisions. With a growing economy and technological base, the frontier is continually expanding, with technology itself as the focus of concern. The well-being of society is subject to decisions about the allocation of resources to technology, to healthcare, and to other goods and services.

Both allocative and production efficiency focus on providing guidance for what might be an optimal allocation of resources and associated costs relative to desired outputs (e.g., health and healthcare). The theoretical underpinnings for determining the optimal distribution of resources to produce these desired ends are described in the next section.

Criteria for Optimal Allocation

Examples of resource misallocation and inefficient production of healthcare can be documented (as will be shown in Chapter 5). Nonetheless, the optimal allocation of resources and production

Figure 4.1 Production Possibility Frontier

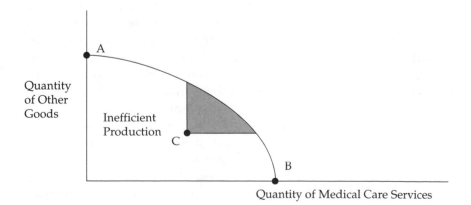

Quantity of Medical Care Services

methods is not known. Three major problems confront analysts and policymakers attempting to evaluate healthcare resource allocation issues. The first problem is limited theoretical and empirical information on how to analyze the effects of resource-allocation decisions on social well-being. Social well-being or social welfare is simply the sum of individual utilities attained by individuals in society (Stokey and Zeckhauser 1978). Second is the related problem of limited information on the relationship between healthcare utilization and health. Third, both market and regulatory systems have proven to be highly imperfect mechanisms for allocating resources in the healthcare sector of the economy.

Philosophers have long sought to develop theories and practical guides to define and measure social welfare. Vilfredo Pareto (1848–1923)[2] provided much of the underpinnings of welfare economics, a collection of analytic devices and concepts for evaluating resource allocation decisions. Central to this work is the Pareto optimum, which occurs when all mutually beneficial exchanges have been made such that no one person can be made better off without making someone else worse off. With freedom to trade, rational individuals or their proxies make all trades that they believe benefit them. However, there are many possible Pareto optimum allocations, depending on the distribution of income. Identifying and achieving the one that maximizes social well-being involves trade-offs between winners and losers and knowledge of a social welfare function.

A social welfare function describes a decision maker's preferences among alternative combinations of individual utilities (Stokey and Zeckhauser 1978). It describes how the decision maker would trade off gains in utility by some people for losses by others. For example, how is social welfare affected by allocating fewer state dollars to public education and more to Medicaid for low-income families? To answer this question requires that individual preferences be combined and aggregated to provide a ranking of welfare, or likely public benefit, for society as a whole.

Arrow (1963) has demonstrated that development of such a function at the overall societal level is not possible. It has been shown in theory, however, that competitive markets can yield a Pareto optimum (Stokey and Zeckhauser 1978). Informed rational consumers make mutually beneficial trades, and competition forces producers to seek efficient methods of production and to respond to consumer preferences.

Given the uncertainty, complexity, and importance of health-care, societies have developed mechanisms for making resource allocation decisions. These include *need*, which primarily undergirds regulatory-based approaches, and *consumer demand*, which under-lies market-based approaches.

Need

Need, as defined by health professionals (Jeffers, Bognanno, and Bartlett 1971), has formed the basis for government-imposed ap-proaches to healthcare resource allocation. Need for medical care exists when someone is better off with a treatment than without it, and the improvement is measured in terms of a person's health (Williams 1974). Therefore, unless healthcare professionals deem a treatment to be effective and the patient values its outcome, the treatment is not "needed."

While need is a useful concept for determining the care pa-tients require, there are severe conceptual and practical problems with using need as a basis for resource allocation. First, there is no objective basis on which to rank health needs and to compare them with other needs of individuals and populations. Second, even with this restrictive definition, needs appear to be insatiable, and thus still require rationing. When some needs are met, the healthcare industry defines new areas not previously addressed by medicine. Third, the relationship between providing healthcare services and reducing health needs is often unclear if not nonexistent (see Chapter 3 for a detailed discussion of this issue). Fourth, resources provided to meet need as defined by health professionals or government agencies may go unutilized because the population does not demand them (e.g., preventive services) (Feldstein 1988).

Consumer demand

Consumer demand—what consumers are willing and able to buy at alternative prices—is another important criterion for allocating resources. Need, as perceived by the consumer, is a major but not the sole determinant of demand for healthcare. Rational consumers compare the marginal value benefit and marginal cost associated with alternative uses of their limited money and time resources, and make allocation decisions in their own best interest.[3]

Consumer demand, as the basis for allocational decisions, underlies much of economic theory. The concept of demand is represented in Figure 4.2 as a demand (D) curve. It shows the quantities of a good or service, for example, routine doctor visits (horizontal axis), that an individual is willing and able to purchase at alternative prices (vertical axis) during a given period of time. Consumers are assumed to be well informed about prices and services and to attempt to make choices that maximize their well-being. A host of factors affect the position and slope of the demand curve, including consumer income, preferences, need, and the prices of other related goods and services. The typical demand curve is downward sloping because (1) as price falls consumers are able to buy more; (2) the service is less costly relative to other substitute services (i.e., services that serve the same ends, such as outpatient and inpatient surgery for minor problems); and (3) the marginal value of the service to the consumer falls as more is consumed in a given period of time. The demand curve represents the marginal value of the service to the consumer at alternative levels of consumption (Q), and the market price (P) represents the marginal cost of the service to the consumer. By consuming at the level (Q') corresponding to that level at which a given price (P') intersects the demand curve (point E'), the consumer maximizes well-being. For quantities of doctor visits that exceed Q', given the price P', marginal cost is greater than marginal benefit (D), making the consumer worse off.

Market demand is merely the aggregation of the individual demands of market participants. While demand is an individual concept and depends on individual behavior, it is aggregations of individuals that form markets. Prices and quantities of goods and services are then determined by the operation of supply and demand in markets.

Assumptions of a Competitive Market

In a competitive market, supply represents the amount of a good or service that suppliers are willing to sell at alternative prices during

Figure 4.2 Individual Demand Curve

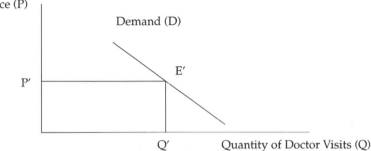
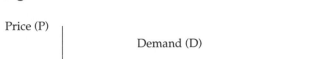

Price (P)

Demand (D)

E′

P′

Q′   Quantity of Doctor Visits (Q)

a given period of time (Figure 4.3). The curve is positive or upward sloping, meaning that greater quantities are supplied at higher prices. The position of the supply curve depends on technology (i.e., the ability to transform inputs into output), the prices of inputs such as wages and rents, and the objectives of suppliers (i.e., whether they are attempting to maximize profits or services or some combination). For example, technological innovation in electronics has markedly increased productivity and allowed producers to offer the same products at lower prices, a shift to the right in the supply curve. Similarly, increases in wages and other input costs would require higher prices for the same number of units, resulting in a shift to the left in the supply curve. Market supply is the aggregation of individual supply of market participants.

The intersection of market supply and demand determines the equilibrium (E′), market price (P′), and quantity of services (Q′) for a given period of time (Figure 4.4). This is the model that undergirds the market approach to healthcare reform. As an application of theory, it is a simplification of reality, and any application must deal with the disparities between the model and the real world of healthcare. Consumer choice and self-regulating market forces are assumed in such a model.

By rapidly adjusting to changes in consumer preferences, incomes, resource scarcity, and technology, competitive markets generally provide a flexible mechanism for solving the basic economic problems of what, how, and for whom a good or service is produced.

Figure 4.3   Individual Supply Curve

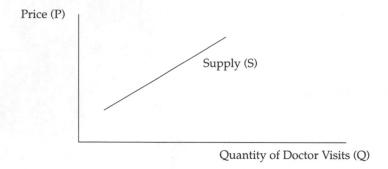

Figure 4.4   Market Demand and Supply

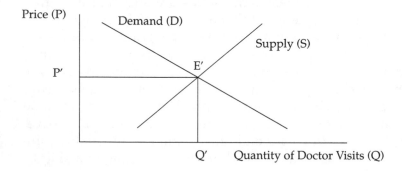

For many goods, and possibly for routine healthcare, consumers appear to be the best judge of their needs and desires relative to other uses of their resources.[4] Under competitive market conditions, producers who fail to respond to consumer demand, who charge prices above the market rate, or who use inefficient production methods are forced out of business, and consumers individually allocate resources to maximize their own well-being, leading the system toward a Pareto optimum allocation of resources.

Assumptions of Healthcare Market

Healthcare, however, diverges from some fundamental properties of a perfectly competitive market. See Rice (1997) for a thorough critique of the use of competitive markets to achieve healthcare goals for society. The basic conditions of a competitive market are (1) free entry to and exit from the market by buyers and sellers; (2) many well-informed buyers and sellers, no one of whom is large enough to influence market price; and (3) no collusion among buyers and sellers, that is, they act independently. Many healthcare market areas are too small to support competition, especially for services of specialists and hospitals. Historically, the market has been characterized by price discrimination and collusion (Kessel 1958), ostensibly to protect consumers and provide access for those who cannot pay. Asymmetry of information puts consumers at a disadvantage vis-à-vis providers, and entry by providers is strictly limited by licensing and regulation of the professions and facilities (Fuchs 1972).

The competitive model therefore does not fully apply to healthcare because of several inherent market limitations. There are significant externalities (i.e., instances in which one person's consumption or production affects another person's well-being). For example, a person who obtains immunizations to prevent infectious diseases provides benefits to others by reducing their risk of contracting the disease. Private markets tend to underinvest in these types of services because benefits to third parties are not directly incorporated in market demand by those who seek services. Similarly, people seem to care that others have access to basic healthcare, and therefore benefit when others gain access to care that would otherwise not be available. Markets alone have no mechanism for translating this value into the desired result.

Another problem with a private healthcare market is so-called supplier-induced demand—that is, the lack of independence between demand and supply. Provider interests may affect consumer demand due to the large disparity of information between provider and consumer and the fact that a third party often pays for a substantial portion of services rendered (Reinhardt 1987). Thus, the provider, who is generally not financially disinterested, has a major influence over consumer demand, greatly diminishing the independent role of consumer choice in the market for healthcare services. Due to these problems, as well as other monopoly elements such as the lack of free entry and exit to the industry by producers, price collusion among producers, and the fact that the available distribution of income may exclude some groups from healthcare, the market fails to achieve satisfactory allocation and distribution of healthcare resources.

The tools of efficiency analysis, grounded in theories of the competitive market, do provide, however, a conceptual point of reference and a set of methodologies for examining the extent to which the operation and outcomes of healthcare markets achieve optimal efficiency—either in the production of health or healthcare.

Key Methods of Assessing Efficiency

Economic analysis is typically divided into microlevel and macrolevel. The microlevel examines the behavior of individuals, firms, and markets. It therefore encompasses the three health services research levels defined earlier within the clinical perspective on effectiveness: patient, institution, and system. Macroeconomics focuses on the economy as a whole. Of concern are aggregate measures of employment, economic growth, foreign trade, and inflation. Analogous macrolevel concerns in healthcare are the life expectancy of the population, infant mortality rate, disability-adjusted life years, and the growth in healthcare expenditure, particularly as they compete with other health-producing investments. This parallels the population perspective on health outcomes at the community level (as shown in Figure 2.1).

Microlevel

The principal methods employed in microlevel analyses of efficiency include (1) estimating production functions; and (2) cost-effectiveness, cost-benefit, and related cost-utility analyses.

Production functions

Economists have developed a comprehensive theoretical model of production efficiency, expressing how the total, average, and marginal costs of a given product or commodity change under a given set of assumptions regarding the relationship between inputs and outputs (i.e., the production function), the cost of inputs, and technology. For example, inputs for ambulatory healthcare may include nurse and physician time, and outputs may be defined in terms of services rendered or their effect on the health of patients. Input costs include nurse and physician earnings, rents, and the cost of supplies. Technology is defined broadly as the information and techniques required to transform inputs into outputs. The cost functions represent the minimum total and unit costs attainable for alternative combinations of inputs and the size of the production units.

It is possible to determine the cost-minimizing mix of inputs for any level of output and the cost-minimizing size of the production unit (Byrns and Stone 1987). Even when producers have the "right" combination of inputs and size, they may fail to achieve maximum output. This may be due to poor management, low employee motivation, or other unspecified production problems and is referred to as x-inefficiency (Leibenstein 1966). X-inefficiency occurs whenever a firm produces less than the maximum possible output from given resources. Production and cost functions can be empirically estimated for any production process and level of analysis, although they will be less precise in areas where output is often difficult to define and measure (e.g., healthcare). Production and cost models have been applied to physician, hospital, and insurance services to determine the extent to which production efficiency has been achieved and how it may be enhanced.

Similarly, production functions have been applied in the context of allocative efficiency analyses concerned with determining the optimal allocation of resources to improve the health of individuals and communities. Summaries of selected studies are provided in Chapter 5.

Cost-effectiveness, cost-benefit, and cost-utility analysis

Other efficiency analysis methods frequently applied in healthcare are cost-effectiveness analysis (CEA), cost-benefit analysis (CBA), and cost-utility analysis (CUA) (Drummond et al. 1997). (See Table 4.1 for a comparison of these methods.) CEA is a systematic analysis of the effects and costs of alternative methods or programs for achieving the same objective (e.g., saving lives, preventing disease, or providing services). CEA is used to determine production efficiency and effects are measured in non-monetary units. CBA is a systematic analysis of one or more methods or programs for achieving a given objective and measures both benefits and costs in monetary units. CUA is conducted when effects are weighted by utility measures denoting the patient's or member of the general public's preference for, or the overall desirability of, a particular outcome (Gold et al. 1996).

CBA can determine whether a program is worth establishing, in the sense that its benefits are greater than its costs (i.e., allocative efficiency), while CEA compares the cost of alternatives in achieving a common objective (i.e., production efficiency) without determining whether the objective itself is worth achieving. For example, what are the costs and associated savings of annual screening and treatment for diabetic retinopathy for persons in the United States? A broader view might compare this program to other medical (e.g., chronic disease self-management program) or public health alternatives (e.g., population-based health risk reduction programs). Programs with the highest net benefit are most allocatively efficient. Society is made worse off by adopting projects for which the costs outweigh benefits, and better off by adopting projects for which benefits most outweigh costs. While it is not practical to rank all possible competing uses of resources to achieve the optimal resource allocation, projects can be considered on an incremental basis.

CEA can be used as both a complement to and a substitute for CBA. For example, to evaluate the retinopathy program, one would first determine the most efficient way to screen for the problem, given several available technologies. These production efficiency results would then feed into the CBA to address the allocation question: How much, if any amount, should society invest in screening and treating diabetic retinopathy? Alternatively, it may be determined that the program would not have net economic benefits because of the population affected, but may yield health benefits and should be compared with other programs in terms of cost per quality-adjusted life year (QALY) gained. Effectiveness can then be measured in terms of increases in QALYs, and compared to other activities on the basis of cost per QALY, which would move the analysis toward a cost-utility approach. Instead of monetary values,

Table 4.1   Comparisons of Cost-Effectiveness, Cost-Benefit, and Cost-Utility Analysis

Type of study	Measurement/ valuation of cost in both alternatives	Identification of consequences	Measurement/ valuation of consequences
Cost-effectiveness analysis	Dollars	Single effect of interest, common to both alternatives, but achieved to different degrees (e.g., two technologies to screen for diabetic retinopathy).	Natural units (e.g., life years gained, disability, etc.)
Cost-benefit analysis	Dollars	Single or multiple effects not necessarily common to both alternatives, and common effects may be achieved to different degrees by the alternatives (e.g., dollars saved from investment in diabetic retinopathy screening compared to chronic care self-management program).	Dollars
Cost-utility analysis	Dollars	Single or multiple effects, not necessarily common to both alternatives, and common effects may be achieved to different degrees by the alternatives (e.g., quality-adjusted life years added from investment in diabetic retino-pathy screening compared to chronic care self-management program).	Healthy days or (more often) quality-adjusted life years

Source: Adapted from *Methods for the Economic Evaluation of Health Care Programmes* by M. F. Drummond et al. 1997. By permission of Oxford University Press.

life years would be valued, or quality-adjusted, according to utility values, or how people feel about time spent in alternative health states ranging from states they feel would be worse than death to being completely healthy (Torrance and Feeny 1989; Torrance et al. 1996). For example, while being completely healthy may be assigned a utility value of 1, the condition of blindness may be assigned a value of 0.6. If an otherwise healthy person could avert blindness for one year, the gain would be 0.4 QALYs.

Use of CBA and CUA has largely focused on medical care services as opposed to non-medical health investments (Blumenschein
and Johannesson 1996; Segal and Richardson 1994). In response
to cost pressures associated with managed care and government
policies, the application of CEA has been greatly expanded in the
pharmacy area. As a consequence, a new field of pharmacoeconomics has emerged, in which economic evaluation methods are
used to examine alternative drug treatments and to identify the
costs and benefits of these treatments (Drummond et al. 1992; Oster
and Epstein 1987). Australia, Canada, and the United Kingdom, for
example, have developed guidelines for economic evaluations of
pharmaceuticals as a basis for determining which might be included
in national or provincial drug formularies (CCOHTA 1995; Lovatt
1996; Rovira 1996).

In the United States, the economic evaluation of pharmaceuticals has become an area of increasing interest with the growth in
managed care (Power 1996). Alan Hillman has presented a series of
guidelines for economic analysis of healthcare technology, including
pharmaceuticals (Hillman 1996). The Food and Drug Administration also has issued draft guidelines that would establish standards
for cost-effectiveness claims by pharmaceutical companies.

Expanded government funding of medical effectiveness, outcomes research, and clinical guidelines provides information to
carry out further economic evaluation of healthcare services
(AHCPR 1991). AHCPR established Patient Outcome Research
Teams (PORTs) to carry out broad investigations of alternative services or procedures for managing specific clinical conditions (see
Chapter 3).

Effectiveness information can also feed into policy models designed to integrate issues of quality of life, patient functional status,
and costs. Kaplan and Anderson (1988) developed a measure that integrates the health benefit and utility frameworks for the evaluation
of healthcare programs. Specifically, their measure integrates point-
in-time estimates of function, transition among functional levels
over time, utilities of health states, and mortality. It has been applied
to several prevention and treatment program evaluations.

Oregon policymakers applied CUA, if not the exact methods,
to the allocation of scarce health resources. The Oregon program attempted to rank health services according to their potential benefits,

with services being limited by the total budget that is politically allocated. In this way more persons could obtain basic coverage, but some services judged to be of less value were not covered (Eddy 1991; Hadorn 1991). The economic evaluation of services was limited by political considerations and therefore the methods were not rigorously applied (Tengs 1996). This may simply reflect the fact that the allocation of public resources is ultimately a political decision, and political factors may override strictly economic considerations.

Macrolevel

The principal macrolevel approaches to efficiency analysis are based on international comparisons of the performance of healthcare systems in different countries (OECD 1995). While there are major problems with comparisons at the system level, such as measurement of health outcomes, cultural and demographic differences, and data comparability, such comparisons do serve to raise questions about the efficiency and equity of health systems and to stimulate inquiry into reasons for major observed differences (Schieber and Poullier 1990).

Researchers at the OECD have collected data and attempted to develop standardized international health accounts for the organization's 24 member countries. Because of interest in the population health perspective and the difficulty in measuring health outcomes in ways that are very sensitive to healthcare inputs (this point is elaborated in Chapter 2), these comparisons rely on aggregate measures of life expectancy, infant mortality, and cause of death–specific mortality. Simple correlations between healthcare spending per capita and aggregate health measures are examined along with differences in input prices, the production structure of the health sector (e.g., amount spent on hospitals and doctors), input volumes, administrative costs, and appropriateness of care.

Recently, analysts have emphasized the need to broaden the policy framework beyond healthcare to include the social and physical environment, and to focus more on primary prevention and health promotion services that are usually underfunded due to the large expenditure on medical care treatment. Healthcare purchasers in a few countries (e.g., Canada, United Kingdom, Ireland, Iceland, and New Zealand) have established health goals for the population and are searching for alternative ways of achieving those health goals, including preventive healthcare and more effective integration of health and other policy issues such as education, housing, and social policy. Methods of allocative efficiency analysis have been applied in making these decisions (OECD 1995).

Summary and Conclusions

The principal objectives of this chapter were (1) to define efficiency; and (2) to describe how it might be assessed. To address the first objective, the major types of efficiency analyses—allocative and production efficiency—and the theoretical assumptions underlying them were presented. With population health as the goal, allocative efficiency concerns attainment of maximum population health from the limited resources that society has available for that objective during any given period of time. This requires that societies maximize efficiency by choosing the "right" most-valued mix of medical and non-medical services and by producing them at minimum cost.

Analysts have developed both micromethods and macromethods for efficiency assessment. Micromethods include the normative microeconomic theories of markets, including production and cost functions as applied to healthcare. Also, the techniques of CBA, CEA, and CUA are used to examine the efficiency of healthcare production and efficiency in the mix of specific healthcare services and programs. Extensive data on the OECD countries permit international comparisons at the macrolevel in terms of spending, utilization, and health indicators for the population (OECD 1997).

Chapter 5 provides a selected summary of evidence on the efficiency of the U.S. and other healthcare systems, discusses the major policy strategies for improving efficiency, and delineates and applies efficiency criteria to an assessment of Medicaid managed care.

Notes

1. Spending for environmental activities (e.g., air and water pollution abatement, sanitation and sewage treatment, water supplies) is excluded from the national health accounts (Levit et al. 1991).

2. For a detailed explanation of Pareto's work, see Kohler (1990), pp. 484–519.
3. "Marginal" refers to the next unit of a good or service that the consumer is considering. This differs from the average total value of all units consumed. A "rational" consumer would not purchase the next unit of a good or service if he or she perceived the benefit of that next unit to be less than the cost of the unit.
4. Even for sophisticated tertiary care, doctors have long acknowledged, if not always fostered, the patient's right to be part of the decision-making team when alternative courses of action are contemplated that include alternative levels of risk, benefit, and costs. Patient values are now being fully integrated with clinical information in patient outcome studies (Barry et al. 1988).

References

Agency for Health Care Policy and Research. 1991. *Report to Congress: Progress of Research on Outcomes of Health Care Services and Procedures*, AHCPR Pub. No. 91-0004. Rockville, MD: Agency for Health Care Policy and Research.

Arrow, K. J. 1963. *Social Choice and Individual Values*. 2nd ed. New York: John Wiley & Sons.

Barry, M., A. Mulley, F. Fowler, and J. Wennberg. 1988. "Watchful Waiting Versus Immediate Transurethral Resection for Symptomatic Prostatism: The Importance of Patients' Preferences." *Journal of the American Medical Association* 259: 3010–17.

Behrman, J. R., and B. L. Wolfe. 1989. "Does More Schooling Make Women Better Nourished and Healthier? Adult Sibling and Fixed Effects Estimates for Nicaragua." *Journal of Human Resources* 24: 644–63.

Berger, M. C., and J. P. Lee. 1989. "Schooling, Self Selection, and Health." *Journal of Human Resources* 24: 433–55.

Blumenschein, K., and M. Johannesson. 1996. "Economic Evaluation in Healthcare: A Brief History and Future Directions." *Pharmacoeconomics* 10 (2): 114–22.

Byrns, R. T., and G. W. Stone. 1987. *Economics*. 3rd ed. Glenview, IL: Scott, Foresman and Co.

Canadian Coordinating Office for Health Technology Assessment. 1995. Report From the Canadian Coordinating Office for Health Technology Assessment (CCOHTA): "Guidelines for Economic Evaluation of Pharmaceuticals: Canada." *International Journal of Technology Assessment in Health Care* 11: 796–7.

Culyer, A. J. 1992. "The Morality of Efficiency in Health Care: Some Uncomfortable Implications." *Health Economics* 1: 7–18.

Davis, K., G. F. Anderson, D. Rowland, and E. P. Steinberg. 1990. *Health Care
Cost Containment*. Baltimore: The Johns Hopkins University Press.

Drummond, M. F., B. S. Bloom, G. Carrin, A. L. Hillman, H. C. Hutchings,
R. P. Knill-Jones, G. de Pouvourville, and K. Torfs. 1992. "Issues in
the Cross-National Assessment of Health Technology." *International
Journal of Technology Assessment in Health Care* 8: 671–82.

Drummond, M. F., B. O'Brien, G. L. Stoddart, and G. W. Torrance. 1997.
Methods for the Economic Evaluation of Health Care Programmes. New
York: Oxford University Press.

Eddy, D. M. 1980. *Screening for Cancer: Theory, Analysis, and Design*. Englewood Cliffs, NJ: Prentice Hall.

———. 1991. "Clinical Decision Making: From Theory To Practice: What's
Going on in Oregon?" *Journal of the American Medical Association* 266:
417–20.

Evans, R. G., M. L. Barer, and T. R. Marmor, eds. 1994. *Why Are Some People
Healthy and Others Not? The Determinants of Health of Populations*. New
York: Aldine De Gruyter.

Evans, R. G., and G. L. Stoddart. 1990. "Producing Health, Consuming
Health Care." *Social Science and Medicine* 31: 1347–63.

Feldstein, P. 1988. *Health Care Economics*. 3rd ed. New York: John Wiley &
Sons.

Folland, S., A. C. Goodman, and M. Stano. 1997. *The Economics of Health
and Health Care*. 2nd ed. Upper Saddle River, NJ: Prentice Hall.

Fuchs, V. 1972. "Health Care and the United States Economic System: An
Essay in Abnormal Physiology." *Milbank Memorial Fund Quarterly* 50:
211–44.

Gold, M. R., J. E. Siegel, L. B. Russell, and M. C. Weinstein. 1996. *Cost-
Effectiveness in Health and Medicine*. New York: Oxford University
Press.

Grossman, M. 1972. "On the Concept of Health Capital and the Demand
for Health." *Journal of Political Economy* 80: 223–55.

Hadorn, D. C. 1991. "Setting Health Care Priorities in Oregon: Cost-
Effectiveness Meets the Rule of Rescue." *Journal of the American Medical Association* 265: 2218–25.

Hillman, A. L. 1996. "Summary of Economic Analysis of Health Care
Technology: A Report on Principles." *Medical Care* 34 (Supplement):
DS193-DS196.

Hillman, B. J., C. A. Joseph, M. R. Mabry, J. H. Sunshine, S. D. Kennedy,
and M. Noether. 1990. "Frequency and Costs of Diagnostic Imaging
in Office Practice: A Comparison of Self-Referring and Radiologist-

Referring Physicians." *The New England Journal of Medicine* 323: 1604–08.

Hsiao, W. C., P. Braun, D. Dunn, E. R. Becker, M. DeNicola, and T. R. Ketcham. 1988. "Results and Policy Implications of the Resource-Based Relative Value Study." *The New England Journal of Medicine* 319: 881–88.

Jeffers, J. R., M. F. Bognanno, and J. C. Bartlett. 1971. "On the Demand Versus Need for Medical Services and the Concept of 'Shortage'." *American Journal of Public Health* 61: 46–64.

Kaplan, R. M., and J. P. Anderson. 1988. "A General Health Policy Model: Update and Applications." *Health Services Research* 23: 203–35.

Kessel, R. 1958. "Price Discrimination in Medicine." *Journal of Law and Economics* 1 (1): 20–53.

Kohler, H. 1990. *Intermediate Microeconomics: Theory and Applications.* 3rd ed. Glenview, IL: Scott, Foresman and Co.

Kottke, T. E., M. L. Brekke, and L. I. Solberg. 1993. "Making 'Time' for Preventive Services." *Mayo Clinic Proceedings* 68: 785–91.

Leibenstein, H. 1966. "Allocative Efficiency Vs. 'X-Efficiency'." *American Economic Review* 56: 392–415.

Levit, K. R., H. C. Lazenby, C. A. Cowan, and S. W. Letsch. 1991. "National Health Expenditures 1990." *Health Care Financing Review* 13 (1): 29–54.

Levit, K. R., H. C. Lazenby, and L. Sivarajan. 1996. "Health Care Spending in 1994: Slowest in Decades." *Health Affairs* 15 (2): 130–144.

Lovatt, B. 1996. "The United Kingdom Guidelines for the Economic Evaluation of Medicines." *Medical Care* 34 (Supplement): DS179-DS181.

Lubitz, J., and R. Prihoda. 1984. "The Use and Costs of Medicare Services in the Last 2 Years of Life." *Health Care Financing Review* 5 (3): 117–31.

Luft, H. S., and M. R. Greenlick. 1996. "The Contribution of Group- and Staff-Model HMOs To American Medicine." *Milbank Quarterly* 74: 445–67.

National Center for Health Statistics. 1997. *Health, United States, 1996–97 and Injury Chartbook.* Hyattsville, MD: Public Health Service.

Organization for Economic Cooperation and Development. 1995. *New Directions in Health Care Policy*, Health Policy Series No. 7. Paris, France: OECD.

———. 1997. *OECD Health Data 1997.* Paris, France: OECD.

Oster, G., and A. M. Epstein. 1987. "Cost-Effectiveness of Antihyperlipemic Therapy in the Prevention of Coronary Heart Disease: The Case of Cholestyramine." *Journal of the American Medical Association* 258: 2381–87.

Pear, R. 1997. "New Options Include Shift into Preventive Benefits, and Slightly Higher Costs." *New York Times.* 30 July (Section A): 13.

Power, E. J. 1996. "Current Efforts in Standards Development: United States." *Medical Care* 34 (Supplement): DS200-DS207.

Reinhardt, U. E. 1987. "Comment On: A Clarification of Theories and Evidence on Supplier-Induced Demand for Physicians' Services." *Journal of Human Resources* 22: 621–23.

Rice, T. 1997. "Can Markets Give Us the Health System We Want?" *Journal of Health Politics, Policy and Law* 22: 383–426.

Rovira, J. 1996. "Standardization of the Economic Evaluation of Health Technologies: European Developments." *Medical Care* 34 (Supplement): DS182-DS188.

Schieber, G. J., and J. P. Poullier. 1990. "Overview of International Comparisons of Health Care Expenditures." *Health Care Systems in Transition: the Search for Efficiency*, Social Policy Series No. 7. Paris: OECD.

Scitovsky, A. A. 1988. "Medical Care in the Last Twelve Months of Life: The Relation Between Age, Functional Status, and Medical Care Expenditures." *Milbank Quarterly* 66: 640–60.

Segal, L., and J. Richardson. 1994. "Efficiency in Resource Allocation." In *Economics and Health: Proceedings of the 16th Australian Conference of Health Economists*. Edited by A. Harris, 231–55. Sydney, Australia: University of New South Wales.

Stokey, E., and R. Zeckhauser. 1978. *A Primer for Policy Analysis*. New York: W.W. Norton.

Tengs, T. O. 1996. "An Evaluation of Oregon's Medicaid Rationing Algorithms." *Health Economics* 5: 171–81.

Thompson, R. S. 1996. "What Have HMOs Learned about Clinical Prevention Services? An Examination of the Experience at Group Health Cooperative of Puget Sound." *Milbank Quarterly* 74: 469–509.

Torrance, G. W., and D. H. Feeny. 1989. "Utilities and Quality Adjusted Life-Years." *International Journal of Technology Assessment in Health Care* 5: 559–75.

Torrance, G. W., D. H. Feeny, W. J. Furlong, R. D. Barr, Y. Zhang, and Q. Wang. 1996. "Multiattribute Utility Function for A Comprehensive Health Status Classification System: Health Utilities Index Mark 2." *Medical Care* 34: 702–22.

U.S. Department of Health and Human Services. 1990. *Prevention '89/90: Federal Programs and Progress*. Washington, D.C.: U.S. Government Printing Office.

U.S. Preventive Services Task Force. 1989. *Guide To Clinical Preventive Services: Report of the U.S. Preventive Services Task Force*. Baltimore, MD: Williams and Wilkins.

Waldo, D. R., and H. C. Lazenby. 1984. "Demographic Characteristics and Health Care Use and Expenditures by the Aged in the United States: 1977–1984." *Health Care Financing Review* 6 (1): 1–29.

Webster, J. R., and C. Berdes. 1990. "Ethics and Economic Realities: Goals and Strategies for Care Toward the End of Life." *Archives of Internal Medicine* 150: 1795–97.

Williams, A. H. 1974. "Need As A Demand Concept (With Special Reference To Health)." In *Economic Policies and Social Goals: Aspects of Public Choice*. Edited by A. J. Culyer, 60–76. London: Robertson.

Wolfe, B. L., and J. R. Behrman. 1987. "Women's Schooling and Children's Health: Are the Effects Robust With Adult Sibling Control for the Women's Childhood Background?" *Journal of Health Economics* 6: 239–54.

Efficiency: Evidence, Policy Strategies, Criteria, and an Application

The major questions addressed in this chapter ask (1) What policy strategies are available to achieve efficiency? (2) What is the evidence regarding the efficiency of these strategies? and (3) What criteria should be used in judging the efficiency of policy alternatives?

This chapter first describes the theoretical assumptions and specific strategies for achieving efficiency that underlie both market-maximized and market-minimized healthcare systems. Secondly, evidence is provided regarding the allocative efficiency of healthcare systems in improving health outcomes at the macrolevel based on the performance of the U.S. healthcare system compared to selected Western nations. Microlevel evidence on production efficiency focuses on physicians, hospitals, and health plans. The final section presents efficiency criteria for evaluating alternative health policies and applies those criteria to the evaluation of Medicaid managed care.

Policy Strategies Relating to Efficiency

Anderson (1989, 19) has noted that countries in the developed world vary along a continuum, from left to right, of market-minimized to market-maximized organization and financing of their healthcare sectors:

> On the right-hand side of the continuum, one is likely to believe in cash indemnity for health services and financial controls on patients.

This view regards providers of services as essentially autonomous sellers of services; patients, as it were, hire a physician to manage their service needs. On the left-hand side of the continuum, with the highly structured and completely government-owned health service, there would be no charge to the patient at the time of service. Charges to the patient at that time, no matter how small they were, would be regarded as an undesirable barrier to access to services for prevention, early diagnosis, and treatment. At the right-hand extreme, patients are assumed to know their self-interest well enough not to be inhibited by charges at the time of service.

While all countries seek to achieve equity, efficiency, and overall cost control in their health sectors, each has a unique approach to addressing these basic economic and social issues. The market-minimized systems tend to rely more on direct government or quasi-government controls to achieve the desired results, while market-maximized models rely primarily on the private market to allocate resources, and use the government to subsidize care for the most vulnerable segments of the population. Each country's approach to healthcare may depend largely on its culture, history, and political situation (Swint 1990). The theoretical foundations for the market-maximized and market-minimized strategies, and implications of each for the formulation of health policy, are reviewed in the sections that follow.

General Efficiency Strategies

Market-maximized models

Paul Feldstein (1988) used a qualitative method to evaluate the allocative efficiency of the healthcare sector from a market perspective. The assumption of consumer power in the marketplace and the criterion of maximum consumer well-being form the basis of his economic evaluation. The various sectors (e.g., insurance, hospital care, and physician care) are examined in terms of the degree to which observed behavior is consistent with the predictions derived from the basic economic model of the competitive market. For example, do producers strive to minimize the cost of production, and are the mix and quality of goods and services guided by consumer choices? When inconsistencies occur, the basic assumptions of the competitive model are reexamined and altered in an attempt to better explain observed behavior. Feldstein found distortions in the insurance and healthcare markets that have led to misallocation of resources and inefficient production methods. Cost-based reimbursement of hospitals resulted in non-price competition, excess capacity, and high cost. These problems have been addressed through government policy changes and market reform. For example, Medicare PPS reversed the economic incentives facing hospitals for beneficiaries, and health plans based on the principles of managed care are forcing hospitals to compete on price to serve health plan enrollees.

Enthoven (1990) proposed managed competition as a comprehensive solution to market failure in the healthcare sector in the United States. This approach depends on market incentives to motivate health plans and providers to be efficient and responsive to consumer needs and demands. Private sponsors of health benefits (e.g., employers) and public sponsors (e.g., state government agencies) would aggressively monitor and manage competition among health plans in the healthcare market. Employers would play their traditional role as suppliers of health benefits, and a public agency or agencies designated by the state would serve as a broker for self-employed and other persons who chose to obtain health insurance through the state sponsor. Fixed contributions (with a limit on tax deductibility) from sponsors would provide incentives for cost-conscious choice by consumers. By spending their own after-tax dollars beyond the employer contributions, consumers would determine the growth in healthcare spending in the United States.

In 1992, President Clinton selected managed competition as the strategy for achieving universal coverage and cost control. Failure of that federal legislative effort left the states and the private sector to deal with the problem. Because of the apparent success of managed care and competition in controlling cost, the private sector and most states continue to expand enrollment of beneficiaries in managed care, and many states are also establishing rules and regulations to control some of the negative consequences of healthcare competition (Jensen et al. 1997). States are serving in the sponsor role for Medicaid managed care patients and the federal government has established mechanisms for Medicare beneficiaries to enroll in competing risk-based health plans. Still lacking in most states are regional purchasing cooperatives, limits on tax deductibility of health insurance, mandatory provision of health insurance benefits or payments by all employers, and a means to finance and enroll all of the uninsured. Various states' approaches to these and related issues will be reviewed in Chapter 9.

Market-minimized models

Williams (1990) contrasted the market-maximized approach with a public-sector political framework that is also concerned with production efficiency. However, in the political framework, the electorate judges allocative efficiency by the extent to which the healthcare system improves the health status of the population in relation to the resources allocated to the system, and priorities are determined by social judgments of need. European nations with social insurance systems or tax-financed national health systems have traditionally used this approach to healthcare resource allocation. In such systems, solidarity is promoted over individual rights and choice.

National Health Services in Britain and New Zealand exemplify systems that use a needs-based approach to establish the allocation of resources to the health sector and the type of services to be provided. Internal markets are developed to achieve efficiency of production (Glennerster 1995; Street 1994). The goal in establishing an internal market is to provide incentives for efficient production and allocation of resources while retaining overall control of spending and tax-based financing of healthcare and maintaining or improving equity in access to care. These markets separate the responsibility for ensuring that patients receive care from the responsibility for the direct provision of that care. Under this system a health authority uses its budget to purchase services from other health authorities, general practitioners, private hospitals, nursing homes, and local government social service departments.

These authorities identify healthcare needs and priorities for their area and determine the best way to spend funds allocated by the central government to meet area health needs and priorities. General practitioner groups are also responsible for the health needs of their patients and are encouraged to be conscious of the costs of their clinical decisions. Physician groups receive budgets to provide primary care services and purchase selected secondary health services (e.g., diagnostic services, elective surgical procedures, and prescription drugs) for their registered patients.

In both the United Kingdom and New Zealand, providers compete to supply services demanded by purchasers. Hospitals no longer receive a global budget to provide services; rather, they have increased autonomy and are encouraged to compete among themselves and with private providers for contracts with district authorities, thereby minimizing costs and focusing on enhanced patient satisfaction. The central government retains authority over general health policy and total public health expenditures.

All systems represent some mix of market elements and non-market controls. The United States, which may be the most market-oriented system, implemented administered price systems for federal beneficiaries under the Medicare program. The resource-based relative value fee scale (RBRVS) for physician services was developed to complement the prospective payment diagnosis-related group (DRG)–based fee system for hospitals. In addition, work continues on medical effectiveness studies, guidelines, and methodological improvements for cost-effectiveness studies that will yield information for better public and private decisions on resource allocation (Gold et al. 1996).

The precise strategies employed to assure efficiency in the respective systems differ, but include efforts to control both the prices and volume of healthcare services, through the methods of paying providers and of managing and overseeing utilization, respectively.

Specific Efficiency Strategies

Payment methods

Alternative methods of paying physicians and hospitals provide different incentives regarding efficiency (D'Intignano 1990). Market-minimized models tend to rely more on global budgets and strict fee controls, while market-maximized models encompass a range of alternatives, including fee-for-service, salary, capitation, and prospective payment.

The United States has many different payment methods and sources operating simultaneously, while other countries have a primary method for hospital and physician reimbursement and funnel payment through relatively few channels. For example, physicians in the United States are paid by local, state, and federal agencies; by over 1,500 insurers; and by direct out-of-pocket payments from patients. Methods of payment include fee-for-service, salary, and capitation. Until recently, fee-for-service based on usual and customary fees was the dominant payment method in the United States. While fee-for-service provides an incentive for high productivity, it also leads to inflation and a proliferation of procedures with low marginal value relative to their cost (Moloney and Rogers 1979). Canada and Germany have also relied on fee-for-service payment for physicians, but fees were strictly controlled. Germany also developed fixed negotiated budgets for ambulatory care for the period from 1989 to 1992 that were nonetheless unsuccessful in controlling the accelerating rates of increase in ambulatory expenditures (Schwartz and Busse 1996). In 1993, Germany introduced further global budget controls on physician and pharmaceutical expenditures (Henke, Murray, and Ade 1994).

Per diem prices, prospective payment by DRGs, and prepayment are the primary methods for paying for hospital services in the United States. Each method provides different financial incentives for the hospital and has different implications for efficiency (Dowling 1974). Although traditionally hospitals have been paid per diem rates plus fees for individual ancillary services, with the passage of PPS under the Medicare program in the United States in 1983, the U.S. system of paying for hospital services began to assume more market-minimized methods of financing. That system was designed to pay a fixed amount per episode of hospital care defined by one of 483 diagnostic groups. It provided an incentive for hospitals to encourage doctors to reduce length of stay and to provide hospital services more efficiently, because each hospital could retain any surplus in payments over costs. Peer review organizations were to monitor the necessity of admissions and the adequacy of care to offset the incentive to admit more patients, to underserve them, and to discharge them prematurely.

Canada has global hospital budgets and regional health planning to control the cost of hospital care and the diffusion of medical technology, and many provinces have also introduced caps on physician spending. In Germany, hospitals are financed through all-inclusive per diems negotiated between hospitals and the regional associations of sickness funds (Jonsson 1990). Rates, as well as capital spending, are subject to approval by the state. The state pays for capital spending based on statewide hospital planning.

During the 1980s and early 1990s, many countries focused their efforts to control healthcare expenditures on global budgets or budget caps. The key to cost control in these macromanaged systems is having a dominant source of payment that fixes the budget for a given period of time. Growth in the budget is generally limited by growth in the economy. Thus, the Canadian and German systems rely on control of the funds available to physician and hospital providers rather than on the mixture of market incentives and controls present in the United States.

With the increasing use of capitation and prospective payment methods, the United States has taken on more of the characteristics of market-minimized models for paying providers, while countries that have traditionally been more market-minimized are increasingly looking to the United States for innovative ways to control the rising cost of both physician and hospital services in their own countries.

Utilization management

The market-maximized model that dominates approaches to controlling cost and resource allocation in the United States has been characterized as micromanagement, in contrast to the macromanagement strategy practiced in other countries (Reinhardt 1990). Micromanagement tends to rely on incentives such as copayments for consumers and capitation payment for providers in competing managed care health plans, whereas macromanagement relies on controls such as fee schedules, global budgets, and limits on diffusion of technology to achieve health system objectives.

In the market-based U.S. healthcare delivery system, emphasis is on affecting the behavior of individual providers and patients with a mix of incentives and controls. Thus, in managed care plans, there are elaborate methods for utilization review, selective contracting, capitated payment of providers, and practice guidelines.

For patients, there are provider gatekeepers and control of referrals, copayments, coverage limits, limits on provider choice, and associated financial penalties for not complying with plan requirements. Competition is introduced through an array of health plan choices for those with public or private insurance.

The key to macromanagement is limiting the sources of payment and controlling the payment amounts. Regional planning to limit the physical facilities and assure fair distribution, thereby providing the constraints within which providers work is one example of macromanagement. The system results in queues for expensive high-technology procedures and equipment, forcing physicians to allocate services based on the urgency of the cases.

Evidence regarding the success of market-maximized models in comparison with the success of market-minimized models will be discussed in the section that follows.

Evidence Relating to Efficiency

Allocative Efficiency

As indicated in Chapter 4, allocative efficiency is most essentially concerned with maximizing health, given constrained resources. Three general health policy strategies that reflect a concern with allocative efficiency were reviewed, related to investing in (1) medical versus non-medical policy alternatives; (2) preventive services; and (3) mix or types of treatment, in relationship to health improvements. Specific microlevel evidence, based on related microlevel methods (e.g., health production functions and cost-effectiveness analysis), is presented with respect to the likely allocative efficiency of these alternatives. Macrolevel evidence is provided on the comparative experiences of the United States and other countries, to provide a sense of whether market-maximized or minimized models of healthcare system design might be more successful in optimizing allocative efficiency.

Microlevel

Medical versus non-medical alternatives. A basic conclusion of Chapter 3 was that personal healthcare provides a contribution to population health that is modest compared to those of human biology, environment, and behavior. Thus, critics have long been concerned that modern developed countries allocate too many resources to the delivery of personal health services and too few to broader public health and social interventions at the population level (Fuchs 1974; McKeown 1990).

Folland, Goodman, and Stano (1997, 98–99) have provided an overview of the contributions of medical and non-medical interventions to health, grounded in the concept of a production function for health—that is, the relationship of inputs to health outputs. They conclude that the production function for health tends to exhibit diminishing marginal returns to healthcare, particularly in developed countries. Historical declines in mortality rates may be most accurately attributed to improved environment and nutrition, rather than to medical care per se. Studies have demonstrated that the marginal product of healthcare in reducing mortality in the United States does not differ significantly from zero, although it is higher for certain groups, such as the elderly. As indicated in Chapter 4, lifestyle and education as measured by years of schooling appear to be significantly related to the population health status. The findings, based on estimating the production function for health, argue for a broader focus on public health and non-medical interventions to serve the allocative efficiency, as well as the population effectiveness, objective.

Preventive services. Economic evaluations of the cost-effectiveness of specific prevention-oriented interventions provide another important type of evidence for making resource allocation decisions. The Harvard study of 500 life-saving programs (Tengs et al. 1995) surveyed the literature on the cost-effectiveness of life-saving interventions in the United States. Life-saving interventions were defined as any behavioral or technological strategy that reduced the probability of premature death among a specified target population.

Programs were categorized by sector, including healthcare, residential, transportation, occupational, and environmental; and by three levels of prevention, including primary, secondary, and tertiary. The 587 interventions ranged from those that save more resources than they consume to interventions that cost more than 10 billion dollars per year of life saved. The median intervention cost

$42,000 per year of life saved, while the median medical intervention cost $19,000, injury reduction $48,000, and toxin control $2,800,000, respectively, per year of life saved.

Cost-effectiveness also varied by sector; the median intervention in the transportation sector costs $56,000 per year of life saved, and residential sector $36,000, occupational sector $346,000, and environmental sector $4,207,000, respectively, per year of life saved. Overall, primary prevention programs were less cost-effective ($79,000 per year of life saved) compared to secondary and tertiary prevention (about $23,000 per year of life saved). However, in medicine, primary prevention programs cost only $5,000 per life-year saved, compared to about $23,000 for secondary and tertiary programs.

Since this research represented a synthesis of existing studies, there were significant methodological limitations: the validity of the conclusions is dependent on the accuracy of data and analyses in the original studies; due to publication bias the studies represented a nonrandom sample of life-saving programs; and some benefits and effects were not measured (e.g., efforts to save lives of some people may have reduced injuries in others and environmental programs may improve the quality of life as well as save some lives). The study does, however, illustrate the potentially large variation within and between sectors and levels of prevention and, therefore, the potential efficiency gains associated with targeting limited resources at those programs that achieve the greatest health improvement per dollar of investment.

Mix or types of treatment. The RAND Health Insurance Experiment addressed the allocative efficiency of coinsurance in the context of the U.S. healthcare financing and delivery system. The study examined the effect of copayments on utilization and expenditures for healthcare services, and the extent to which increases in utilization associated with "free" care affected health status. The basic finding was that free care, compared to higher copayment levels, resulted in a 50 percent increase in expenditure with no significant effect on the health status of the typical person. Those, however, who were sick, poor, or both at the time of enrollment obtained significant health status benefits from increased utilization. Reducing the price to the "typical" consumer below the cost of production results in consumption of services for which the marginal value is below the marginal cost of production with little or no effect on health. This is the basic condition of resource misallocation—resources would provide more benefit if allocated elsewhere.

From the Health Insurance Experiment findings, Manning et al. (1987) estimated that out of the $200 billion the under-65 population of the United States spent on healthcare in 1984, a $37 billion to $60 billion welfare loss—the allocation of resources to procedures or services with minimal or no benefits—would have been incurred by moving from the 95 percent copayment plan with a $1,000 maximum out-of-pocket expenditure to the free plan. This is the estimated amount of overspending that would have occurred under the free plan given the low marginal value of the added healthcare services that would have been consumed. The authors note that some of the strong assumptions required to obtain this estimate might not hold and therefore might lead to an overestimate of loss. However, this is probably more than offset by the fact that the estimate ignores the incentives to employ new technologies associated with more generous insurance plans. New technology is often used in ways that produce low marginal benefits for patients relative to cost, thereby adding to welfare loss.

The Health Insurance Experiment established a baseline of the probable magnitude of inefficiencies in the U.S. system and identified some areas for potential savings. For example, Siu et al. (1986) found that the introduction of cost sharing had an impact on both appropriate and inappropriate hospital admissions. The percentage of hospital admissions deemed inappropriate (22 percent) was only slightly lower than the proportion of inappropriate hospital admissions for free care (24 percent). This information suggests that significant portions of hospital admissions are inappropriate and potentially avoidable. The welfare loss estimate given by Manning et al. (1987) was based on the 1984 structure of the U.S. healthcare system with its mix of regulatory and competitive features. The estimate also does not represent a forecast of the effects of fundamental restructuring of the healthcare delivery and financing system to approximate systems in Canada, Europe, or the present-day United States. While other systems provide first-dollar coverage, they also include budget caps, volume controls, and stringent control over capital expenditure on healthcare technology and facilities.

Compared to 1984, the current U.S. system is more competitive, and utilization and cost are more constrained by managed care.

Comparing U.S. spending, utilization, coverage, and health outcomes with those of other democratic industrialized countries provides an important macrolevel perspective on the U.S. healthcare system. Although observed differences may be a function of a variety of factors, they nonetheless pose questions, as well as point to answers, regarding ways in which present and future system performance might be improved (Schieber and Poullier 1990).

Macrolevel

The 24 member countries of OECD include democratic countries that range from economic powers, such as the United States, Germany, and Japan, to smaller countries with more modest economic achievement, such as Greece and Portugal.

Table 5.1 provides data by country on the role of the public sector in the provision of health insurance coverage and payment for healthcare services. Until the market reforms of 1991, the United Kingdom represented the extreme of market-minimization with a national health service; government ownership of hospitals; direct employment of hospital physicians, nurses, and allied health workers; and central budgetary control. The market-maximized extreme is represented by the United States, with a majority of private hospitals and private physicians and other health workers; private insurance covering a majority of the population; out-of-pocket payment representing 20 percent of expenditures; and a plethora of payors without coordination of payment. Between these two extremes, but leaning more toward market-minimization, are the Scandinavian countries and France. Countries leaning more toward market mechanisms, although far left of the United States on the continuum, are Australia, Canada, Germany, Switzerland, and Japan.

Relative to the United States, the Canadian system has high utilization of inpatient days and constraints on high-cost surgical and diagnostic procedures (see Table 5.2). The system suffers from the "bed blocker" phenomenon. Older individuals, whose condition does not require the high intensity of care available in hospitals, have lengths of stay on the order of 50 to 60 days. Germany appears to have a similar experience, with even higher inpatient utilization

Table 5.1   Public Coverage against Cost of Medical Care and
Average Percentage of Bill Paid for by Public
Insurance: Selected Countries, 1995

Country	Percent of Population with Public Coverage		Percent Paid by Public Insurance	
	Hospital Care	Ambulatory Care	Hospital Care	Ambulatory Care
United Kingdom	100%	100%	99%	88%
Finland	100	100	82	90
Norway	100	100	100	—
Sweden	100	100	98	74
France	99	98	92	57
Australia	100	100	79	84
Canada	100	100	90	72
Germany	92	92	98	90
Switzerland	99	99	100	78
Japan	100	100	93	—
United States	46	45	55	—

Source: Organization for Economic Cooperation and Development 1997.

rates. Differences in average length of stay may reflect different
policies regarding the use of hospitals for long-term and geriatric
care (Organization for Economic Cooperation and Development
[OECD] 1997). Consultations and visits per capita were also higher
in Germany and Canada than in the United States (see Table 5.2)
This may reflect the relatively high out-of-pocket payments at the
point of service in the United States—traditionally the highest such
payments among the developed nations.

All three countries experienced a compound annual growth in
per capita healthcare expenditure on the order of 10 percent per year
until about 1990 (see Table 5.3). Since the early 1990s, Canada has
been more successful in controlling healthcare costs than has the
United States and Germany.

Although global budgets may control the rate of increase in
spending, they do not necessarily lead to either greater allocative efficiency or greater production efficiency. In the process of controlling
total costs, perverse incentives may be created for both allocation
and production. Hospitals may pressure physicians to keep beds

Table 5.2 Use of Inpatient Healthcare in Selected Countries

Year	Hospital Bed Days/ Person Per Year			Hospital Admission Rates (% of Population) Per Year			Average Length of Stay in Inpatient Institutions			Consultations and Visits Per Capita		
	U.S.	Canada	Germany	U.S.	Canada	Germany	U.S.	Canada	Germany	U.S.	Canada	Germany
1970	2.3	2.0	3.6	15.5%	16.5%	15.4%	14.9	11.5	24.9	4.6	—	—
1975	1.9	2.0	3.6	16.7	16.5	16.9	11.4	11.2	22.2	5.1	4.9	10.9
1980	1.7	2.1	3.6	17.1	15.0	18.8	10.0	13.1	19.7	4.8	5.6	11.4
1985	1.4	2.2	3.5	15.2	14.8	19.9	9.2	13.8	18.0	5.2	6.2	—
1990	1.2	2.0	3.1	13.7	13.6	19.0	9.1	13.0	16.7	5.5	6.7	—
1995	1.1	1.9	2.9	12.4	—	20.7	8.0	12.2	14.2	—	—	6.4

Source: Organization for Economic Cooperation and Development 1997.

Table 5.3   Healthcare Expenditures in Selected Countries

Year	Percent of GDP			Per Capita Outlays in U.S. $			Per Capita Inpatient Outlays in U.S. $		
	U.S.	Canada	Germany	U.S.	Canada	Germany	U.S.	Canada	Germany
1970	7.2%	7.1%	5.7%	341	279	194	150	146	59
1975	8.2	7.2	8.0	582	518	606	273	280	199
1980	9.1	7.3	8.1	1,051	779	1,187	512	415	387
1985	10.7	8.4	8.5	1,733	1,127	966	805	576	324
1990	12.7	9.2	8.2	2,689	1,878	2,118	1,185	910	724
1995	14.2	9.7	10.4	3,644	1,857	3,089	1,578	847	1,121

Source: Organization for Economic Cooperation and Development 1997.

full to justify a continuation or expansion of the hospital budget. More efficient, innovative outpatient delivery may lag because of the lack of incentives to develop new services. Recognition of these issues has contributed to concern about the ability of global budgets to continue to control healthcare expenditure increases. Concerns have also been expressed about the ability of these health delivery systems to respond to changing patient needs and demand for healthcare. Spending constraints, for example, have resulted in queues in Canada for coronary artery bypass graft (CABG) surgery, radiation therapy, and knee replacement surgery (Coyte et al. 1994; Naylor 1991; Naylor et al. 1993, 1995).

Because reforms in the United Kingdom and New Zealand have been introduced only recently, information on the impact of internal markets is limited. District and regional authorities have been encouraged to define health needs and priorities for their residents (Cooper 1994; Robinson, R. 1996). In some cases, competitive bidding has been limited and purchasers have continued historical arrangements for the provision of services or have focused on more limited incremental changes in resource allocation decisions. Administration costs have increased (OECD 1995a). Some providers have experienced financial difficulties, necessitating the closure of beds and the merger of facilities (e.g., selected London hospitals and rural hospitals in New Zealand), reductions in staffing, and, in some cases, transitional or additional funding support from the central government.

Analysis of general practitioner (GP) fund holding in the United Kingdom indicates that hospital services have become more responsive to the needs of GPs, including improved information, response time, and access to services (Robinson, R. 1996) although the wait-times have also been influenced by additional targeted NHS funding (Maynard and Bloor 1996). There is no clear evidence regarding physician referral rates and prescribing patterns (Harrison and Choudhry 1996), quality of care, and patient satisfaction. Preliminary reports suggest selection bias in the recruitment of physician practices to fund holding—fund holding attracted large and well-organized practices (Baines and Whynes 1996). However, there is no consistent evidence of "cream-skimming" (i.e., selecting healthier patients) or insufficient patient service as GP fund holders have sought to increase their own returns (Harrison and Choudhry 1996). The differences in the organization and utilization of services between the United States and other Western country healthcare systems are also likely to be mirrored in differences in their costs and population health outcomes. Table 5.4 shows a comparison among seven of the major industrialized OECD member countries. With 14.2 percent of its GDP directed to healthcare in 1996, the United States spent 3.7 percentage points more than the second-ranked country, Germany. The U.S. per capita healthcare expenditure was $3,708 in 1996, almost 1.5 times greater than France, about twice the per capita health expenditure in Canada, and 2.7 times more than the seventh-ranked country, the United Kingdom. This large expenditure gap was apparently not offset by health outcome advantages for the United States, which had the highest infant mortality level of the seven countries and life expectancy figures that were lower than all of the other countries (OECD 1997). Furthermore, the United States was the only country of the seven with a significant population lacking health insurance—over 40.6 million people (NCHS 1997).

Overall, then, the U.S. healthcare system, which represents the market-maximized end of the health policy continuum, appears to be faring poorly in comparison to other countries in terms of allocative efficiency—that is, maximizing health benefits in the aggregate relative to the magnitude of aggregate healthcare expenditures. This confirms the microlevel evidence on allocative efficiency presented earlier in this chapter, which documented that the marginal product of expenditures for healthcare in terms of health improvements is small relative to the contribution of other non-medical social, economic, and public health investments.

Table 5.4 Comparative Expenditures and Health Indicators for Seven Industrialized Countries

Country	Healthcare Expenditures as Percentage of GDP, 1996	Healthcare Expenditures Per Capita in US $, 1996	Population Uninsured, 1995	Percentage of Population Eligible for Public Insurance for Hospital Care, 1995	Infant Mortality Per 1,000 Live Births, 1995	Life Expectancy at Birth in Years, 1995 Male	Life Expectancy at Birth in Years, 1995 Female
United States	14.2%	3708	39.7 million	46%	8.0	72.5	79.2
Canada	9.2	1796	0	100	6.0	75.3	81.3
France	9.6	2550	0	99.5	5.0	73.9	81.9
Germany	10.5	2036	0	92.2	5.3	73.0	79.5
Italy	7.6	1597	0	100	6.2	74.4	81.4
Japan	—	—	0	100	4.3	76.4	82.8
United Kingdom	6.9	1365	0	100	6.0	74.3	79.7

Source: Organization for Economic Cooperation and Development 1997.

In addition to concern about misallocating resources to services that provide low benefit relative to cost, there is concern in the United States and other countries that healthcare services of given quality are not being produced at minimum cost; efficiency strategies can also be judged by this criterion. While the least-cost production scale and methods are difficult to determine for medical services, several studies have produced evidence of inefficient production. The evidence regarding the production efficiency within the United States and other countries is reviewed next.

Production Efficiency

Healthcare services can be provided in many different ways with different combinations of personnel, facilities and equipment, production levels, and sites of service delivery. Production efficiency is achieved when production units are of optimal size and the mix of inputs is such that the marginal output per dollar of cost is equal across all inputs. Only then is the cost minimized for a given level of output of health services.

Economists and other health services researchers have conducted numerous studies of production efficiency, concentrating on (1) general administrative costs of health systems; (2) the size and mix of personnel within physician practices, as well as the method of paying physicians; (3) the optimal bed size for hospital care, the mix of inpatient and outpatient service delivery, and the role of payment methods on hospital costs; and (4) the utilization and cost impact of managed care (Ludbrook 1987). Evidence regarding each of these dimensions will be reviewed in the discussion that follows.

Administration

One result of micromanagement is very high administrative costs: one estimate places such costs at 24 percent of healthcare costs in the United States versus 11 percent in Canada (Woolhandler and Himmelstein 1991, 1997). Systems that both supply and finance care in the public sector, such as those in Canada and the United Kingdom, appear to have lower administrative costs. Such costs are greater in insurance-based systems such as those in the United States and Germany (OECD 1995b); in Canada administration is simplified by having one or few sources of payment and sets of rules. With global hospital budgets and fixed fee schedules, there is little need for close monitoring of provider behavior.

Physician services

Personnel mix. Reinhardt (1972), Smith, Miller, and Golladay (1972), and Brown (1988) took different analytical approaches to the optimal use of physician aides, but arrived at the same general conclusion: physicians could raise the productivity of their practices and lower the cost per office visit by employing more aides. Kindig (1996) also reported that managed care organizations were able to increase a physician's panel size by 50 percent by adding a non-physician provider.

An array of studies have documented that the growth of managed care in the future will have a significant impact on physician requirements. Generally, the number of physicians required will decline while the percentage of primary care specialists is expected to grow (Ginzberg and Ostow 1997; Greenberg and Cultice 1997; Kindig 1996; Reinhardt 1996).

Economies of scale. Studies on economies of scale (i.e., the tendency of average cost to decline as the scale of production increases) in physician practice conclude that group practice is more efficient than the traditional solo practice of medicine (Lee 1990). Reinhardt (1975), for example, found that physicians in group practices generated 5.0 percent more patient visits and 5.6 percent more patient billings than physicians in solo practices. A case study by Newhouse (1973) documented that slight economies of scale accrued to group practices, but that the savings were offset by higher costs associated with x-inefficiency. Because of sharing arrangements, individual physicians were less likely to conserve resources.

Survivor analysis has also been used to test for economies of scale in physician practice. In this type of analysis, the fastest-growing size of practice for a given period of time is judged most efficient. The documented growth of large multispecialty group practice arrangements in the United States since the mid-1960s further attests to the production efficiency of this mode of practice

(Frech and Ginsburg 1974; Havlicek 1996; Marder and Zuckerman 1985).

Medical practice and technology have changed dramatically during the last 25 years, permitting many more surgical and diagnostic services to be done in an outpatient setting. Capital required to provide more sophisticated outpatient services can be financed and efficiently used in group practice settings. In addition to the production efficiencies of group practice, high practice start-up costs, greater competition in a period of growing supply and budget restraints, and national and state health policies that favor HMOs all point to continued growth in group medical practice.

Physician payment. The RBRVS physician payment counterpart to the PPS for hospitals under Medicare was intended to reduce the rate of increase in physician expenditures under that program. There is some evidence that these policies have reduced the rate of increase in physician costs and have redistributed payments from procedural to primary care services. The difficulty lies in separating the effects of the RBRVS from other major changes taking place in healthcare. The change to managed care may be more important in explaining the rising incomes of generalists and the falling incomes of most specialists (Gonzalez 1996).

Overall, Medicare expenditure projections prepared by the Congressional Budget Office suggest that expenditures for physician service will remain constant through 2002, whereas spending for Medicare overall is projected to increase at an average annual rate of 8 to 9 percent through 2002 (PPRC 1997). These trends suggest that the RBRVS payment system may be playing a role in restraining physician expenditure under the Medicare program, as well as in inducing some reallocation of care from specialty to primary care.

Hospital services

Economies of scale. Considerable research has been conducted on the degree to which community hospitals are subject to economies of scale. In ways similiar to methods of physician services analysis, the methods of hospital cost function analysis have been somewhat crude, because measures of input and output do not take account of the great complexity of hospital-based care (Berki 1972; Cowing,

Holtmann, and Powers 1983). Nevertheless, Feldstein (1988) concluded that slight economies of scale were taking place, with the optimum-sized community hospital at between 200 and 300 beds. While hospitals in the United States are increasing in size, the average number of beds per hospital is still less than 200 (NCHS 1997).

Hansen and Zwanziger (1996) estimated cost functions to assess marginal costs of hospital outputs and to compare marginal costs between the United States and Canada based on 1981 and 1985 data. From this analysis, it appeared that economies of scale were not present in the American hospitals. Acute care marginal costs increased as output increased in California and New York hospitals in 1981 and, for the most part, in 1985. On the other hand, acute care marginal costs in Canada decreased as hospital size increased suggesting that Canadian acute care hospitals—except for very large hospitals—realized modest economies of scale.

A more important issue for hospitals, and one that also raises the quality question, is the efficient size of a given service or department within the hospital (Grannenmann, Brown, and Pauly 1986). Luft, Bunker, and Enthoven (1979) have shown a positive relationship between volume of heart surgery and outcome. Hannan et al. (1991) also found that annual surgeon volume and annual hospital volume were significantly and inversely related to mortality for CABG surgery. Thus, in cases where higher service volume results in improved outcomes, efficiency can be improved by producing services at a lower cost per unit and by achieving more positive outcomes. Whether determined by regulation or market competition, such specialized services should be regionalized. Medicare, for example, instituted a program to regionalize heart surgery in "centers of excellence," and large private-sector HMOs such as Kaiser and Group Health of Puget Sound have traditionally regionalized delivery of costly, infrequent procedures.

Payment methods. While extremely difficult to demonstrate conclusively, PPS has generally been judged successful in containing hospital costs under Medicare without harming patients (Kahn et al. 1990; Russell 1989). However, one result of PPS was rapid expansion in outpatient hospital services, home care, and long-term care. Although hospitals profited initially under PPS, subsequent restrictions on payment increases reduced operating profit margins to near zero by 1993 (American Hospital Association 1996; Guterman, Ashby, and Greene 1996). Cost-cutting strategies subsequently improved margins to about 8 percent by 1996 (Guterman, Ashby, and Greene 1996). Schwartz and Mendelson (1991) have shown that hospital cost-containment strategies in the 1980s, including PPS, did not affect the underlying increase in hospital costs in the United States. Reductions in the rate of growth in Medicare expenditures were offset by an increase in non-Medicare spending.

Health plans

While input mix and economies of scale are important issues, the extent of service use by the population and the intensity of care are more important determinants of healthcare expenditure. These have been affected by significant changes in the financial and organizational structure of the healthcare system induced by managed care and related market competition (AMA 1990). Evidence regarding the dynamics and impacts of managed care on state, national, hospital, and employer expenditure trends will be reviewed.

State- and national-level expenditures. Research has suggested that managed care plans have reduced the overall rate of growth in healthcare costs by inducing price competition and reducing costs. Comparative state and national data confirmed that the development of managed care and competition was restraining the growth of medical care costs. Zwanziger and Melnick (1996) compared the cumulative growth in total real per capita health expenditures and in selected components of health expenditures for several states and the United States as a whole between 1980 and 1991. California was the state with the most highly developed managed care and the most competition during that period. Maryland, New York, and other northeastern states were among states with less competition and more regulation. California's healthcare cost growth rates were substantially lower. For example, the total percentage growth was 63 percent for the United States, 39 percent for California, and 59 percent for Maryland during that period. Comparable figures for hospital services were 54 percent, 27 percent, and 34.1 percent, respectively. California fared even better in the areas of physician services and drugs. These differences were accompanied by slower growth in full-time equivalent hospital employees per patient in California (0.5 percent) compared to the United States (1.4 percent). Based on a related study of the growth of managed care in California and Minnesota, Zwanziger and Melnick (1996) found that a one percentage point increase in out-of-pocket premium differential was associated with an 8.6 percent decrease in enrollment-based market share.

These state and national healthcare expenditure trends do suggest, if not unarguably, that managed care is playing a role in abating cost growth in the heavily market-maximized U.S. healthcare system (Levit, Lazenby, and Sivarajan 1996).

Hospital expenditures. Evidence confirming the likely role of managed care in accounting for these trends is provided by research on the role of managed care in reducing overall hospital expenditures. J. C. Robinson (1996) examined the impact of HMOs on hospital capacity, utilization, and expenditures in California between 1983 and 1993 and reported that hospital expenditures grew less rapidly (44 percent) in markets with high HMO penetration than in markets with low HMO penetration. The majority of the reduced growth rates of hospital expenditures was the result of reduced volume and mix of services (28 percent), although some was due to reduction in intensity of service (10 percent) and reduced bed capacity (6 percent). The number of inpatient surgical procedures declined more quickly in markets with high HMO penetration and the volume of outpatient procedures increased more slowly in these markets. There was a significant reduction in inpatient psychiatric days in high HMO markets compared to low HMO markets. J. C. Robinson (1996) also argued that the sustained impact of HMOs on hospital expenditures is most likely to be realized from consolidations of hospitals and reductions in excess capacity by hospital systems.

Conrad and his colleagues' research (Conrad et al. 1996) confirmed the impact of various hospital managed care strategies on cost per hospital discharge. Their analysis suggested that the proportion of hospital revenues derived from case or capitation payment was consistently associated with lower costs per discharge. Similarly, hospital approaches to providing resource use information to clinicians and formal care management were related to lower costs per discharge and efficiency.

Employer expenditures. Large employers (those with 200 employees or more) attribute much of their success in slowing the growth of healthcare costs to the managed care and competition strategy pursued during the past decade. After an annual percentage of growth in the upper teens in the cost per employee for health benefits during the period 1988 to 1990, costs began to decline and were negative 1.1 percent in 1994, followed by two years of low growth of about 2 percent per year (Foster Higgins 1994). Wickizer and Feldstein (1995) used premium data to study the competitive effects of HMOs on indemnity plan premiums between 1985 and 1992. The degree of HMO participation in the market was found to have a significant and negative effect on the rate of growth in indemnity insurance premiums (5.9 percent growth in indemnity plan premiums rather than 7.0 percent with a 25 percent increase in HMO penetration). On the other hand, Feldman, Dowd, and Gifford (1993) found that including an HMO option in employment-based health insurance plans actually increased the average family premium by $25.14, as compared with premiums for plans offering only traditional fee-for-service indemnity insurance. Findings regarding the impact of managed care on employee premiums, then, remain mixed.

Plan-level utilization. Studies of the impact of HMOs on patterns of utilization of hospital and physician services provide evidence of the dynamic through which HMOs produce the system and institutional impacts on expenditures just reviewed. Based on a review and synthesis of early research on HMOs, Luft (1981) concluded that they provided care for 10 percent to 40 percent less than comparable fee-for-service systems; the quality was no worse on average; and most of the savings were due to fewer hospital admissions. Through randomization into one large well-established HMO, the RAND Health Insurance Experiment supported Luft's conclusion. They found savings of 25 percent with no adverse health effects on the general population, although persons who were initially sick and poor at the beginning of the experiment did fare better under the free fee-for-service plan than in the HMO.

A later synthesis of research on HMOs and other forms of managed care by Luft and his colleagues in the mid-1990s (Miller and Luft 1994) confirmed that HMOs had lower hospital admission rates, shorter hospital lengths of stay, lower utilization of expensive procedures, and greater utilization of preventive services than traditional indemnity plans. Overall, enrollee satisfaction with services was lower in HMOs than in traditional fee-for-service plans, but HMO enrollees reported greater satisfaction with costs. The relatively high level of HMO enrollee satisfaction and somewhat greater use of ambulatory physician services by HMO enrollees was confirmed by subsequent empirical research (Blendon et al. 1994; Mark and Mueller 1996).

In summary, growth in managed care and competition has altered dramatically the economic incentives in healthcare. Providers have been induced to consider adopting more efficient means of production, reducing prices, and providing care demanded by consumers and payors. Physician practice continues to move toward more efficient personnel mix and scale; the average size of hospitals is increasing; very expensive and difficult services are being regionalized; and the numbers of HMO systems and HMO enrollments are increasing. These changes have reduced the rate of growth in cost, especially to employers. Indicators of improved health outcomes and expanded coverage for the population are lacking. Other democratic developed countries appear to have been more successful at controlling spending, insuring their populations, and achieving health outcomes in the past. Whether they are truly more efficient or not is impossible to determine from aggregate data. Even so, attaining cost-control and access goals are important social achievements. Health services research can play a significant role in documenting the extent to which the emerging dominance of managed care in the United States is likely to improve the performance of the U.S. healthcare system in this regard. In Chapter 7, emerging models of community-oriented managed care, which point to a promising wedding of managed care and population health–oriented principles, are reviewed as innovative alternatives for both enhancing access and improving health.

Criteria for Assessing Policy Alternatives in Terms of Efficiency

Policymakers strive to provide the right mix of regulation and market competition that will provide incentives and controls for consumers and their physicians in choosing efficient amounts and types of healthcare services, and for providers in adopting efficient practices to deliver those services.

When evaluating policies or programs for efficiency concerns, several criteria might be applied (see Table 5.5). These relate to both the macrolevel and microlevel of analysis and concern both allocation and production issues. First, a state or nation is concerned about spending an appropriate fraction of gross domestic (or state) product on the health sector. Given the lack of any objective method to determine the allocation of resources that maximizes the well-being of the population, deciding what is "appropriate" is a political judgment. For many nations during the past 15 years, a guiding principle was that health spending should not increase faster than the rate of growth in national income or wages. This criterion reflects a judgment based on assessment of the health needs and the effectiveness of additional spending on health services—a growing share of national income spent on healthcare is not spent in the best interest of the society. This judgment of the appropriate share of income going to healthcare will differ by state and over time, depending on the dominant political and economic circumstances.

Second, allocative efficiency requires a mix of health services that maximizes a combination of positive health outcomes and consumer satisfaction for the available share of resources expended on health services. A judgment must be made concerning the existing allocation of resources and whether it should be altered to obtain greater health and well-being for the society. The evidence reviewed earlier on the allocative efficiency of the U.S. healthcare system, for example, suggested that it suffers from an overinvestment in secondary and tertiary treatment and an underinvestment in population health–oriented disease prevention, health promotion, and health protection strategies, relative to the observed, as well as to the likely, health return on these investments.

Third, production costs should be minimized for health services in the interests of production efficiency. The output of the production process should consider the health of the individuals receiving care, their satisfaction with the method of service delivery, and any health consequences to others who may be indirectly affected by health programs. Costs should include the direct cost of services plus indirect time costs incurred by participants and

Table 5.5   Criteria for Assessing Health Policies in Terms of
Efficiency

Issue	Criteria	Indicators
Macro–Cost Control	• Spend an appropriate fraction of gross state product on the health sector.	• Health spending should not increase faster than the rate of growth in income in the state.
Allocative Efficiency	• Assure a mix of health services that maximizes a combination of health outcomes and consumer satisfaction for the available share of resources expended on health services.	• A majority of new health spending should be directed to disease prevention, health promotion, and improvement in the social and physical environment for persons likely to achieve the greatest gains from such investment.
Production Efficiency	• Produce health services at minimum cost.	• Produce services at a cost at or below nationally recognized benchmarks of cost per unit of service.
Dynamic Efficiency	• Search for technological and organizational advances which raise the productivity of given resources.	• Encourage research and development of new health services and efficient ways to organize and deliver them.

other affected parties (OECD 1992). Service quality and cost should therefore be compared to the comprehensive national benchmarks deemed to be the most efficient producers of the services in question. A number of organizations have developed information on standards of performance for healthcare providers (Cleverly 1997; HCIA–MERCER 1996) and health plans (HEDIS 1996).

For example, the HCIA–MERCER project ranks the top 100 hospitals in the United States according to several factors including risk-adjusted mortality, complications, length of stay, expense per adjusted discharge, profitability, and productivity. HEDIS was developed primarily for employers that required performance information for making a selection from competing managed health plans. The HEDIS instrument was subsequently adapted for use by the Medicaid program. It covers effectiveness of care, availability, satisfaction with care, cost of care, use of services, and plan-descriptive information.

Finally, a search should be made for technological and organizational advances that raise the productivity of given resources (i.e., dynamic efficiency). Policies should therefore encourage development of and experimentation with new services and with more efficient ways to organize and deliver healthcare. Innovative alternatives can be identified and evaluated through comparative research of variant policies or programs across the United States or within individual states. International comparative research may alert policymakers to the lessons that other countries may have to teach.

An Application of Efficiency Criteria: Medicaid Managed Care

Healthcare for the poor is one aspect of the U.S. system that has suffered from inefficiency. Medicaid managed care has emerged as a dominant policy intervention at the state level in an attempt to improve both the efficiency and access of healthcare services to the poor in the United States (Rowland et al. 1995). The efficiency criteria just reviewed will be applied in identifying the sources of inefficiency and in determining the likely success of Medicaid managed care in addressing them.

Macro–Cost Control

Data show that the national growth rate of Medicaid expenditures declined in the 1990s from the rates experienced in the late 1980s. Average annual Medicaid expenditure growth rates were 22.4 percent for 1988–1992, 9.5 percent for 1992–1995, and 3.3 percent for 1995–1996 (Holahan and Liska 1996). Thus, states appear to be succeeding in the goal of containing the growth in Medicaid expenditures. This may not, however, be attributed to the development of Medicaid managed care. Expenditure growth in the late 1980s was fueled by enrollment expansions and general medical inflation. Furthermore, while 38.6 percent of all beneficiaries were enrolled in managed care plans in 1996—a fourfold increase since 1991—Medicaid managed care represented only about five percent of total Medicaid spending

in 1994 (PPRC 1997). Managed care enrollees are drawn disproportionately from low-income children and adults, who account
for about 75 percent of Medicaid beneficiaries but only about one-
third of total program spending. The elderly and disabled account
for most of the spending. Since their expenditure rates have also
declined and they have not been enrolled in managed care, factors
other than managed care, such as a decline in general inflation, are
contributing to the reduction in expenditure growth.

The evidence on macro–cost control at the state level is mixed.
The analysis of evaluations of 12 Medicaid managed care programs
showed that seven reported a decrease of 5 to 15 percent in costs to
state Medicaid agencies when compared with traditional Medicaid
plans. Two reported increases in costs; the rest reported unchanged
or unknown cost effects (Hurley, Freund, and Paul 1993). Oregon's
managed care program was estimated to save $8.78 per beneficiary
per month compared with the costs expected under traditional fee-
for-service program between 1988 and 1990. Arizona's program
achieved substantial savings over a nine-year period. Medicaid
managed care programs in Georgia, Michigan, and Tennessee, on
the other hand, cost more than traditional fee-for-service Medicaid
(Hurley, Freund, and Paul 1993).

Allocative Efficiency

There is no indication or pretense that Medicaid managed care has
been primarily intended to assume a broad population perspective
on improving the health of affected populations. There is, however,
limited evidence that such programs have resulted in a shift from
costly and inappropriate emergency room use to less costly primary
care, which tends to be more prevention-oriented in focus.

Much of the research on Medicaid managed care is based on
evaluations of Arizona's Medicaid program, the Health Care Financing Administration (HCFA) Medicaid Competition Demonstration
Projects of the 1980s, and assessments of 25 Medicaid managed care
programs in 16 states by Robert Hurley and his colleagues (Freund
et al. 1989; Freund and Hurley 1995; Hurley, Freund, and Paul 1993).
In every HCFA Medicaid Competition Demonstration site except
Missouri, the probability of seeing a specialist at least once during
the year declined by more than 30 percent for both adults and

children (Freund and Lewit 1993). In 9 of 12 evaluations of Medicaid managed care programs, emergency room visits decreased; the results from the other three evaluations were unknown. For example, an evaluation of four HCFA programs found that emergency room use dropped between 30 and 45 percent for adults and between 27 percent and 37 percent for children. The decline occurred in both capitated and primary care case management PCCM plans. Use of immunizations and prenatal care was unaffected, while changes in well child care and gynecological exams varied across studies. Use of preventive care remained low for both fee-for-service and managed care Medicaid enrollees.

Production Efficiency

The cost of providing services to Medicaid enrollees has not been compared to a national benchmark. HEDIS (1996) data on utilization and healthcare cost per member per month are not available for Medicaid populations. However, several studies have provided tentative evidence of the prospect for greater production efficiency in Medicaid managed care compared to fee-for-service alternatives. For example, in a comparison between satisfaction with and use of healthcare among New York City Medicaid beneficiaries in five managed care plans and that of beneficiaries enrolled in conventional Medicaid, Sisk et al. (1996) found that the managed care enrollees reported higher levels of satisfaction, had a greater likelihood of a usual source of care (i.e., of seeing the same clinician), and shorter appointment and office waiting times than traditional Medicaid program recipients. There was no difference in utilization of inpatient stays, emergency department visits, or office or clinic visits. Therefore, there were no apparent cost savings associated with managed care. Efficiency may have been enhanced, however, since access and satisfaction were improved by the managed care plan, while the cost of care remained the same as in the traditional program.

A randomized trial–based evaluation of a Florida prepaid managed care program further confirmed that the staff model HMO was able to lower members' likelihood of using care (Buchanan, Leibowitz, and Keesey 1996). The amount of services received, once care was initiated, was the same in the prepaid and fee-for-service

Medicaid. The authors found that the HMO attracted sicker-than-average enrollees, so this reduced utilization translated into Medicaid program savings. The authors note that for utilization by two vulnerable groups—children with at least one preexisting condition and blacks—the managed care plan provided as much care as the fee-for-service Medicaid plan. This study provides only qualified evidence of production efficiency, however, because it contained no assessment of the health effect differences between the two groups.

The RAND Health Insurance Experiment, described previously (Manning et al. 1987), found that those enrolled in the HMO experienced less hospitalization, which resulted in expenditure being only 72 percent of that in the free fee-for-service plan. This did not result in worse health outcomes for the average person. However, limited evidence suggested that those HMO enrollees who were both poor and in poor health incurred a higher rate of bed days and serious symptoms relative to individuals with similar economic and physical conditions who were enrolled in the free fee-for-service plan. Therefore, managed care plans may not be more efficient for the poor unless special attention (e.g., case management and outreach services) is given to their special healthcare needs.

A significant and related policy impact of the increasing dominance of Medicaid managed care is that the movement of Medicaid recipients into managed care plans has resulted in a significant increase in competition for Medicaid enrollees among health plans. This, in turn, has had a major impact on traditional "safety net" providers, prompting some of these providers to pursue vertical and horizontal integration, managed care contracting, and marketing to attract other patient groups (Lipson and Naierman 1996). Neither the efficiency nor the access consequences of these changes have been fully assessed.

Dynamic Efficiency

Managed care tends to be innovative in organizing and delivering healthcare services compared to the traditional fee-for-service system. Managed care programs have led the way in the development and use of outpatient surgery, telephone counseling, triage systems, nurse practitioners and physician assistants, extended care beds, and preventive care. With capitation payment and a defined population to which they are responsible, managed care plans have the incentive to consider population-level interventions to improve the health of their enrollees (Lairson et al. 1997). Models that attempt to integrate features of managed care and more population health–oriented principles will be reviewed in Chapter 7.

In summary, only mixed evidence exists that Medicaid managed care is contributing significantly to healthcare cost control at the national and state levels and that the allocation of resources within Medicaid is being improved by shifting care from episodic acute services in the emergency room and hospital outpatient departments to primary care in community settings. Specific studies suggest the potential both for improved patient satisfaction, with no detrimental effects on health, and lower cost. The source of cost savings and the long-term implications for the health status of low-income populations are unclear. While managed care plans have the incentives and the potential to address health problems at the population level, Medicaid policy is disrupting systems of medical education and traditional safety net providers. Attempts to improve efficiency and control cost also have important equity consequences that will be examined more fully in the chapters that follow.

Summary and Conclusions

Three major questions are addressed in this chapter: (1) What policy strategies are available to achieve efficiency? (2) What is the evidence regarding the efficiency of these strategies? and (3) What criteria should be used in judging the efficiency of policy alternatives?

In response to the first question, national healthcare systems can be positioned on a continuum ranging from market-maximized demand-based systems of healthcare to market-minimized need-based systems. The former is characterized by individual choice by consumers, non-universal coverage, private insurance, numerous sources of payment, high out-of-pocket payment, the private practice of medicine, and the private ownership of healthcare facilities, many of which are operated on a for-profit basis. The interaction of supply and demand forces within a market context, however imperfect, guides the allocation of resources within healthcare and between healthcare and other sectors. Market-minimized systems are characterized by community need–based determinations, universal and public coverage, relatively few sources of payment, low out-of-pocket payments, public practice or public control of private practice, and public ownership or control of healthcare facilities operated on a not-for-profit basis. Professional and bureaucratic determinations of need guides the allocation of resources to and within the health sector.

National healthcare systems generally have some combination of regulatory and market aspects. Many payment schemes (e.g., prospective payment of hospitals by DRGs) and utilization management schemes (e.g., managed care tools) have been developed to enhance efficiency.

In response to the second and third questions posed at the beginning of the chapter, the evidence regarding the efficiency of these strategies, particularly the market-maximized strategy that dominates in the United States, will be reviewed in its relationship to the criteria for assessing efficiency outlined earlier (see Table 5.5): macrocontrol of healthcare costs, allocative efficiency, production efficiency, and dynamic efficiency.

Macro–Cost Control

The United States eschews the proven macro-approach that stabilized health spending in Canada and western Europe as a percent of gross domestic product, by exerting direct government and community control over healthcare spending (OECD 1995b). The United States continues to develop an unstructured market that minimally regulates insurers and gives providers and consumers strong incentives for making efficient decisions at the microlevel. Cost control achieved through the macro-approach does not necessarily translate directly into efficiency, but micro-incentives have yet to demonstrate long-term cost control, making allocative efficiency uncertain.

Allocative Efficiency

Considerable evidence exists that the United States fails to achieve maximum value from the resources allocated to healthcare services, and that it may perform less well than many other developed countries. Indicators include evidence on variability in the use of services; the lack of effectiveness and appropriateness of many healthcare procedures; substantial underinvestment in selected preventive services, including prenatal care; a focus on procedure-oriented care that is costly and may add little to health at the margin; high rates of spending; and a relatively poor showing on many indicators of the U.S. population's health compared to that of other countries.[1]

Production Efficiency

Additionally, numerous studies have documented that hospital, physician, and insurance services are not produced in the most efficient manner, and comparative data suggest that prices and associated incomes are set higher than necessary to attract the required resources to healthcare. Evidence includes excess capacity, a lack of attention to the most efficient personnel mix, and a failure to take advantage of potential economies of scale.

Dynamic Efficiency

As evidenced by the data comparing the healthcare investment experiences of different countries reviewed earlier, U.S. policymakers can perhaps begin to discern new answers to the troubling question of how best to inprove the efficiency of the U.S. healthcare system. This effort at discernment can begin with a study of alternative models that have been developed on a state, regional, or national basis, and by development of a program to measure their effects on population health costs (Roos et al. 1996). Health services researchers and policy analysts can contribute to the fund of knowledge by assessing ways in which other countries have dealt with (1) the role of environmental, social, behavioral, and medical determinants of health in the formulation of health policy; (2) the design of population-oriented data systems directed toward assessing these policies; and, finally, (3) the extent to which the effectiveness, efficiency, and equity objectives of health policy have been or are likely to be achieved.

Note

1. This is not to imply that all preventive services are cost-effective. See Russell (1986) for an economic critique of preventive programs.

References

American Hospital Association. 1996. *Hospital Statistics: Emerging Trends in Hospitals.* 1995–1996 ed. Chicago: American Hospital Association.

American Medical Association. 1990. *Medical Group Practice in the United States: Survey of Practice Characteristics.* Chicago: American Medical Association.

Anderson, O. W. 1989. *The Health Services Continuum in Democratic States: An Inquiry into Solvable Problems.* Chicago: Health Administration Press.

Baines, D. L., and D. K. Whynes. 1996. "Selection Bias in GP Fundholding." *Health Economics* 5: 129–40.

Berki, S. 1972. *Hospital Economics.* Lexington, MA: Lexington Books.

Blendon, R. J., R. A. Knox, M. Brodie, J. M. Benson, and G. Chervinsky. 1994. "Americans Compare Managed Care, Medicare, and Fee-For-Service." *Journal of American Health Policy* 4 (3): 42–47.

Brown, D. M. 1988. "Do Physicians Underutilize Aides?" *Journal of Human Resources* 23: 342–55.

Buchanan, J. L., A. Leibowitz, and J. Keesey. 1996. "Medicaid Health Maintenance Organizations: Can They Reduce Program Spending?" *Medical Care* 34: 249–63.

Cleverly, W. O. 1997. *Essentials of Health Care Finance.* 4th ed. Gaithersburg MD: Aspen Publishers, Inc.

Conrad, D., T. Wickizer, C. Maynard, T. Klastorin, D. Lessler, A. Ross, N. Soderstrom, S. Sullivan, J. Alexander, and K. Travis. 1996. "Managing Care, Incentives, and Information: An Exploratory Look Inside the 'Black Box' of Hospital Efficiency." *Health Services Research* 31: 235–59.

Cooper, M. H. 1994. "Jumping On the Spot—Health Reform New Zealand Style." *Health Economics* 310: 69–72.

Cowing, T. G., A. G. Holtmann, and S. Powers. 1983. "Hospital Cost Analysis: A Survey and Evaluation of Recent Studies." In *Advances in Health Economics and Health Services Research.* Edited by R. M. Scheffler, and L. F. Rossiter, 257–304. Vol. 4. Greenwich, CT: Jai Press.

Coyte, P. C., J. G. Wright, G. A. Hawker, C. Bombardier, R. S. Dittus, J. E. Paul, D. A. Freund, and E. Ho. 1994. "Waiting Times for Knee-Replacement Surgery in the United States and Ontario." *The New England Journal of Medicine* 331: 1068–71.

D'Intignano, B. M. 1990. *Incentives in Health Care Management.* Zurich, Switzerland: Second World Congress On Health Economics.

Dowling, W. 1974. "Prospective Reimbursement of Hospitals." *Inquiry* 11: 163–80.

Enthoven, A C. 1990. "What Can Europeans Learn from Americans?" *Health Care Systems in Transition: The Search for Efficiency*, Social Policy Series No. 7. Paris, France: OECD.

Feldman, R., B. Dowd, and G. Gifford. 1993. "The Effect of HMOs On Premiums in Employment-Based Health Plans." *Health Services Research* 27: 779–810.

Feldstein, P. 1988. *Health Care Economics*. 3rd ed. New York: John Wiley & Sons.

Folland, S., A. C. Goodman, and M. Stano. 1997. *The Economics of Health and Health Care*. 2nd ed. Upper Saddle River, NJ: Prentice Hall.

Foster Higgins. 1994. National Survey of Employer Sponsored Health Plans, 1994 [Online]. Available: http://www.insweb.com/research/facts/health001.htm [12/15/97].

Frech, H. E., and P. B. Ginsburg. 1974. "Optimal Scale in Medical Practice: A Survivor Analysis." *Journal of Business* 47 (1): 23–36.

Freund, D. A., and R. E. Hurley. 1995. "Medicaid Managed Care: Contribution to Issues of Health Reform." *Annual Review of Public Health* 16: 473–95.

Freund, D. A., and E. Lewit. 1993. "Managed Health Care for Children and Pregnant Women: Promises and Pitfalls." *The Future of Children* 3: 92–123.

Freund, D. A., L. F. Rossiter, P. D. Fox, J. A. Meyer, R. E. Hurley, T. S. Carey, and J. E. Paul. 1989. "Evaluation of the Medicaid Competition Demonstrations." *Health Care Financing Review* 11 (2): 81–97.

Fuchs, V. 1974. *Who Shall Live?* New York: Basic Books.

Ginzberg, E., and M. Ostow. 1997. "Managed Care: A Look Back and a Look Ahead." *The New England Journal of Medicine* 336: 1018–20.

Glennerster, H. 1995. "Internal Markets: Context and Structure." In *Health Care Reform Through Internal Markets*. Edited by M. Jerome-Forget, J. White, and J. Wiener, 17–26. Washington, D.C.: IRPP.

Gold, M. R., J. E. Siegel, L. B. Russell, and M. C. Weinstein. 1996. *Cost-Effectiveness in Health and Medicine*. New York: Oxford University Press.

Gonzalez, M L, ed. 1996. *Socioeconomic Characteristics of Medical Practice in 1996*. Chicago: American Medical Association.

Grannenmann, T. W., R. S. Brown, and M. V. Pauly. 1986. "Estimating Hospital Costs: A Multiple-Output Analysis." *Journal of Health Economics* 5: 107–27.

Greenberg, L., and J. M. Cultice. 1997. "Forecasting the Need for Physicians in the United States: The Health Resources and Services Administration's Physician Requirements Model." *Health Services Research* 31: 723–37.

Guterman, S., J. Ashby, and T. Greene. 1996. "Hospital Cost Growth Down." *Health Affairs* 15 (3): 134–39.

Hannan, E. L., H. Kilburn, H. Bernard, J. F. O'Donnell, G. Lukacik, and E. P. Shields. 1991. "Coronary Artery Bypass Surgery: The Relationship Between Inhospital Mortality Rate and Surgical Volume After Controlling for Clinical Risk Factors." *Medical Care* 29: 1094–107.

Hansen, K. K., and J. Zwanziger. 1996. "Marginal Costs in General Acute Care Hospitals: A Comparison Among California, New York and Canada." *Health Economics* 5: 195–216.

Harrison, S., and N. Choudhry. 1996. "General Practice Fundholding in the UK National Health Service: Evidence to Date." *Journal of Public Health Policy* 17: 331–46.

Havlicek, P. L. 1996. *Medical Groups in the U.S.: A Survey of Practice Characteristics*. Chicago: American Medical Association.

HCIA–MERCER. 1996. 100 Top Hospitals for 1996 [Online]. Available: http://www.hcia.com/newsletters/100top/intro.html [12/17/97].

HEDIS. 1996. HEDIS 3.0: Executive Summary [Online]. Available: http://www.ncqa.org/hedis/30exsum.htm [11/21/97].

Henke, K. D., M. A. Murray, and C. Ade. 1994. Global Budgeting in Germany: Lessons for the United States. *Health Affairs* 13 (4): 7–21.

Holahan, J., and D. Liska. 1996. *Where Is Medicaid Spending Headed?* Washington, D.C.: Kaiser Commission on the Future of Medicaid.

Hurley, R. E., D. A. Freund, and J. E. Paul. 1993. *Managed Care in Medicaid: Lessons for Policy and Program Design*. Chicago: Health Administration Press.

Jensen, G. A., M. A. Morrisey, S. Gaffney, and D. K. Liston. 1997. "The New Dominance of Managed Care: Insurance Trends in the 1990s." *Health Affairs* 16 (1): 125–36.

Jonsson, B. 1990. "What Can Americans Learn from Europeans?" *Health Care Systems in Transition: The Search for Efficiency*, Social Policy Series No. 7. Paris, France: OECD.

Kahn, K. L., L. V. Rubenstein, D. Draper, J. Kosecoff, W. H. Rogers, E. B. Keeler, and R. H. Brook. 1990. "Comparing Outcomes of Care Before and After Implementation of the DRG-Based Prospective Payment System." *Journal of the American Medical Association* 264: 1984–88.

Kindig, D. A. 1996. "Strategic Issues for Managing the Future Physician Workforce." In *Strategic Choices for a Changing Health Care System*. Edited by S. H. Altman, and U. E. Reinhardt, 149–82. Chicago: Health Administration Press.

Lairson, D. R., G. Schulmeier, C. E. Begley, L. A. Aday, Y. Coyle, and C. H. Slater. 1997. "Managed Care and Community-Oriented Care: Conflict or Complement." *Journal of Health Care for the Poor and Underserved* 8: 36–55.

Lee, R. H. 1990. "The Economics of Group Practice: A Reassessment." In *Advances in Health Economics and Health Services Research*. Edited by R. M. Scheffler, and L. F. Rossiter, 111–29. Vol. 11. London: JAI Press.

Levit, K. R., H. C. Lazenby, and L. Sivarajan. 1996. "Health Care Spending in 1994: Slowest in Decades." *Health Affairs* 15 (2): 130–144.

Lipson, D. J., and N. Naierman. 1996. "Effects of Health System Changes On Safety-Net Providers." *Health Affairs* 15 (2): 33–48.

Ludbrook, A. 1987. Economic Appraisal and Planning Decisions for Health Technologies. In *Economic Appraisal of Health Technology in the European Community*. Edited by M. F. Drummond, 120–135. Oxford: Oxford Medical Publications.

Luft, H. S. 1981. *Health Maintenance Organizations: Dimensions of Performance*. New York: John Wiley & Sons.

Luft, H. S., J. P. Bunker, and A. C. Enthoven. 1979. "Should Operations Be Regionalized? The Empirical Relation Between Surgical Volume and Mortality." *The New England Journal of Medicine* 301: 1364–69.

Manning, W. G., J. P. Newhouse, N. Duan, E. B. Keeler, A. Leibowitz, and M. S. Marquis. 1987. "Health Insurance and the Demand for Medical Care: Evidence from a Randomized Experiment." *American Economic Review* 77: 251–77.

Marder, W. D., and S. Zuckerman. 1985. "Competition and Medical Groups: A Survivor Analysis." *Journal of Health Economics* 4 (2): 167–76.

Mark, T., and C. Mueller. 1996. "Access to Care in HMOs and Traditional Insurance Plans." *Health Affairs* 15 (4): 81–87.

Maynard, A., and K. Bloor. 1996. "Introducing a Market to the United Kingdom's National Health Service." *The New England Journal of Medicine* 334: 604–8.

McKeown, T. 1990. "Determinants of Health." In *The Nation's Health*. 3rd ed. Edited by P. R. Lee, and C. L. Estes, 6–13. Boston: Jones and Bartlett.

Miller, R. H., and H. S. Luft. 1994. "Managed Care Plan Performance Since 1980: A Literature Analysis." *Journal of the American Medical Association* 271: 1512–19.

Moloney, T. W., and D. E. Rogers. 1979. "Medical Technology—A Different View of the Contentious Debate over Costs." *The New England Journal of Medicine* 301: 1413–19.

National Center for Health Statistics. 1997. *Health, United States, 1996–97, and Injury Chartbook*. Hyattsville, MD: Public Health Service.

Naylor, C. D. 1991. "A Different View of Queues in Ontario." *Health Affairs* 10 (3): 110–128.

Naylor, C. D., C. M. Levinton, S. Wheeler, and L. Hunter. 1993. "Queueing for Coronary Surgery During Severe Supply-Demand Mismatch in a Canadian Referral Centre: A Case Study of Implicit Rationing." *Social Science and Medicine* 37: 61–67.

Naylor, C. D., K. Sykora, S. B. Jaglal, S. Jefferson, and the Steering Committee of the Adult Cardiac Care Network of Ontario. 1995. "Waiting for Coronary Artery Bypass Surgery: Population-Based Study of 8517 Consecutive Patients in Ontario, Canada." *The Lancet* 346: 1605–9.

Newhouse, J. P. 1973. "The Economics of Group Practice." *Journal of Human Resources* 8 (1): 37–56.

Organization for Economic Cooperation and Development. 1992. *The Reform of Health Care: A Comparative Analysis of Seven OECD Countries*, Health Policy Series No. 2. Paris, France: OECD.

———. 1995a. *Internal Markets in the Making*, Health Policy Series No. 6. Paris, France: OECD.

———. 1995b. *New Directions in Health Care Policy*, Health Policy Series No. 7. Paris, France: OECD.

———. 1997. *OECD Health Data 1997*. Paris, France: OECD.

Physician Payment Review Commission. 1997. *Annual Report to Congress, 1997*. Washington, D.C.: Physician Payment Review Commission.

Reinhardt, U. E. 1972. "A Production Function for Physician Services." *Review of Economics and Statistics* 54 (1): 55–66.

———. 1975. *Physician Productivity and the Demand for Health Manpower: An Economic Analysis*. Cambridge, MA: Ballinger Publishing Company.

———. 1990. "What Can Americans Learn from Europeans?" *Health Care Systems in Transition: The Search for Efficiency*, Social Policy Series No. 7. Paris, France: OECD.

———. 1996. A Social Contract for the 21st Century Health Care: Three-Tier Health Care With Bounty Hunting. *Health Economics* 5: 479–99.

Robinson, J. C. 1996. "Decline in Hospital Utilization and Cost Inflation Under Managed Care in California." *Journal of the American Medical Association* 276: 1060–1064.

Robinson, R. 1996. "The Impact of the NHS Reforms 1991–1995: A Review of Research Evidence." *Journal of Public Health Medicine* 18: 337–42.

Roos, N. P., C. Black, N. Frohlich, C. DeCoster, M. Cohen, D. J. Tataryn, C. A. Mustard, L. L. Roos, F. Toll, K. C. Carrière, C. A. Burchill, L. MacWilliam, and B. Bogdanovic. 1996. "Population Health and Health Care Use: An Information System for Policy Makers." *Milbank Memorial Fund Quarterly* 74: 3–31.

Rowland, D., S. Rosenbaum, L. Simon, and E. Chait. 1995. *Medicaid and Managed Care: Lessons from the Literature*. Kaiser Commission on the Future of Medicaid.

Russell, L B. 1986. *Is Prevention Better Than Cure?* Washington, D.C: The Brookings Institution.

―――. 1989. *Medicare's New Hospital Payment System: Is It Working?* Washington, D.C.: The Brookings Institution.

Schieber, G. J., and J. P. Poullier. 1990. "Overview of International Comparisons of Health Care Expenditures." *Health Care Systems in Transition: The Search for Efficiency*, Social Policy Series No. 7. Paris, France: OECD.

Schwartz, F. W., and R. Busse. 1996. "Fixed Budgets in the Ambulatory Care Sector: The German Experience." In *Fixing Health Budgets: Experience from Europe and North America.* Edited by F. W. Schwartz, H. Glennerster, and R. B. Saltman, 93–108. Chilchester: John Wiley & Sons.

Schwartz, W. B., and D. N. Mendelson. 1991. "Hospital Cost Containment in the 1980s: Hard Lessons Learned and Prospects for the 1990s." *The New England Journal of Medicine* 324: 1037–42.

Sisk, J. E., S. A. Gorman, A. L. Reisinger, S. A. Glied, W. H. DuMouchel, and M. M. Hynes. 1996. "Evaluation of Medicaid Managed Care: Satisfaction, Access, and Use." *Journal of the American Medical Association* 276: 50–55.

Siu, A. L., F. A. Sonnenberg, W. G. Manning, G. A. Goldberg, E. S. Bloomfield, J. P. Newhouse, and R. H. Brook. 1986. "Inappropriate Use of Hospitals in a Randomized Trial of Health Insurance Plans." *The New England Journal of Medicine* 315: 1259–66.

Smith, K. R., M. Miller, and F. L. Golladay. 1972. "An Analysis of the Optimal Use of Inputs in the Production of Medical Services." *Journal of Human Resources* 7: 208–55.

Street, A. 1994. "Purchaser/Provider Separation and Managed Competition: Reform Options for Australia's Health System." *Australian Journal of Public Health* 18: 369–79.

Swint, J. M. 1990. *International Summit on the Economic Impact of Health Care Systems*, Houston: Health Policy Institute, University of Texas Health Science Center.

Tengs, T. O., M. E. Adams, J. S. Pliskin, D. G. Safran, J. E. Siegel, M. C. Weinstein, and J. D. Graham. 1995. "Five Hundred Life-Saving Interventions and Their Cost-Effectiveness." *Risk Analysis* 15: 369–90.

Wickizer, T. M., and P. J. Feldstein. 1995. "The Impact of HMO Competition On Private Health Insurance Premiums, 1985–1992." *Inquiry* 32: 241–51.

Williams, A. H. 1990. "Ethics, Clinical Freedom and the Doctor's Role." In *Competition in Health Care: Reforming the NHS.* Edited by A. J. Culyer, A. K. Maynard, and J. W. Posnett, 178–91. London: Macmillan Press.

Woolhandler, S., and D. U. Himmelstein. 1991. "The Deteriorating Administrative Efficiency of the U.S. Health Care System." *The New England Journal of Medicine* 324: 1253–58.

———. 1997. "Costs of Care and Administration at For-Profit and Other Hospitals in the United States." *The New England Journal of Medicine* 336: 769–74.

Zwanziger, J., and G. A. Melnick. 1996. "Can Managed Care Plans Control Health Care Costs?" *Health Affairs* 15 (2): 185–99.

Chapter 6

Equity: Concepts and Methods

Overview

The fundamental questions posed in this chapter are (1) What is equity? and (2) How should equity in healthcare be assessed? Chapter 7 asks (3) To what extent has equity been achieved?

With the failure of universal health insurance reform in the United States and the emerging dominance of managed care in the medical care market place, concerns with equity have surfaced along an array of dimensions. A growing number of Americans are uninsured. Both public and private managed care plans often seek to exclude particularly high-risk groups. Policies and procedures, such as mandatory enrollment or "gag rules" regarding what providers are allowed to tell patients, are put into place in both the public and private sectors with little or no input from those most affected by them. Traditional safety net providers in many communities face financial instability and risks of closure. Health and healthcare inequalities persist in areas ravaged by social, economic, and healthcare disinvestment.

A variety of approaches have been developed and applied in health services research and policy analysis to assess equity. They have focused primarily on potential or realized barriers to access to medical care; the extent to which subgroup variations exist in the utilization of medical care services relative to need; and the conceptual foundations of distributive justice and associated individual rights required to assure equity (Aday and Andersen 1981; Aday et al. 1993).

These conventional conceptualizations have, however, failed to encompass the weight of the empirical evidence regarding the limited role of medical care relative to other inputs or sectors for improving health, and the corollary concerns with the common good and health of populations and communities. They have also failed to acknowledge or accommodate emerging philosophical criticisms of the distributive justice and associated individual rights framework as a basis for judgments of equity, as well as criticisms of the fairness of the deliberative processes and procedures in policy debates on the allocation of public and private resources.

An implicit assumption underlying the perspective on equity presented here is that the conventional lenses for viewing equity have failed to penetrate the origins of, or envision other promising remedies for, the persistent health and healthcare inequalities that plague our national conscience. An explicit aim is to provide a broader and deeper vision of the foundations of fairness undergirding the formulation and evaluation of health policy. New and innovative paradigms, or defining frameworks, of justice and their implications for conceptualizing and measuring equity will be presented to address the questions posed at the beginning of this chapter: what is equity, and how should equity in healthcare be assessed? The chapter that follows addresses the question: to what extent has equity been achieved?

Conceptual Framework and Definitions

Contrasting Paradigms of Justice

Three primary philosophical traditions that have focused primarily on individuals, institutions, or the community in judging justice may be used to illuminate the correlates and indicators of equity in health and healthcare (see Table 6.1) (Daly 1994; Habermas 1996; Mulhall and Swift 1992):

Table 6.1   Contrasting Paradigms of Justice

Focus	Individuals	Institutions	Community
Theory	**Liberalism** Personal well-being Individual freedom	**Deliberative Democracy** Public governance Popular sovereignty	**Communitarianism** Common good Social solidarity
Policies	**Minimalist State** Individual rights	**Responsive State** Civic participation	**Responsible State** Public welfare
Paradigms	**Distributive Justice** What can I justly claim?	**Deliberative Justice** Who decides and how?	**Social Justice** What's good for us?

The distinctions between the individual and community perspectives are most deeply lodged in the debate between liberal and communitarian values. The liberal political tradition focuses on the norms of personal well-being and individual freedom. Policies grounded in this tradition have been concerned with protecting or assuring individual rights, and its underlying *distributive justice* paradigm. Rights are those benefits to which one has a claim, based on assessing what might be a fair distribution of benefits and burdens. This encompasses a consideration of both negative and positive rights—that is, noninterference and freedom of choice, as well as a positive conferring of specific material or nonmaterial benefits. The question of equity posed from this point of view is, What can I justly claim?

This framework has often guided policy debates regarding universal health insurance, Medicaid and Medicare reform, and the impact of immigration and welfare reform on the most vulnerable (Chapman 1994). The rising costs of medical care, the failure of universal healthcare reform at the national level, and the growing dominance of managed care in both the public and private sectors have raised significant questions regarding to whom and to what extent benefits of coverage might be extended, as well as how corresponding costs should be allocated. Increasing emphasis is being placed on consumer choice, personal responsibility, experience rating, actuarial fairness, and free riders. The answer to the question "What can I justly claim?" is more and more sharply focused on the attributes and actions of the I.

Communitarian sentiments are based on norms of the common good, social solidarity, and protection of the public welfare. The concept of justice on which this perspective is based is concerned with the underlying social, economic, and environmental underpinnings of inequity. Rather than focusing on conferring or assuring positive or negative rights or benefits to individuals, this paradigm encompasses a broader consideration of public health and the social and economic interventions required to enhance the well-being of groups or communities as a whole. The essential question of justice posed from this perspective is, What's good for us?

The *social justice* paradigm is reflected in traditional public health policy and practice, with its emphasis on the public welfare and the use of medical police power (e.g., public health regulations, inspections, quarantines, etc.) to protect the population's health (Beauchamp 1985, 1988). Critics have argued, however, that public health planning and practice have focused less on what communities may view as good for them, and more on what public health professionals determine communities need, based on agency or administratively driven data-gathering or needs-assessment activities (Kretzman and McKnight 1993; Labonte 1993, 1994; Rissel 1994; Robertson and Minkler 1994; Wallerstein and Bernstein 1994). In many communities the consequence is that the social, economic, and environmental issues that determine the health of the public are not adequately addressed, and the capacities of affected populations to ameliorate them are untapped or, at worst, undermined.

These criticisms of the distributive justice paradigm as applied to medical care and the social justice model underlying public health mirror the array of criticisms that have been raised about liberal and communitarian theories (Daly 1994; Habermas 1996; Mulhall and Swift 1992). The dominance of the liberal paradigm in shaping health and social policy in the United States has, it is argued, served to weaken communal sentiments, such as civility and reciprocity; sacrificed considerations of the public good to serve private interests; promoted self-centeredness; and blamed the victim for circumstances that likely were created by society or others. On the other hand, communitarianism is charged with weakening private autonomy, or the ability of the public to make rational, informed choices, due to the increasing bureaucratization of public institutions and attendant shift of individuals served by these institutions into the role of dependent clients.

Contemporary social theorists, most notably German philosopher Jürgen Habermas, have addressed the weaknesses of the liberal and communitarian traditions by arguing for a new synthesis for the foundations for fairness, based on a theory of deliberative democracy. Policies attuned to this perspective address the extent to which norms of civic participation appear to guide decision making. The question of justice posed from this point of view is, Who decides and how? The foundation for the enlargement of *deliberative justice* is the growth and promotion of a public sphere of secondary associations, social movements, and an array of civil and political forums for influencing the formal policymaking process. The deliberative justice paradigm recognizes and attempts to resolve conflicts rooted in the other dominant paradigms of fairness through rational discourse on the part of affected groups and individuals. Such discourse is oriented primarily toward mutual understanding. Habermas argues that strategic or technical-rational aims of decision makers at either the macrolevel or microlevel (e.g., implementing a state Medicaid managed care program or achieving patient adherence to therapeutic regimens) are unlikely to be orchestrated and achieved unless affected stakeholders (e.g., providers, patients, and taxpayers) have the opportunity to present and have their points of view heard and respected in the process.

The discussion that follows presents an expanded framework of equity, incorporating elements of the deliberative, distributive, and social justice paradigms, and the relationships implied among them, as a foundation for guiding health services research on the equity of healthcare provision.

An Expanded Conceptual Framework of Equity

Figure 6.1 displays how the conceptual framework for guiding health services research and policy analysis introduced in Chapter 1 might reflect and integrate the deliberative, distributive, and social justice paradigms. The unshaded boxes *without* shadows represent a conceptual model of equity of access to medical care developed by Ronald Andersen, Lu Ann Aday, and their colleagues to guide the conduct of national and community surveys of access; this method is rooted in the distributive justice paradigm (Aday and Andersen 1981; Aday, Andersen, and Fleming 1980). The shaded boxes represent components that are reflective of the broader social justice paradigm, grounded in research on the social-structural factors that influence the health and healthcare needs of vulnerable populations (Aday 1993; Beauchamp 1976). The explicit addition of the equity, effectiveness, and efficiency concepts to the framework, reflected in the unshaded boxes *with* shadows, points out the importance, as well as the interrelationship, of these factors in ultimately influencing the health of individuals and communities.

The original access framework begins with the role of health policy in influencing the characteristics of the health delivery system and the population to be served by it. A new dimension in the expanded model is the deliberative justice character of health policy that focuses on the institutions and procedures through which policy is formulated and implemented. Placing the governing norm of deliberative justice above health policy in the expanded framework is intended to convey that conflicts between the disparate paradigms of distributive justice and social justice that have tended to guide medical care and public health policy, respectively, must be effectively addressed if the health and well-being of individuals and communities are to be enhanced. Assuring that those most affected by health policy decisions at both the macrolevel and microlevel are involved in shaping them constitutes the means for doing so. The deliberative paradigm has not been explicitly explored as a basis for the equity of health policy. It is, however, implicit in the focus on consumer involvement and community participation in the design and implementation of private and public health programs in the United States and other countries (Green 1986; Wallerstein 1992; Wallerstein and Bernstein 1994).

The unshaded, unshadowed boxes in Figure 6.1, encompassing the delivery system, population at risk, and realized access, define the major distributive justice components of the conceptual framework that has guided much of health services research on access to medical care (Aday and Andersen 1981; Aday, Andersen, and Fleming 1980). Relevant characteristics of the health system include the availability, organization, and financing of services. Predisposing characteristics of the population at risk include those that describe the propensity of individuals to use services, including

Figure 6.1   An Expanded Conceptual Framework of Equity

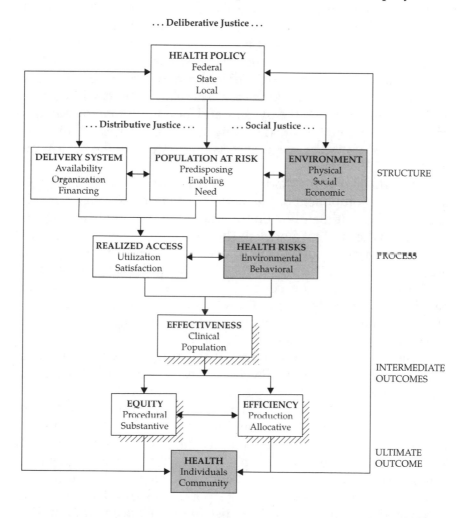

basic demographic characteristics (e.g., age, sex), social structural variables (e.g., race and ethnicity, education, employment status, and occupation), and beliefs (e.g., general beliefs and attitudes about the value of health services, and/or knowledge of disease). Enabling characteristics include the means individuals have available to them for the use of services. Both financial resources, such as family income or insurance coverage, as well as organizational resources, such as having a regular source or place to go for care, specific to the individuals and their families are relevant here. Need refers to health status or illness as a predictor of health service use. The need for care may be perceived by the individual and reflected in reported disability days or symptoms, for example, or may be evaluated by a provider and reflected in actual diagnoses or complaints.

Realized access refers to the objective and subjective indicators of the actual process of seeking care. These are, in effect, indicators of the extent to which the system and population characteristics predict the demand for care (i.e., how much care is used, if any) and how satisfied potential or actual consumers are with the healthcare system.

As indicated by the shaded boxes in Figure 6.1, in the expanded social justice component of the model, there is an explicit acknowledgment of the ultimate outcome of interest that was only implicit or assumed in the original model: the health and well-being of individuals and communities. The model acknowledges that the physical, social, and economic environment in which individuals live and work can also have consequences for their access to health and healthcare. The model also indicates that the environment directly influences the likelihood of exposures to significant environmental and behavioral health risks.

The social justice component of the model may be viewed as focusing on the community level of analysis. It primarily examines the characteristics of the physical, social, and economic environment; the population residing within it; and the health risks the population experiences as a consequence. The distributive justice component of the model relies on individuals as the ultimate unit of analysis. Their attributes and behavior may, however, be aggregated to reflect the characteristics of patients within a given health system or delivery organization or of the population resident within a designated geographic area. The distributive justice paradigm has led to an emphasis on the equity of the medical care delivery system, while the social justice paradigm is reflected in public health and in social and economic policies directly or indirectly related to health.

The goal of health policy, as indicated in the expanded equity framework, is to contribute to improving the health of individuals and communities. The ultimate test of the equity of health policy from the social justice perspective is the extent to which disparities or inequalities in health among subgroups of the population are minimized (Whitehead 1992). Substantive equity is reflected in sub-group disparities in health. Procedural equity refers to the extent to which the structure, process, or procedures intended to reduce these disparities may be judged to be fair, grounded in norms of deliberative, distributive, and social justice. The normative import of these procedural factors for substantive equity can be empirically judged by the extent to which these factors are predictive of inequalities in health across groups and communities. The expanded framework of equity (Figure 6.1) is intended to provide normative and empirical guidance for assessing both substantive and procedural equity.

Based on the synthesis and integration of the theoretical underpinnings of substantive and procedural equity reviewed here, the answer to the first question posed at the beginning of this chapter—what is equity?—may be summarized as follows: equity is concerned with health disparities and the fairness and effectiveness of the procedures for addressing them. The response to the second question—how should equity in healthcare be assessed?—is this: examine and account for health disparities.

The effectiveness of medical and non-medical investments in producing health is essentially an empirical question. The fairness of the means for doing so is a normative one. The expanded framework, however, implies that health policymaking must take into account norms of distributive and social justice, and that conflicts between affected stakeholders grounded in these contrasting norms must be resolved through deliberative discourse if the resultant policies are ultimately to contribute to improving health and minimizing health disparities. Both the effectiveness and equity criteria demand it.

Key Methods of Assessing Equity

Conceptual Frameworks

Conceptual frameworks provide useful analytic guidance for selecting empirical indicators and generating hypotheses about interrelationships between them. The framework Aday, Andersen, and their colleagues developed for the study of access has guided a great deal of research on equity (Aday and Andersen 1981). Integral to that framework is the value judgment that the system would be deemed fair or equitable if need-based criteria, rather than resources such as insurance coverage or income, were the main determinants of the amount of care sought. As indicated earlier (and displayed in Figure 6.1), the developers have continued to extend their framework to encompass social and environmental factors, as well as access to medical care, as factors that ultimately influence health, and to acknowledge the interdependence of the equity, effectiveness, and efficiency norms in assessing the performance of health policies and programs (Aday 1993; Andersen 1995; Andersen and Davidson 1996).

Other frameworks have been developed that are useful in exploring the distributive, social, or deliberative justice paradigms in the context of the growth of managed care. In general, frameworks grounded in the distributive justice paradigm may be seen as primarily turning inward, assessing the fairness of the healthcare system for the patients directly served by the system. Social justice–oriented frameworks direct attention outward to the community to assess the equity of health and health risks of the population who reside within the community. Conceptual approaches to equity influenced by the deliberative justice paradigm attempt to enhance the dialogue between those who design and those who are affected by health policies, in order to develop more effective policies.

Frameworks grounded in these respective paradigms of justice, their relationship to the expanded framework of equity (Figure 6.1), and the defining focus of each will be reviewed in the discussion that follows.

Distributive justice

Docteur, Colby, and Gold (1996) have developed an access framework that identifies a variety of components that are relevant in influencing and assessing access for managed care enrollees. The framework includes the structural, financial, and personal determinants of patients' plan selection; the associated characteristics of the health plan delivery system itself; the influence of these patient and plan characteristics on plan choice and subsequent use of services; the mediators and determinants of the continuity of plan enrollment; and the ultimate clinical and equity outcomes for enrollees and users. This framework then focuses the lens of distributive justice on the availability, organization, and financing of services within a particular delivery system and the utilization and satisfaction of individuals and their families who choose to enroll in it.

Social justice

Aday's (1993) framework for the study of vulnerable populations delineates the social and economic factors determinant of health risks and argues for community and individual levels of analyses in exploring the correlates of vulnerability to poor health. Her perspective argues for the development of a broader continuum of health services, encompassing prevention-oriented services, long-term community-based services, and acute medical care services (displayed in Figure 1.1 in Chapter 1) to address the health and healthcare needs of the most vulnerable. The U.S. Public Health Service and WHO Year 2000 Objectives and accompanying empirical and programmatic emphases also provide guidance for identifying and tracking the indicators and predictors of subgroup disparities in health (NCHS 1995; WHO 1994).

Stephen Shortell, based on his and his colleagues' research on organized, or integrated, healthcare delivery systems, has argued convincingly for the importance of a population health–oriented perspective in designing and assessing these systems. Health services research has documented the evolution and adoption of this perspective as managed care markets mature and extend further into the communities they serve (Shortell, Gillies, and Anderson 1994; Shortell et al. 1996). A focus on the health of populations and the integrated array of programs and services needed to address the health needs of the most vulnerable provides conceptual and analytic guidance for assessing the extent to which the health of communities as a whole is enhanced in the evolving managed care environment. (These issues are discussed in the context of the criteria for assessing the effectiveness of healthcare in Chapter 3.)

Deliberative justice

Community participation and empowerment have ostensibly been central components of the design of social and health programs in the United States as well as in other countries. The extent to which individuals affected by these initiatives have been fully involved in shaping them, however, has often been less than fully realized in practice. Rissel (1994), Robertson and Minkler (1994), and Wallerstein and Bernstein (1994), for example, documented that public health and health promotion professionals have often imposed interventions they deem necessary on selected target communities or populations without either soliciting or fully taking into account the wants of the affected groups and individuals. Program developers may claim that communities have been involved in shaping such interventions when in fact there has been little or only token participation on the part of affected groups.

Habermas's discourse theory provides a template for examining the nature of these exchanges and the aims and actions of the institutional and individual actors involved in them. For Habermas, communication directed toward a mutual understanding between affected parties can best establish the foundations of trust and collaboration needed for solving their common problems despite their potentially different points of view (Habermas 1995, 1996). Opportunities for analyzing the form and quality of participation may range from the microcosm of the patient-physician relationship, to the design of consumer-oriented healthcare programs and neighborhood services or community-wide needs assessment and program development efforts, to broader social change–oriented movements that have important impacts on the health of individuals and communities (e.g., environmental justice, AIDS advocacy, etc.) (Charles and DeMaio 1993; Labonte 1993, 1994; Waitzkin, Britt, and Williams 1994). The fairness of healthcare programs and policies may be judged by the extent to which affected parties are involved in shaping them, assessed through qualitative interviews or more structured quantitative scales of participation to key informants. (Some of these approaches will be discussed later in this chapter in reviewing selected empirical indicators of equity.)

The discussion that follows reviews how the dimensions of equity reflected in these respective frameworks would be operationalized in the conduct of health services research to assess the extent to which equity has been achieved.

Criteria and Indicators of Equity

Table 6.2 summarizes empirical indicators of equity in relationship to the primary dimensions of the expanded equity framework (Figure 6.1) and to the related criteria of justice underlying them. Data may be gathered to descriptively assess dimensions of procedural and substantive equity, as well as to conduct analytic or evaluative research, exploring those factors which are most predictive of the persistent substantive inequities mirrored in subgroup variations in health. The ultimate test of equity is the extent to which these disparities are minimized. The challenge to analytic and evaluative public health and health services research is determining how best to design studies and gather data to assess the factors most likely to influence this endpoint and the health policy interventions suggested as a consequence. Later in this chapter and in Chapter 7, the methods and empirical evidence for assessing the extent to which these criteria have been realized and their import for reducing health disparities will be presented.

Health policy

Criterion: participation.   Habermas's discourse theory is most directly concerned with the extent to which those likely to be affected by decisions participate in shaping them (Habermas 1996). The defining normative underpinning for Habermas's theory is grounded in his discourse principle: "Only those norms are valid to which all affected persons could agree as participants in rational discourse(s)" (Habermas 1996, xxvi). "Rational discourse" in this case refers to communication directed toward mutual understanding, rather than strictly ends-oriented communication directed toward instrumental (i.e., technical-rational or strategic) aims. Habermas's discourse principle is grounded in fundamental democratic ideals, in which the power to govern is ultimately vested in the people and exercised by them directly or indirectly through a system of representation, involvement in a public political sphere, and free elections. The discourse principle characterizes policy or development activities that are oriented toward gaining a reasonable consensus about the definition of the problem and the best possible ways to

Table 6.2   Criteria and Indicators of Equity

Dimensions	Criteria	Indicators
PROCEDURAL EQUITY		
Deliberative Justice		
Health Policy	Participation	Type and extent of affected groups' participation in formulating and implementing policies and programs
Distributive Justice		
Delivery System	Freedom of choice	
• Availability		Distribution of providers
• Organization		Types of facilities
• Financing		Sources of payment
Realized Access	Cost-effectiveness	
• Utilization		Type and volume of services used
• Satisfaction		Public opinion, patient opinion
Distributive & Social Justice		
Population at Risk	Similar treatment	
• Predisposing		Age, sex, race, education, etc.
• Enabling		Regular source, insurance coverage, income, etc.
• Need		Perceived, evaluated
Social Justice		
Environment	Common good	
• Physical		Toxic, environmental hazards
• Social		Social capital (family structure, voluntary organizations, social networks)
• Economic		Human and material capital (schools, jobs, income, housing)
Health Risks	Need	
• Environmental		Toxic, environmental exposures
• Behavioral		Lifestyle, health promotion practices
SUBSTANTIVE EQUITY		
Health	Need	
• Individuals		Clinical indicators
• Community		Population rates

address it on the part of the stakeholders most likely to be affected by the resulting policy. Communication grounded in mutual respect between stakeholders is essential to assuring the realization of this principle in the formulation of policy at the microlevel or macrolevel. For Habermas, the foundations of trust and collaboration required to be successful in addressing more instrumental aims are established through such "communicatively rational" discourse. These norms of deliberative justice would be attended to at the microlevel in forging effective patient-physician relationships, in shaping culturally sensitive service provision at the institutional level, and in assuring the full participation of affected populations in the design of health policies and programs at the system and community levels.

This philosophical and programmatic thrust, as well as the parallel participatory action research agenda, developed in the writings of Brazilian social activist Paulo Freire (1970), are intended to encourage researchers and policymakers to more fully listen to and learn from communities. Communication with and the involvement of affected parties in the design and implementation of programs are seen as essential. This emphasis acknowledges that by giving voice to concerns in their own syntax and semantics, affected parties learn together how best to address their concerns. This perspective is manifest in the formulation and implementation of community-based health education and health promotion initiatives (Wallerstein 1992; Wallerstein and Bernstein 1994).

Norman Daniels (1996, 10) has argued for incorporating the norms of "deliberative democracy" in developing managed care policies and procedures. By that, he means that participation on the part of affected parties (e.g., patients and providers) must be assured in decision making regarding the protection of normal functioning of a given population within defined constraints (e.g., limited resources). This perspective would, for example, oppose the "gag rule" that inhibits physicians providing full information to patients about their treatment options; make explicit the rationale for decisions about covering new technologies and provide an opportunity for public discussion of this rationale; and streamline and make less adversarial patient grievance and dispute resolution procedures.

Indicators: participation.   Empirical indicators of deliberative justice attempt to express the type and extent of involvement of affected groups' participation in formulating and implementing policies and programs. Arnstein (1969) conceptualized a ladder of citizen participation, with each respective rung representing a gradient ranging from nonparticipation to tokenism to increased levels of citizen power and control. Charles and DeMaio (1993) incorporated this and other dimensions reflecting the perspective being adopted (i.e., that of a user versus a policymaker) and the decision making domain (i.e., individual treatment, overall service provision, or macro policy formulation) in constructing a framework for assessing lay participation in healthcare decision making. Promoting lay participation and empowerment has been a particular focus of health education and health promotion activities in the United States, Canada, and other countries (Green 1986; Labonte 1993, 1994; Robertson and Minkler 1994). Related indicators with particular relevance in the managed care context focus on the nature and quality of communication between patients and providers, the extent to which norms of "deliberative democracy" guide the development of organizational policies and procedures, and the magnitude of trust healthcare consumers have for providers or organizations (Daniels 1996; Mechanic 1996; Waitzkin, Britt, and Williams 1994).

Delivery system

Criterion: freedom of choice.   The freedom-of-choice norm emphasizes the importance of personal autonomy in determining who receives what care. This criterion conforms most closely to Nozick's libertarian theory of justice, which emphasizes that equity is rooted in the freedom to possess and use one's property and resources as one chooses (Nozick 1974). People are entitled to what they have as long as they acquire or transfer it through just means—that is, through their own labor or as a result of a gift, an inheritance, or a voluntary exchange with others. Further, the state should not interfere with or attempt to regulate these transactions. Instead, the "invisible hand" governing the free marketplace should be allowed to operate unhindered. The only appropriate intrusions would be made to correct situations in which there is clear historical evidence that the property or resources some people possess were not acquired through just means. Such evidence is often difficult to assemble or document, however. This perspective endorses policies that maximize consumer preferences (i.e., choice and satisfaction) in the medical care marketplace. Proponents of this approach endorse the operation of market-based forces of supply and demand for the allocation of healthcare.

Indicators: freedom of choice.   Empirical indicators of access based on the freedom-of-choice norm are the distribution and availability of healthcare resources to consumers. For example, personnel- (e.g., primary care physicians or specialists) and facility- (e.g., hospitals or hospital beds) to-population ratios and related inventories of healthcare personnel or providers (e.g., HMOs, PPOs) in a given target, or market, area are indicators of the basic supply of providers and delivery sites available to consumers.

Lists of preferred providers affiliated with employer-sponsored health insurance plans also effectively define the range of enrollees' choices for a regular source of medical care. Other indicators of the extent to which patients' decisions may be constrained include data on the hours of clinic operation and provider availability at night, on weekends, or in emergencies; the average distance to the nearest medical facility and the available modes of transportation for getting there; and the average time it takes to get an appointment, as well as the waiting time to see a physician or other provider once on site.

Characteristics of the system of financing in an area—such as the type and scope of benefits provided by major employers, and the local public or private arrangements for people who have no third-party coverage—also dictate the options consumers can realistically afford. Substantial cost-sharing provisions or uncovered healthcare expenses also can result in decisions to forgo goals or sacrifice personal resources intended for other uses—such as an elderly woman using her and her husband's life savings (or "spending down"), so he can qualify for nursing home coverage under Medicaid.

Realized access

Criterion: cost-effectiveness.   Utilitarians advocate access to those services for which the measured benefits (e.g., in terms of health, well-being, or productivity) would be maximized relative to the costs necessary to provide them (Culyer 1992). Utilitarian theory has its origins in the writings of David Hume, Jeremy Bentham, and John Stuart Mill (Dougherty 1988). It is principally consequentialist or ends-oriented. The value of any decision or action is judged by its consequences; the principal goal is to maximize utility or individual preferences. Based on the utilitarian theory of judging the rightness or wrongness of actions by the balance of benefits and burdens produced, CEAs, CBAs, and associated CUAs (discussed in Chapter 4) have become an increasing focus in weighing the types of programs that should be funded and the categories of services to be covered under public or private insurance schemes, and in determining whether the services actually being used are appropriate, effective, and satisfactory to consumers.

Indicators: cost-effectiveness. Components of the costs and benefits of care are reflected in the type and comprehensiveness of services received and the level of patient satisfaction relative to some standard. The Institute of Medicine Committee on Monitoring Access to Personal Health Care Services, for example, developed a set of indicators of services likely to have beneficial health consequences if used—including an array of preventive services (e.g., prenatal care, immunizations, or breast cancer screening), as well as timely and appropriate care for acute or chronic illness (Institute of Medicine 1993). The U.S. Public Health Service Year 2000 Objectives for the Nation also encompass a series of goals regarding the use of preventive services (NCHS 1995). These provide foundations for systems of monitoring the extent to which these services are received. A variety of scales for measuring satisfaction with medical care, physicians, and hospitals have been employed extensively in developing report cards or other reports on provider performance (Gold and Wooldridge 1995). These scales and the standardized reporting systems being developed offer an opportunity to assess the extent to which effective care has been rendered from the point of view of patients or the general public.

Population at risk

Criterion: similar treatment. The similar treatment criterion emphasizes that age, sex, race, income, or type or amount of insurance coverage should not dictate that people with similar needs enter different doors (e.g., private physicians' offices versus hospital emergency rooms) or be treated differently in terms of the type or intensity of services provided. This criterion is a defining tenet of the egalitarian concept of justice. From an egalitarian point of view, the perspective that all individuals are of equal worth and should be treated equally is of primary importance. As Robert Veatch (1981) pointed out, egalitarianism may focus on either procedural or substantive equality (i.e., similarity in treatment or outcome, respectively). Procedural equality assures equal opportunity for every individual to obtain care, regardless of personal characteristics, such as age, gender, race, income, type of coverage, or whether one lives in the city or suburbs. Substantive equality emphasizes minimizing the health status differentials or variations between groups, such as disparities in infant mortality between black and white populations. Considerations of equity from an egalitarian point of view focus on how to narrow or eliminate these disparities in health and medical care.

Egalitarian norms have also been central to the social justice paradigm in the context of examining varying exposures to health risks as a function of environmental, social, or economic conditions. Research on environmental justice has, for example, documented that toxic and hazardous waste sites are more likely to be located in racially segregated or socioeconomically disadvantaged neighborhoods (Brown 1995; Bullard 1994).

Indicators: similar treatment. The similar treatment norm attempts to evaluate intergroup differences that may indicate inequalities in health or access to care. The convenience and characteristics of the places people go for medical care provide data on whether there is differential treatment of individuals in these different settings. Non-medically motivated transfers of patients, or "dumping," principally as a function of fiscal rather than physical diagnostics, or so-called "wallet biopsies," are indicative of inequity under the similar treatment norm. Certain institutions or providers assuming a disproportionate burden of uncompensated care for the medically indigent population calls into question whether they are assuming more than their fair share from an egalitarian point of view. Health inequalities and the factors that give rise to them also surface as issues under the similar treatment norm. To the extent that differential exposures or access to resources for obtaining services give rise to these inequalities, they would be judged to be inequitable from this perspective (Musgrove 1986; Whitehead 1992).

Environment

Criterion: common good.   The concept of the common good is grounded in communitarian theory and focuses on the community as the unit of analysis (Daly 1994; Mulhall and Swift 1992). The primary normative referents are the well-being, or welfare, of communities and the criteria of social solidarity, or unity, and the common good. These norms find expression in more universal modes of financing medical care; in traditional public health policy and practice, with its emphasis on promoting and protecting the health of the public; and in investments in the array of institutions and resources such as families, schools, businesses, and government that are essential for maintaining the health and vitality of communities as a whole. The role of interventions is not on altering individual actions and motivations, but on the distal, foundational roots of health problems, such as the social-structural correlates of health and healthcare inequalities rooted in the physical, social, and economic environments in which individuals live and work. Health risks in the physical environment include toxic and environmental contaminants transmitted through the air, soil, or water in a given neighborhood or community. The social environment encompasses a look at the social resources, or social capital, that may be available to individuals, associated with the family structure, voluntary organizations, and social networks that both bind and support them. The economic environment encompasses both human and material capital resources, reflected in the schools, jobs, income, and housing that characterize the community (Aday 1993).

Indicators: common good.   Empirical indicators related to the common good encompass a look at the array of social status, social capital, and human and material capital resources available to the population-at-risk in a given area, as well as the significant physical environmental exposures that are likely to exist. Assuring health protection is one of the U.S. Public Health Service Year 2000 Objectives for the Nation, which is measured by a series of environmentally-related health indicators (e.g., unintentional injuries, occupational safety and health, environmental health, food and drug safety) (NCHS 1995). The WHO Year 2000 Health for All sets forth indicators for tracking the social, economic, and physical environments and their influence on health (WHO 1994).

Health risks and health

Criterion: need.   Norman Daniels's needs-based theory of justice points out the factors that are necessary to address minimal human needs for "normal species functioning" (Daniels 1985). Health policy initiatives are justified in terms of their role in assuring that there is a fair equality of opportunity for living a normal life. This perspective prompts consideration of what such needs might be, and of the basic decent minimum set of services that should be provided to meet them. Daniels suggests the following for consideration: adequate nutrition and shelter; sanitary, safe, unpolluted living and working conditions; exercise, rest, and other features of a healthy lifestyle; preventive, curative, and rehabilitative personal medical services; and non-medical personal and social support services. The basis for deciding what goods and services might be included and how they could be fairly distributed remains controversial, however.

John Rawls's contractarian theory is based on an argument regarding what reasonable people would decide if they were asked to come together to derive a fair set of criteria for distributing societal goods, operating under the hypothetical assumption that they could by chance be in any position in a society in which such criteria would be applied—including the least socially or economically advantaged (Rawls 1971). Rawls reasoned that under these circumstances, the following criteria would be endorsed, in order of importance: (1) maximize everyone's rights to liberties compatible with a similar system of liberty for everyone; (2) assure fair equality of opportunity for people with similar abilities and skills; and (3) make sure that those who are the worst off benefit. The first two criteria have a strong egalitarian orientation, and the third emphasizes that if any group "counts" more than another, it is those who are worst off, financially or otherwise. This perspective focuses on those least able to buy care or be cured.

Daniels's needs-based theory, as well as the difference criterion recognizing the needs of the least well-off within contractarian theory, lend support to a primary focus on meeting basic needs. Assessing who needs care may be both difficult and expensive (Braybrooke 1987). Economic theory argues that expressed demand is the most rational basis for allocating scarce medical care resources. Needs may, in fact, be quite subjective and ungovernable, unless constrained by some sense that people are willing to pay to have their tastes and preferences satisfied. Further, societal or professional consensus may be required to determine which needs to meet when resources are limited. Needs assessments have been an important component of public health–oriented planning and program development activities at the community level. Contemporary needs assessments focus on inventorying the assets, as well as the problems, that exist in the target communities of concern (Kretzmann and McKnight 1993).

Indicators: need.   Indicators of equity from the perspective of need attempt to assess the magnitude of health risks and health disparities in a population. Sometimes survey respondents are asked questions to obtain their subjective perceptions of the extent to which their needs have been met: "During the past year, did you or a family member need to see a doctor but not see one for some reason? If so, why?" Other indicators of need summarize respondents' objective reports of the number of physician visits relative to the number of disability days they experienced in the year (i.e., the use-disability ratio) or compare the number of people who actually contacted a physician for a set of symptoms with the number of people that a panel of physicians thought should have seen one (i.e., the symptoms-response ratio) (Aday, Andersen, and Fleming 1980).

The social justice perspective on substantive equity, based in the need criterion, is concerned with subgroup variations in health. The primary goals of the U.S. Public Health Service Year 2000 Objectives for the Nation include increasing the span of healthy life for all Americans, as well as reducing health disparities between and among groups (NCHS 1995). Indicators of mortality, morbidity, and years of potential life lost or quality years of life gained are illustrative of the types of indicators that could be used to trace trends and subgroup variations reflective of the extent to which needs are actually met.

In summary, an array of empirical indicators might be developed and used in assessing the equity of health policy design and implementation. Health services research and policy analysis can assist in the conceptualization and measurement of these indicators, and in determining what factors appear to be most predictive of the ultimate equity outcome of interest—reducing subgroup disparities in health.

Data Sources

As implied in the expanded conceptual framework of equity (Figure 6.1), studies of equity could focus on the delivery system as a whole, particular institutions within it, groups of patients, the communities that are the target of health policy initiatives, or various combinations of these levels and their interrelationships. Further, studies could be carried out at the national, regional, state, or local level. Such studies may entail collecting new, or primary, data, as well as using data collected for other purposes, or secondary data. Both quantitative and qualitative data may be needed to fully capture the array of factors reflected in the expanded framework of equity. The data sources used in health services research conducted at the community, system, institution, and patient levels were summarized in Table 1.1 in Chapter 1. The sources of primary and secondary data that are particularly relevant for examining the various dimensions of equity are reviewed in the discussion that follows.

Community

Environment.   Environmental indicators focus on the community itself or definable geographic areas within it as the unit of analysis. They are explicitly intended to reflect the structural or environmental context in which residents live and work that significantly affects health risks or health. The WHO Healthy Cities and Healthy Communities movement has, for example, identified a range of community-level variables related to air and water quality, housing availability and quality, and economic development that can be used in profiling the health and well-being of communities (U.S. Health Corporation 1994; WHO 1988). These data are available from planning agencies, business censuses, U.S. census data on household characteristics, and local public health environmental surveillance systems. Qualitative studies using participant or nonparticipant observation methods may also be useful for profiling the social and environmental context that may affect the health or healthcare of individuals within a designated neighborhood or ethnic group.

Population. Population-based studies include individuals who do not use a given delivery system or institution as well as those who do. The denominator for population-level analyses represents individuals residing in a designated geographic area. Surveys are particularly useful in measuring the attitudes or barriers that preclude targeted individuals or subgroups from seeking care. A number of large-scale, national surveys have examined access and trends over time for the U.S. population as a whole. These include the Robert Wood Johnson Foundation surveys, the AHCPR National Medical Care Expenditure surveys, and the continuing NCHS National Health Interview Survey. Such surveys are, however, complex and expensive to conduct (Aday 1996). State or local agencies may lack the resources and expertise for conducting such studies. Qualitative or semi-structured interviews and focus groups may also be instructive in profiling the health and healthcare experiences of a population at risk, as well as informing the design or interpretation of more structured surveys of a representative sample of the target population.

Public health population surveillance systems, disease registries, Census or vital statistics data, and synthetic estimates based on national sources are some of the major types of secondary data used in profiling the health and healthcare of a population at the state or local level. Small area estimation procedures make use of data gathered at the national level on utilization rates for certain age, gender, or racial groups to impute what the estimates are likely to be at the state or local level given the age, gender, and racial composition of the state or community (NCHS 1979). Managed care plan enrollment files also provide data on the denominator of individuals residing in a given geographic area who are eligible to use plan services.

System

Descriptors at the system level focus on the availability, organization, and financing of services as aggregate, structural properties.

Secondary data sources are most often used for this type of analysis. The Bureau of Health Professions, within the Health Resources and Services Administration, has, for example, compiled a computerized area resource file that has an array of health and healthcare data by county or metropolitan statistical area. The AMA and the AHA, as well as other provider groups, routinely publish directories, and in some instances have computerized data available on the characteristics and distribution of medical personnel. NCHS collects data on the characteristics and utilization of hospitals, nursing homes, and outpatient medical care practices. HCFA and the Health Insurance Association of America also periodically publish information on the amount and distribution of expenditures by the major public (i.e., Medicare and Medicaid) and private third-party payors. These data sources are particularly useful for describing the delivery system at the national level and, to some extent, at the state level (NCHS 1997).

The Community Tracking Study, conducted by the Center for Studying Health System Change with support from the Robert Wood Johnson Foundation, represents a major data collection and analysis effort, drawing upon site visits, consumer surveys, and secondary data sources to monitor and understand the dimensions and impact of healthcare system change in over 60 randomly selected communities, and a random subset of 12 intensive study sites, throughout the United States (Ginsburg 1996; Kemper et al. 1996).

Public health departments or private providers such as national HMO firms considering entering a market may want either more current or more detailed information on the types of services being provided or the profile of clients seen by facilities in a given area than is available from existing sources. In this case, the interested agencies or organizations could collect primary data based on interviews with key community informants, telephone requests to providers for brochures describing their services, or full-fledged surveys of providers to gather data on the programs and services being offered and the clients being served. The NCQA HEDIS data system provides a profile of the organizational and financing features of participating plans (National Committee for Quality Assurance 1997).

Chapters 4 and 5 reviewed an array of indicators from the OECD and other sources for describing and comparing the healthcare systems in different countries.

Institutions

Secondary data used most often by institutions or organizations for assessing access to a particular facility include enrollment, encounter data, claims, and medical records. Financial records provide an indication of the level of uncompensated or undercompensated care the facility provides, and for what types of patients and services. Other institutional sources, such as clinic logbooks or emergency room referral records, are used in conducting studies of the magnitude and profile of unscheduled walk-in visits and of non-medically motivated transfers within an institution. Surveys might also be conducted of administrators, providers, or patients to provide data on the operation of the institutions relevant to access or availability issues.

Patients

Patient surveys are the major sources of primary data for evaluating access at the institutional level. Patient surveys tap individuals' subjective perceptions of their experiences at a given facility (e.g., how long they had to wait to be seen), which may or may not agree with more objective institutional records or data sources (e.g., average clinic waiting time estimates). These subjective perceptions are, however, more reflective of the extent to which people actually are satisfied and loyal users of a facility than are objective, records-based indicators. A variety of standardized instruments have been developed and utilized for this purpose, such as the NCQA HEDIS, Patient Judgment System, and Press-Ganey satisfaction questionnaires (Aday 1996). Focus groups and ethnographic interviews conducted with patients may also assist in explaining problems providers have encountered in dealing with certain types of patients, or in designing more culturally sensitive or consumer-oriented services.

Patient origin studies use patient address and zip code information to determine the areas from which most patients are drawn. Patient record data could also serve as the basis for generating profiles of the demographic composition (i.e., age, sex, and race) or the major presenting complaints of patients seen at the facility.

A variety of research designs may be employed in assessing equity at the community, institution, and system levels that also focus on different components of the conceptual framework of equity and their interrelationships (Figure 6.1).

Study Designs

Three major types of health services research designs may be drawn upon to define and clarify the objective of equity and how well programs and policies have succeeded in achieving it. These include descriptive, analytic, and evaluative research designs (Aday 1996).

Descriptive

Descriptive research focuses primarily on profiling the discrete indicators of equity. In effect, they reflect data that are collected to operationalize the dimensions represented in the respective boxes in Figure 6.1. (Also see Appendix 7.1.) They can also be used to make normative assessments of procedural or substantive equity, based on the criteria of equity they are deemed to most directly express (Table 6.2). Descriptive analyses may, however, be viewed as essentially identifying the symptoms of a problem. More probing analytic research is required to diagnose the underlying etiology, or origins, of a problem and the likely health and healthcare consequences of the problem.

Analytic

Analytic research is directed toward understanding hypothesized cause and effect relationships between the structure, process, and intermediate outcome components of the model, and ultimately toward the primary outcome of interest—improving the health of individuals and communities. The hypotheses to be explored in such studies are implicit in the arrows between components of the expanded equity framework (Figure 6.1). These studies are useful, for example, in illuminating the impact of policy-relevant variables, such as the type and extent of insurance coverage, on the use of services and associated clinical outcomes.

A particular challenge for public health and health services researchers with respect to future analytic research on the equity objective as defined here is identifying the factors that are most predictive of improved health. Evaluating access to medical care for problems that medical care cannot address does little to prevent or remedy these problems. Analytic research on the correlates and consequences of health and human functioning can help to address questions regarding whether investments in medical care or in other systems or services are the most relevant bases for allocating scarce societal resources.

Evaluative

Evaluative research assesses how well programs and services that have been developed and implemented based on previous descriptive and analytic research have done in achieving a desired equity objective. Evaluative studies rely primarily on experimental or quasi-experimental designs to determine program or policy outcomes. Evaluations of Medicaid and Medicare managed care demonstrations have, for example, provided useful information for assessing the access, quality, and cost impacts of these models for low-income enrollees (Hurley, Freund, and Paul 1993; Langwell and Hadley 1990). Evidence from health services research regarding the equity impact of these innovations will be reviewed in Chapter 7.

Summary and Conclusions

In summary, the answer to the first question posed at the beginning of this chapter—What is equity?—may be summarized as follows: Equity is concerned with health disparities and the fairness and effectiveness of the procedures for addressing them. The response to the second question—How should equity in healthcare be assessed?—is this: Examine and account for health disparities.

This chapter has reviewed major paradigms of justice and their implications for an operational framework for the conduct of health services research on equity. The ultimate dependent variable in that framework and the corollary bottom line for assessing the impact of health policy is the health of individuals and populations (Figure 6.1). The distributive justice paradigm evaluates the characteristics of the system and population that contribute to differentials in the distribution of medical care. The social justice paradigm examines the factors in the social, economic, and physical environment that contribute to disparities in the prevalence of poor health. The deliberative justice paradigm provides the blueprint for the design of more effective health policies at the macrolevel and microlevel by assuring that parties affected by such policies participate in shaping them.

The revised conceptual framework of equity, based on these perspectives, points to more focused, expanded, and explanatory health services research to assess equity. The framework would also be more fully informed by the linkage and integration of concepts and methods from research on effectiveness and efficiency, in addition to equity, in assessing system performance. Health services research would be more focused on improving the health of individuals and communities as the ultimate goal of health policy. The resulting research agenda related to this substantive objective must, of necessity, be grounded in the concepts and methods that underlie the population perspective on enhancing the health of populations and the clinical perspective on improving the outcomes of patients. Health services research would be expanded to encompass broader epidemiological, ecological, and related public health theories, methods, and research questions in understanding the medical and non-medical factors that contribute to health. It would draw upon the studies of allocative efficiency related to what types and what mix of inputs are most likely to be productive of health, and the corollary concerns of production efficiency regarding the most efficient means for producing these inputs. And finally, health services research would be more explanatory in that a greater emphasis would be placed on analytic and evaluative research to generate and explore relevant hypotheses regarding the array of factors, and the relationships between them, that are most likely to contribute to the health of individuals and populations. The conceptual framework of equity presented here (Figure 6.1) is intended to provide guidance for developing this more explanatory and health-centered health services research agenda.

Chapter 7 reviews the available evidence to address the second question posed at the beginning of this chapter: to what extent has procedural and substantive equity in health and healthcare actually been achieved in the United States? The distributive justice paradigm has primarily served to guide health services research on equity. The arguments and evidence presented here are intended to document that norms of deliberative and social justice must also be taken into account if the ultimate health policy goals of improving health and narrowing health disparities are to be achieved.

References

Aday, L. A. 1993. *At Risk in America: The Health and Health Care Needs of Vulnerable Populations in the United States.* San Francisco: Jossey-Bass.
————. 1996. *Designing and Conducting Health Surveys: A Comprehensive Guide.* 2nd ed. San Francisco: Jossey-Bass Publishers.
Aday, L. A., and R. Andersen. 1981. "Equity of Access to Medical Care: A Conceptual and Empirical Overview." *Medical Care* 19 (Supplement): 4–27.
Aday, L. A., R. Andersen, and G. Fleming. 1980. *Health Care in the U.S.: Equitable for Whom?* Beverly Hills, CA: Sage Publications.
Aday, L. A., C. E. Begley, D. R. Lairson, and C. H. Slater. 1993. *Evaluating the Medical Care System: Effectiveness, Efficiency, and Equity.* 1st ed. Chicago: Health Administration Press.
Andersen, R. M. 1995. "Revisiting the Behavioral Model and Access to Medical Care: Does It Matter?" *Journal of Health and Social Behavior* 36: 1–10.
Andersen, R. M., and P. L. Davidson. 1996. "Measuring Access and Trends." In *Changing the U.S. Health Care System: Key Issues in Health Services, Policy, and Management.* Edited by R. M. Andersen, T. H. Rice, and G. F. Kominski, 13–40. San Francisco: Jossey-Bass.
Arnstein, S. 1969. "A Ladder of Citizen Participation." *Journal of the American Institute of Planners* 35 (July): 216–24.
Beauchamp, D. E. 1976. "Public Health As Social Justice." *Inquiry* 13: 3–14.
————. 1985. "Community: The Neglected Tradition of Public Health." *Hastings Center Report* 15 (6): 28–36.
————. 1988. *The Health of the Republic: Epidemics, Medicine, and Moralism As Challenges to Democracy.* Philadelphia: Temple University Press.
Braybrooke, D. 1987. *Meeting Needs.* Princeton, NJ: Princeton University Press.
Brown, P. 1995. "Race, Class, and Environmental Health: A Review and Systematization of the Literature." *Environmental Research* 69: 15–30.
Bullard, R. D. 1994. *"Dumping in Dixie: Race, Class, and Environmental Quality."* 2nd ed. Boulder, CO: Westview Press.
Chapman, A. R. (ed.). 1994. *Health Care Reform: A Human Rights Approach.* Washington, D.C.: Georgetown University Press.

Charles, C., and S. DeMaio. 1993. "Lay Participation in Health Care Decision Making: A Conceptual Framework." *Journal of Health Politics, Policy and Law* 18: 881–904.

Culyer, A. J. 1992. "The Morality of Efficiency in Health Care: Some Uncomfortable Implications." *Health Economics* 1: 7–18.

Daly, M. (ed.). 1994. *Communitarianism: A New Public Ethics.* Belmont, CA: Wadsworth Publishing Company.

Daniels, N. 1985. *Just Health Care.* Cambridge: Cambridge University Press.

———. 1996. "Justice, Fair Procedures, and the Goals of Medicine." *Hastings Center Report* 26 (6): 10–12.

Docteur, E. R., D. C. Colby, and M. Gold. 1996. "Shifting the Paradigm: Monitoring Access in Medicare Managed Care." *Health Care Financing Review* 17 (4): 5–21.

Dougherty, C. 1988. *American Health Care: Realities, Rights, and Reforms.* New York: Oxford University Press.

Freire, P. 1970. *Pedagogy of the Oppressed.* Translated by M. B. Ramos. New York: The Seabury Press.

Ginsburg, P. B. 1996. "The RWJF Community Snapshots Study: Introduction and Overview." *Health Affairs* 15 (2): 7–19.

Gold, M., and J. Wooldridge. 1995. "Plan-Based Surveys of Satisfaction with Access and Quality of Care: Review and Critique." In *Consumer Survey Information in a Reforming Health Care System.* Agency for Health Care Policy and Research, 75–109. Report No. AHCPR Pub. No. 95-0083. Rockville, MD: Agency for Health Care Policy and Research.

Green, L. W. 1986. "The Theory of Participation: A Qualitative Analysis of Its Expression in National and International Health Policies." In *Advances in Health Education and Promotion.* Edited by W. B. Ward, Z. T. Salisbury, S. B. Kar, and J. G. Zapka, 215–40. Vol. 1, Part A. Greenwich, CT: JAI Press.

Habermas, J. 1995. *Moral Consciousness and Communicative Action.* Translated by C. Lenhardt, and S. W. Nicholsen. Cambridge, MA: The MIT Press.

———. 1996. *Between Facts and Norms: Contributions to a Discourse Theory of Law and Democracy.* Translated by W. Rehg. Cambridge, MA: The MIT Press.

Hurley, R. E., D. A. Freund, and J. E. Paul. 1993. *Managed Care in Medicaid: Lessons for Policy and Program Design.* Chicago: Health Administration Press.

Institute of Medicine. 1993. *Access to Health Care in America.* Edited by M. Millman. Washington, D.C.: National Academy Press.

Kemper, P., D. Blumenthal, J. M. Corrigan, P. J. Cunningham, S. M. Felt,

J. M. Grossman, L. T. Kohn, C. E. Metcalf, R. F. St. Peter, R. C. Strouse, and P. B. Ginsburg. 1996. "The Design of the Community Tracking Study: A Longitudinal Study of Health System Change and Its Effects on People." *Inquiry* 33: 195–206.

Kretzmann, J. P., and J. L. McKnight. 1993. *Building Communities from the Inside Out: A Path Toward Finding and Mobilizing a Community's Assets.* Chicago: ACTA Publications.

Labonte, R. 1993. "Community Development and Partnerships." *Canadian Journal of Public Health* 84: 237–40.

———. 1994. "Health Promotion and Empowerment: Reflections on Professional Practice." *Health Education Quarterly* 21: 253–68.

Langwell, K. M., and J. P. Hadley. 1990. "Insights from the Medicare HMO Demonstrations." *Health Affairs* 9 (1): 74–84.

Mechanic, D. 1996. "Changing Medical Organization and the Erosion of Trust." *Milbank Quarterly* 74: 171–89.

Mulhall, S., and A. Swift. 1992. *Liberals and Communitarians.* Oxford, U.K.: Blackwell.

Musgrove, P. 1986. "Measurement of Equity in Health." *World Health Statistics Quarterly* 39: 325–35.

National Center for Health Statistics. 1979. *Small Area Estimation: An Empirical Comparison of Conventional and Synthetic Estimators for States*, Report No. DHEW Publication No. [PHS] 80–1356. Vital and Health Statistics Series 2, No. 82. Washington, D.C.: U.S. Government Printing Office.

———. 1995. *Healthy People 2000-Midcourse Review and 1995 Revisions.* Hyattsville, MD: Public Health Service.

———. 1997. *Health, United States, 1996–97, and Injury Chartbook.* Hyattsville, MD: Public Health Service.

National Committee for Quality Assurance. 1997. HEDIS / Report Cards [Online]. Available: http://www.ncqa.org/hedis/ [01/24/97].

Nozick, R. 1974. *Anarchy, State, and Utopia.* New York: Basic Books.

Rawls, J. 1971. *A Theory of Justice.* Cambridge, MA: Harvard University Press.

Rissel, C. 1994. "Empowerment: The Holy Grail of Health Promotion?" *Health Promotion International* 9: 39–47.

Robertson, A., and M. Minkler. 1994. "New Health Promotion Movement: A Critical Examination." *Health Education Quarterly* 21: 295–312.

Shortell, S. M., R. R. Gillies, and D. A. Anderson. 1994. "The New World of Managed Care: Creating Organized Delivery Systems." *Health Affairs* 13 (5): 46–64.

Shortell, S. M., R. R. Gillies, D. A. Anderson, K. M. Erickson, and J. B. Mitchell. 1996. *Remaking Health Care in America: Building Organized Delivery Systems.* San Francisco: Jossey-Bass.

U.S. Health Corporation. 1994. *U.S. Health Corporation's Healthy Community Initiative: The Healthy Community Assessment Process.* Columbus, OH: U.S. Health Corporation.

Veatch, R. 1981. *A Theory of Medical Ethics.* New York: Basic Books.

Waitzkin, H., T. Britt, and C. Williams. 1994. "Narratives of Aging and Social Problems in Medical Encounters with Older Persons." *Journal of Health and Social Behavior* 35: 322–48.

Wallerstein, N. 1992. "Powerlessness, Empowerment, and Health: Implications for Health Promotion Programs." *American Journal of Health Promotion* 6: 197–205.

Wallerstein, N., and E. Bernstein. 1994. "Introduction to Community Empowerment, Participatory Education, and Health." *Health Education Quarterly* 21: 141 48.

Whitehead, M. 1992. "The Concepts and Principles of Equity and Health." *International Journal of Health Services* 22: 429–45.

World Health Organization. 1994. *WHO Progress Towards Health for All: Statistics of Member States 1994.* Albany, NY: WHO Publications Office.

World Health Organization Healthy Cities Project. 1988. *A Guide to Assessing Healthy Cities: WHO Healthy Cities Paper No. 3.* Copenhagen: FADL.

Chapter 7

Equity: Policy Strategies, Evidence, Criteria, and an Application

This chapter highlights alternative policy strategies for enhancing the equity of healthcare grounded in the expanded conceptual framework of equity introduced in the previous chapter (Figure 6.1), assembles empirical evidence to address the question regarding the extent to which the goal of equity has been achieved in the United States, and reviews how Medicaid managed care is performing with respect to this objective. Findings from health services and public health research are presented regarding the correlates and indicators of equity based on the distributive, deliberative, and social justice paradigms. The criteria for assessing health policy in terms of the equity objective are delineated and applied in this chapter in the context of examining the dimensions of Medicaid managed care, and Chapter 9 applies them to selected state healthcare reform alternatives.

Policy Strategies Relating to Equity

Three primary policy goals may be identified as the focus of strategies for enhancing the equity of healthcare provision that are lodged in the distributive, social, and deliberative justice paradigms respectively: (1) enhance access to medical care; (2) reduce health disparities; and (3) assure affected parties' participation in policy and program design.

The distributive justice paradigm and its attendant concern with assuring equity of access to medical care have tended to dominate equity assessments of health policy in the United States since the mid–1960s. This perspective has focused most notably on the availability, organization, and financing of medical care services by providing support for major federal investments in the training of medical care providers, in the construction of healthcare facilities, and in the coverage of the poor and elderly through Medicaid and Medicare, respectively. It culminated in the early 1990s in a major national universal health insurance reform effort and, in the latter half of that decade, led to a plethora of state healthcare financing reform measures. As indicated in previous chapters, assessments of policy initiatives directed at improving access to medical care often have not gone far enough in considering the extent to which such initiatives ultimately have served to enhance the health of individuals and populations.

The population perspective on the health of communities as a whole and on the medical and non-medical factors that give rise to health disparities challenges health services researchers and policy analysts to consider broader conceptions of equity rooted in the social justice paradigm. Population health concerns have traditionally been the domain of public health policy and service provision. Although the U.S. and international public health communities have undertaken a number of major programmatic initiatives— such as the WHO Year 2000 Objectives and Healthy Community programs—to attempt to ameliorate health disparities, such disparities continue to persist in the United States and other countries, and in some cases have widened across racial and socioeconomic groups. Clinical effectiveness research has documented those investments in medical care that can make a difference, as well as how the effectiveness of medical care can be improved. Population effectiveness research has confirmed that public health, social policy, and economic policy investments are also needed to enhance the health of communities and of the individuals residing within them. Health policy ultimately directed toward improving the health of individuals and of populations, then, demands investments in more comprehensive, integrated, and effective medical and non-medical interventions.

The deliberative justice paradigm compels the parties affected by health policy and program design to participate in shaping them. This translates at the macrolevel to mechanisms such as the assurance that stakeholders' interests as well as those of the general public are reflected in the policy formulation process, and at the microlevel to a fuller involvement of patients and their families in clinical decisions affecting health outcomes. Justice is judged by the extent to which those directly affected directly participate. The implication of the expanded equity framework introduced in the previous chapter (Figure 6.1) is that the ultimate goal of health policy—improving the health of individuals and communities—is not likely to be achieved if the norm of deliberative justice fails to influence the policy formulation process.

The discussion that follows presents evidence regarding the equity of healthcare provision, based on the respective paradigms of justice and accompanying policy strategies.

Evidence Relating to Equity

The review of evidence in this chapter begins with the end point for assessing the equity of the healthcare system based on the expanded equity framework (Figure 6.1)—the extent to which subgroup disparities in health persist. This focus is defined most directly by the social justice paradigm. Evidence regarding the magnitude and correlates of substantive equity reflected in these disparities will be presented first, to set the stage for assessing the extent to which this ultimate and defining equity objective has been achieved. Then, evidence regarding the distributive equity of health services provision will be reviewed, with a particular focus on whether it indicates the amelioration or the exacerbation of health disparities. And finally, evidence related to the deliberative justice paradigm will be inventoried, delineating in particular the broader health services research and policy agendas to which it points. The distributive and deliberative justice dimensions point primarily to evidence regarding procedural equity. The import of these factors for substantive equity is reflected in their likely contribution to minimizing health disparities.

The bulk of the health services research evidence regarding the equity of healthcare provision is rooted in the distributive justice paradigm. Evidence regarding the social justice dimensions of equity is drawn primarily from public health and related social science research documenting the predictors and indicators of health disparities. Although the deliberative justice paradigm has not served to explicitly guide the formulation of health services or public health research on equity, elements of it are implicit in the evidence that is being assembled to assess the ethical and equity implications of managed care–driven system changes.

Social Justice

The social justice dimension of equity encompasses a look at the physical, social, and economic environment; health risks; and associated health disparities between groups. The U.S. Public Health Service and WHO Year 2000 Health Objectives provide a framework and a set of indicators for monitoring progress toward this goal. The findings with respect to selected indicators and environmental and behavioral predictors of health disparities in the United States were reviewed in Chapter 1.

Basically, the evidence documents that disparities between groups—particularly between whites and racial or ethnic minorities—persist and have widened in a number of instances (Aday 1993; NCHS 1997). Very young, minority, poorly educated mothers are much less likely to have adequate prenatal care and are more likely to bear low-birthweight infants. The rates of teenage pregnancy, preterm and low-birthweight babies, inadequate prenatal care, and infant and maternal mortality remain two to three times higher among African-American women than among white women, and these rates show no sign of diminishing. The prevalence of chronic disease increases steadily with age, as does the incidence of death and the magnitude of limitation in daily activity due to chronic disease. At any age, men are more likely to die from major chronic illnesses such as heart disease, stroke, and cancer, than are women, although elderly women living with chronic illness have more problems with carrying out their normal daily routines. African Americans—particularly African-American men—are more likely to experience serious disabilities and to die from chronic illness than are whites. Early in the course of the AIDS epidemic, homosexual or bisexual males were most likely to be affected. In recent years, more and more mothers and children are at risk due to intravenous drug use among women or their sex partners. Higher proportions of African Americans and Hispanics than of whites are likely to be HIV-positive, to develop and die of AIDS, and to have contracted the disease through drug use or sexual contact with drug users. Young adults in their late teens and early twenties—particularly men— are more likely to smoke, drink, and use illicit drugs than are their younger or older counterparts. Native American youth are much more apt to use alcohol, drugs, and cigarettes than are white or other minority youth. Minority substance users are also more likely to develop life-threatening patterns of substance abuse, as evidenced by the higher rates of addiction-related deaths among minority groups. Death rates for cirrhosis and other alcohol-related causes are greater among Native Americans compared to whites or other minorites. A disproportionate number of medical emergencies and deaths due to cocaine abuse occur among minorities—particularly among African Americans.

The physical, social, and economic environments to which individuals are exposed can have a profound effect on their health and healthcare. Although the economy in general strengthened in the last half of the 1990s, sustained trends in the movement of businesses and industries out of central cities have contributed to high unemployment rates, particularly among young inner-city minority males. Men's wages remain higher on average than women's wages and the national minimum wage has not kept pace with inflation, further exacerbating the economic burden on female heads of households with dependents. In addition, men are generally made better off financially by divorce or separation, while women's economic situations usually worsen (Aday 1993; U.S. Department of Commerce 1996).

The percentage of families with children headed by only the mother is increasing among all racial and ethnic groups. The average salaries of working African-American women are lower than those of either white women or African-American men, and the average aid to families with dependent children has continued to decline in real purchasing power. Though more African-American men have entered the workforce in recent years, the rates of unemployment among young African-American men remain high. Lack of employment opportunities, poverty, and the associated problems of crime, substance abuse, and violence plague many inner-city neighborhoods. The socioeconomic status of Hispanic and Native American families resembles that of African Americans more than that of whites. Nonetheless, the reduced number of jobs in the manufacturing and industrial sectors, the growth in the number of minimum wage and part-time jobs in the service sectors, and the increased tax burden on low-income and middle-class taxpayers have also resulted in many working poor families—including white families and those with two breadwinners—experiencing economic difficulties. These aspects of the social and economic environment can have profound consequences for the health and health risks of the most vulnerable (Aday 1993; U.S. Department of Commerce 1996).

A challenge in the design, conduct, and interpretation of research examining these issues is determining the essential meaning of factors such as race and poverty, and the dynamics through which these factors operate to influence health. A particular criticism of the application of these variables is that they are typically used as attitudinal, biological, or behavioral descriptors of individuals—especially in studies based on large-scale surveys or data bases—while insufficient attention is paid to the social-structural, cultural, and environmental contexts that fundamentally shape these individuals' access to health and healthcare. As a consequence, the focus of health policy informed by such research remains aimed at intervention at the individual level, not at the broader social and economic conditions and the systems of opportunity that influence the health risks of socially and economically disadvantaged populations (James 1993; Krieger 1992; LaVeist 1994; Link and Phelan 1995; Muntaner, Nieto, and O'Campo 1996; Williams 1994).

Although the U.S. Public Health Service Year 2000 Objectives for the United States do offer a widely acknowledged and widely utilized set of indicators for tracing the predictors and indicators of health disparities, the formulation of these objectives was constrained by conservative political forces that focused more on individual behavioral rather than on broader public health or social and economic policies to effect change. Although consideration was given to tracking poverty rates and related indicators of social and economic health and well-being in the process of formulating these objectives, these types of measures were eventually excluded from the set of more overtly health-related aims. Environmental risk measures that point to the greater accountability of corporate interests for ameliorating health risks remain the set of indicators for which the least data are available to monitor progress (McBeath 1991).

The weight of the evidence in the United States and other countries documents that health disparities based on social and economic disparities between and among groups persist and have, in fact, widened in some cases. Medical care and public health have been ineffective in significantly narrowing these disparities. These findings indicate the necessity of considering broader roles for medical care and for public health, social, and economic policy to influence health and to reduce persistent racial and income-related health disparities. Aday (1993) points out the importance of the considerations in addressing the fundamental origins of poor physical, psychological, or social health among particularly vulnerable populations (e.g., persons with AIDS, the mentally ill, alcohol and substance abusers, families living with physical or emotional abuse, the homeless, and immigrant and refugee populations). The challenge to both the medical care and the public health communities is to create and extend the partnerships between them, and to create and extend partnerships with other sectors within their communities, to more fully and effectively address persistent or widening subgroup disparities in health.

Distributive Justice

The distributive justice paradigm has dominated the conceptualization and measurement of the equity of the U.S. healthcare system. Illustrative examples and estimates of indicators of equity based on the distributive justice framework are highlighted in Appendix 7.1. The presentation and discussion of findings in the context of this paradigm focus principally on trends in potential access indicators, their relationship to predicting people's actual utilization and their levels of satisfaction with care, as well as likely health consequences.

Delivery system

Availability

- *Potential access.* The major policy concerns regarding the availability of healthcare personnel and resources in an area have shifted over the past 30 years from the number of providers to the location of providers and who exactly is being served. The distribution of providers and, more importantly, the effect of service availability on the decision to seek care have been and continue to be a focus of health policy efforts regarding access. Post–World War II policies supporting medical personnel training and new hospital construction led to overall increases in the number of providers and facilities. These increases were mirrored in steady rises in the traditional provider-to-population and facility-to-population ratios. Wide variability nonetheless persists in the geographic distribution of providers (NCHS 1997). A related issue of availability is the willingness of providers to see patients who are publicly insured or uninsured. Physicians' refusals to see Medicaid clients and strategies by managed care plans to locate in areas that are not readily accessible to these populations create significant barriers to care for low-income, pregnant women—particularly those residing in inner-city areas with large minority populations (Komaromy, Lurie, and Bindman 1995; Mitchell 1991; Perloff et al. 1997; Silverstein and Kirkman-Liff 1995).

• *Realized access.* Research during the 1970s and early 1980s suggested that provider-to-population ratios alone did not determine actual rates of use. Even in areas of ostensible shortage, residents with transportation and financial resources traveled out of the neighborhood or to adjoining towns for care (Chiu, Aday, and Andersen 1981; Kleinman and Wilson 1977). Later research has documented that insurance coverage and the availability of a racially and ethnically diverse provider workforce may be equally or more important than overall physician supply in influencing access to care, especially in high-risk underserved communities (Grumbach, Vranizan, and Bindman 1997).

There has also been heightened concern over the effect of a number of national and local trends on the availability of providers and the resultant utilization patterns of residents in rural and inner-city communities. These include the buyout and conversion of not-for-profit community hospitals by for-profit healthcare corporations; an increase in the closure rates of rural hospitals and of financially stressed safety-net providers serving poor, inner-city populations; and primary-care provider reluctance to locate or to remain in these same areas. In addition, a large proportion of physicians in certain specialties, such as obstetrics-gynecology, have closed their practices to medically indigent and Medicaid patients, due to the low rates of public third-party reimbursement and to heightened fears of medical malpractice liability (Claxton et al. 1997; Gray 1997; *Health Services Research* 1989; Institute of Medicine 1989a, 1989b; National Commission to Prevent Infant Mortality 1988).

- *Health impacts.* The effect of these changes on actual patterns of service use and health depends to a large extent on whether alternative and appropriate service delivery arrangements subsequently become available to the populations previously served by these providers (e.g., through reconfiguring a formerly inpatient-oriented rural hospital to a primary care or emergency care service provider). The lack of an adequate system of primary care in general, and maternity and prenatal care services in particular, for low-income inner-city women and for poor minorities living in isolated rural counties or communities, such as along the Texas-Mexico border, has been found to contribute to their lower rates of use of effective preventive and illness-related care (Warner 1991). Health services research has documented higher rates of avoidable hospitalizations and ambulatory care–sensitive conditions (i.e., disease occurrence that could have been prevented with adequate primary care) in medically underserved areas with lower socioeconomic status (Billings, Anderson, and Newman 1996; Billings et al. 1993; Bindman et al. 1995; Friedman 1994; Institute of Medicine 1993).

Organization

- *Potential access.* The organization and the financing of healthcare in the United States increasingly reflect a multiple-tiered system of benefits including, in descending order of generosity, the privately insured middle and upper class, the elderly who have Medicare only, the Medicaid-eligible indigent or working-class poor population, and individuals and families with neither public nor private coverage. Such disparities have, in some sense, always been a fact of life in the U.S. healthcare system. They emerge as a particular paradox now, however, because as the overall public and private commitment of expenditures for medical care continues to rise, so does the number of Americans who have no or inadequate protection against these burgeoning increases.

Relman (1980) has characterized the U.S. "medical-industrial complex" as a large network of private corporations engaged in the business of supplying medical care to patients for a profit, such as chain hospitals, emergicenters, walk-in clinics, dialysis centers, and home health care companies. The diverse and evolving forms of private medical practice are also increasingly linked to methods of paying for care. These include group practice–based HMOs, individual practice associations (IPAs), PPOs, and POS plans. The organizational distinctions between these different arrangements are becoming increasingly obscure. All of these alternatives have attempted to develop systems of cost-conscious medical practice and methods of reimbursement (Morrison and Luft 1990; Weiner and de Lissovoy 1993). Managed care organizations (MCOs) typically limit consumer choice of providers to participating physicians and emphasize primary care gatekeeper arrangements and less use of specialists. The competition among MCOs has resulted in the reduction of cross-subsidies to the safety-net providers that serve large numbers of the uninsured or medically indigent (Davis and Schoen 1997; Davis, Schoen, and Sandman 1996; Davis et al. 1995; Lipson and Naierman 1996; Schauffler and Wolin 1996).

The growing number of elderly—particularly the oldest old—and the impetus for shortened lengths of hospital stays resulting from DRGs have put increasing pressures on families and other home- and community-based long-term care arrangements. The deinstitutionalization movement in mental health care led to the discharge of large numbers of the mentally ill and a greatly increased burden on community-based mental health services provision (Aday 1993).

- **Realized access.** The major concerns underlying the realized access impact of the increasing corporatization of medical practice relate to the fact that private and for-profit institutions are less likely to serve the poor and medically indigent, and that large-scale, bureaucratic, publicly supported providers are less likely to be convenient and satisfactory to consumers. They are also more subject to close or to be purchased by for-profit entities in an increasingly competitive healthcare environment (Aday 1987; Lipson and Naierman 1996). MCOs primarily enroll employed individuals, especially employees of large firms. Employers and insurers have typically restricted enrollment and coverage for employees' dependents and for particularly vulnerable or high-risk populations (e.g., persons with AIDS) (Davis 1997).

  Both not-for-profit and for-profit private institutions are less likely to serve patients without insurance and have much lower rates of uncompensated and undercompensated care than publicly supported institutions—teaching hospitals in particular (Gray 1986; Sloan, Blumstein, and Perrin 1986). The poor and elderly generally have been underrepresented also in HMO and private insurance plans. Demonstration projects and programs supported by HCFA to enroll the poor and elderly in such arrangements have met with mixed success in terms of access, cost, and quality objectives. In general, Medicaid enrollees expressed less satisfaction with providers than fee-for-service patients at comparison sites. This was particularly the case for enrollees who were assigned a new physician as gatekeeper (Freund and Hurley 1995; Freund et al. 1989; Hurley, Freund, and Paul 1993). Medicare enrollees as a whole were satisfied with their care experiences, although frail and vulnerable HMO enrollees (e.g., the disabled, the oldest old, African Americans, low-income enrollees, and those in fair or poor health) were more likely to report access problems than their counterparts in fee-for-service arrangements (Langwell and Hadley 1989; Nelson et al. 1997). The RAND Health Insurance Experiment documented lower client satisfaction among HMO enrollees than among fee-for-service clients (Wagner and Bledsoe 1990; Ware et al. 1986), and a RAND evaluation of PPOs demonstrated that PPO enrollees generally were also more satisfied than those in HMOs (Hosek et al. 1990). States are increasingly enacting laws to ensure access and to improve the accountability of managed care organizations for the quality and appropriateness of care for managed care enrollees in general and for the most vulnerable enrollees in particular (Gosfield 1997).

- *Health impacts.* Users of publicly supported facilities such as public health clinics, hospital outpatient departments, or emergency rooms often may have to wait hours to be seen when they are ill or injured, or may be told that it will be weeks or even months before they can get an appointment for a routine or prevention-related visit (e.g., for prenatal care) which could have serious health consequences (Berk, Schur, and Cantor 1995; Institute of Medicine 1988, 1993). MCOs' restrictions on gatekeepers and specialty referral patterns may also have health consequences for chronically ill patients, women, or others who require access to a broader array of providers (e.g., obstetrician-gynecologist or cardiologist) to fully monitor and maintain their health (Moore, Fenlon, and Hepworth 1996; Rosenbaum et al. 1995; Weisman 1996). Research based on the Medical Outcomes Study documented that although physical and mental health outcomes did not differ for the average patient seen in HMOs compared to fee-for-service arrangements, elderly, poor, and chronically ill HMO patients experienced poorer physical health outcomes (Ware et al. 1996).

Financing

- *Potential access.* The advent of Medicaid and Medicare in the mid–1960s led to a significant increase in the percentage of personal healthcare (PHC) expenditures paid for by the federal government, which ranged from 9.0 percent in 1960 to 34.5 percent in 1995. Private health insurance also assumed a larger role in financing healthcare through employer-based coverage. The percentage of PHC expenditures by private insurers increased from 21.2 percent in 1960 to 31.5 percent in 1995, while the proportion of out-of-pocket expenditures borne by households or individuals declined from 55.3 percent to 20.8 percent over this same period (Levit et al. 1996).

During the past decade, as the costs of care continued to rise, public and private third-party payors became increasingly interested in reducing the amounts they had to pay for medical care. They have, therefore, imposed stricter eligibility criteria; cutbacks in covered services; fixed, predetermined (i.e., prospective) rates of reimbursement by service or diagnosis, such as DRGs; and greater consumer cost sharing (Levit et al. 1996).

• *Realized access.* Empirical findings related to the major prospective pricing initiative (i.e., reimbursement for hospital services under Medicare on the basis of DRGs) on hospital utilization and expenditures show that admission rates, total days of care, and average length of stay have declined since its introduction. These trends, however, are confounded with trends that were already underway in the organization and delivery of medical care prior to the introduction of DRGs, such as an increased emphasis on ambulatory care. (See the discussion of these trends in Chapters 1 and 5.)

• *Health impacts.* Nonetheless, there is evidence that the elderly have been discharged after shorter stays and in poorer health, largely as a result of providers' responses to the DRG pricing policy. The post-discharge death rates for those in unstable condition were higher after the introduction of DRGs— particularly among those discharged home rather than to a nursing home or to another institutional care setting (Kosecoff et al. 1990). The tendency to discharge such patients when they reach the limit of reimbursable days has also exposed deficiencies in the system of post-hospitalization care for the chronically ill and elderly in many communities, such as inadequate discharge planning, an insufficient number of nursing home beds, lack of community support services, and corollary stresses on the patient's family and on others (Levit et al. 1996; PPRC 1997).

The RAND Health Insurance Experiment documented an inverse relationship between the amount of physician and hospital services consumed and the amount of consumer copayment—the more consumers had to pay, the less medical care they consumed. The office-based medical use rates for children in particular were likely to be lower for those in cost-sharing compared to those in free-care plans (Anderson, Brook, and Williams 1991). Although the Health Insurance Experiment documented minimal overall negative health consequences as a result of plan cost-sharing provisions, the negative effects that were found were primarily among low-income, chronically ill individuals (Lohr et al. 1986). Medical care expenses tend to absorb a much higher proportion of the total income of low-income families than that of families with higher incomes. Policies that encourage greater cost sharing by consumers will undoubtedly lower the overall use of services. The resultant economic and health effects are most likely to fall on the poorest and sickest.

Population at risk

The focus in reviewing evidence on distributive justice at the population-level is the effect of an array of predisposing, enabling, and need factors on the population's use of and satisfaction with medical care. Equity in this context is grounded in the similar treatment norm—variations in medical care utilization should be primarily a function of need, rather than of socioeconomic or related healthcare factors.

Predisposing. Age is significantly associated with all different types of medical care service use, primarily because it is an important indicator of age-associated morbidity. In general, women use more health services than do men; this is to some extent a function of their obstetrics-related care needs, their greater longevity, and the perception that it is more socially acceptable for women to engage in help-seeking behaviors (Aday 1992). As noted earlier, however, substantial availability, organizational, and financial barriers exist for certain categories of women—especially low-income, uninsured, or Medicaid-eligible women—seeking needed prenatal and maternity care services (Gany and de Bocanegra 1996; Miles and Parker 1997; Weisman 1996).

Education is an important predictor of the use of preventive services. Better-educated people are, for example, more likely to have had a general physical, immunizations, tests, and procedures for preventive purposes, and better-educated women are more likely to have sought care early in their pregnancy (NCHS 1997).

The influence of these predisposing factors on utilization has remained relatively stable over time.

Enabling. According to the 1993 NHIS, 5.3 percent of children (i.e., 0–17 years of age) and 17.3 percent of the working-age adult population (i.e., 18–64 years) did not have a usual source of care. Among those who did, a private doctor's office was used most frequently, followed by health centers and similar sites such as company or school clinics, and hospital outpatient departments or emergency rooms. Blacks, Hispanics, the poor, males, and residents of large metropolitan statistical areas were least likely to have a regular source of care or, if they did, were more likely to use clinics or hospital outpatient departments or emergency rooms (Bloom et al. 1997a, 1997b).

The number of Americans lacking public or private insurance on any given day has been estimated to range from 31 to 40 million. The number of those uninsured for some period of time in the last two years is estimated to be even higher—around 53 million (Davis et al. 1995). Those most likely to be uninsured at some point during the year were young adults and children under 18; Hispanics and blacks; and the poor (Hellander et al. 1995). The percentage of those uninsured in 1996 was higher for blacks (23.0 percent) and Hispanics (33.5 percent) than for other racial groups, including whites (13.7 percent) (Beauregard, Drilea, and Vistnes 1997).

Most of the uninsured are workers or the dependents of workers who do not receive health insurance through their jobs. More than half are in families headed by a full-time worker who has been employed for at least a year. The uninsured are more likely to work in small firms or industries such as service or agricultural jobs that do not provide coverage (Davis et al. 1995; Rowland et al. 1994).

Further, almost one in five (18.5 percent) of the nonelderly insured (29 million people) have been estimated to be underinsured or inadequately protected against the possibility of large medical bills. This represents a significant increase from 12.6 percent in 1977 (Farley 1985; Short and Banthin 1995).

The proportion of the poor and near-poor covered by Medicaid reached a peak of 64 percent in the mid–1970s and subsequently declined to around 40 percent in the mid- to late 1980s. Medicaid expansions have attempted to reverse this trend, particularly for low-income women, infants, and children (Friedman 1991). In 1993, 55.2 percent of individuals with family incomes under 100 percent of poverty level had Medicaid coverage. The percent without coverage increased for all other groups above poverty level—principally due to the decline in insurance available from employers (Holahan, Winterbottom, and Rajan 1995).

Need. Assessments of need may be based on patients' self-perceptions of their health, as well as on medical professionals' clinical diagnoses and evaluations. Providers' and patients' evaluations of needs may not always agree. Nonetheless, need—however measured—is consistently borne out to be an important predictor of the use of services, and in particular, of the volume of services consumed. Need is, for example, generally the most important predictor of the number of physician visits for those with at least one visit and of the number of days of care once a patient is admitted to the hospital. For more prevention-oriented or discretionary services, such as dental care, need has been and continues to be less important than other factors, particularly enabling factors such as income or insurance coverage. The utilization of services may be deemed to be equitable to the extent that services are distributed on the basis of need (Aday, Andersen, and Fleming 1980; Andersen et al. 1987).

Realized Access

Utilization. Race, income, having a regular source of care, and insurance coverage are important policy-relevant predictors of the utilization of medical care services.

Despite improvements in the levels of access to medical care among Hispanics, and other minorities, these groups are still less likely to use certain types of services than are whites. Mexican Americans in particular are less likely to have seen a physician or dentist or to have been hospitalized than are whites, blacks, or other categories of Hispanics. Hispanic and Native American women are less likely to have sought care during the first trimester, or in some cases at all, during their pregnancy. The lack of insurance coverage appears to be a particularly important contributor to Hispanics' lower use of medical and dental services (Andersen, Giachello, and Aday 1986; Berk, Schur, and Cantor, 1995; Ginzberg 1991; Lillie-Blanton and Alfaro-Correa 1995; NCHS 1997).

The proportion of women seeking care in the first trimester of their pregnancy, of preschool children who are immunized, and of adults or children who have been to a dentist is much lower among blacks than among whites. The incidence of congenital syphilis and late-stage cancer, both of which are preventable through early intervention, is also higher among blacks (Institute of Medicine 1993).

In the past, people with higher incomes used more medical care services than those with lower incomes. With the enactment of Medicare and Medicaid, the rates of utilization increased greatly among the poor. Nonetheless, income-related use differentials remain. The rates of use of physician and hospital services in general relative to need are lower for the poor—particularly the poor or working poor who have no insurance (NCHS 1997).

In 1994, the percentage of people who saw a doctor during the year was lower for people from families with incomes less than $14,000 (78.0 percent), than for those with family incomes of $50,000 or more (83.7 percent). People with lower incomes were nonetheless in much poorer health than people with higher incomes based on subjective perceptions of health, reported days of limited activity due to illness, and limitations in major activity due to the presence of a chronic condition. Since the introduction of Medicaid and Medicare, the rates of hospital discharges, days of care, length of stay, and the mean number of visits to a physician, once seen, have tended to be higher for those with lower than those with higher incomes—reflecting perhaps their greater need, as well as their greater tendency to delay seeking care until the health problem has worsened (NCHS 1997).

Having a regular source of medical care is a strong and consistent predictor of medical care utilization, particularly of the initial decision to seek care (Ettner 1996; Lambrew et al. 1996). Once entry to the system is gained, having an established provider is a less significant predictor of the subsequent number of visits to a physician or length of hospital stay (Andersen et al. 1987). Questions have been raised about the accuracy of self-reports of a usual source of care, as well as whether a regular source of care is a determinant or a result of using services (Perloff and Morris 1989). Causal models testing the direction of this relationship have confirmed that having an identifiable medical provider does directly influence the decision of whether or not to seek care, though unidirectional models may tend to overestimate this effect (Kuder and Levitz 1985).

The presence and the extent of insurance coverage have been demonstrated to be important predictors of the utilization of medical care services in numerous national and local studies of access (Andersen et al. 1987; Donelan, Blendon, Hill, Hoffman, Rowland, Frankel, and Altman 1996). In addition, there is evidence that patients with private third-party coverage are more likely to receive more intensive and technology-oriented care and to experience better outcomes than those with public coverage or no insurance (Franks, Clancy, and Gold 1993; Hadley, Steinberg, and Feder 1991; Weissman, Gatsonis, and Epstein 1992; Wenneker, Epstein, and Weissman 1990). Studies in states that have dropped large numbers of the poor from the Medicaid program have shown corollary increases in adverse health outcomes, such as higher infant mortality rates (Braveman et al. 1989).

Managed care enrollees have typically had lower hospital admission rates and shorter lengths of stay than those covered under fee-for-service arrangements. Research suggests that they have comparable or somewhat higher physician office visit rates, lower use of expensive tests and procedures, and greater use of preventive services (Miller and Luft 1994).

Satisfaction.   Surveys of public and patient opinion regarding the performance of the medical care system in different countries confirm that U.S. residents are more critical of the system as a whole and much less satisfied with their own particular experiences in getting care than are people in other countries, including the United Kingdom, Canada, and Germany. Around 18 percent of U.S. residents thought that the healthcare system worked pretty well and that only minor changes were needed, in contrast to 29 percent of Canadians and 30 percent of West Germany residents. Twenty-eight percent of U.S. residents thought the system had so much wrong with it that it should be completely rebuilt, compared to 12 percent in Canada and 11 percent in West Germany. U.S. residents also tended to report more problems with actually getting access to care and with the high costs of their care than people living in Canada or West Germany (Blendon, Benson, Donelan, Leitman, Taylor, Koeck, and Gitterman 1995). Minorities in the United States also tend to report more barriers and to rate the healthcare system less highly than do white Americans (Blendon, Scheck, Donelan, Hill, Smith, Beatrice, and Altman 1995).

Satisfaction surveys of managed care enrollees and of people in fee-for-service arrangements have tended to document that managed care patients have lower satisfaction with appointment waiting times, quality, and patient-physician interaction, but have greater satisfaction with costs (Mark and Mueller 1996; Miller and Luft 1994). In particular, managed care enrollees are often dissatisfied with the choices of plans and providers that are available to them (Davis and Schoen 1997; Davis, Schoen, and Sandman 1996; Ullman et al. 1997).

Deliberative Justice

As indicated in the previous chapter, individual and community empowerment and participation have been important components of many international and national health initiatives. There are, however, no standardized or widely applied indicators and scales for measuring this key dimension of deliberative justice. Voter turnout rates and public opinion polls regarding levels of perceived confidence in or ability to influence public officials provide macrolevel evidence of the presence and magnitude of civic participation (Blendon, Benson, Donelan, Leitman, Taylor, Koeck, and Gitterman 1995; Blendon, Scheck, Donelan, Hill, Smith, Beatrice, and Altman 1995). The failure of the Clinton healthcare reform initiatives has been attributed to the dominance of technical-rational experts in the policy formulation process and the lack of a clear public consensus in support of comprehensive reform (Hacker 1996; Skocpol 1996).

Attitudinal scales have been developed to measure the extent to which organization or community members feel a sense of control or influence over the decisions that most directly affect their health and well-being (Israel et al. 1994). Key informant interviews and social network analysis yield data useful for mapping the extent of community activation and involvement in health program design (Wickizer et al. 1993). Rosenbaum et al. (1997) have documented a number of practices on the part of MCOs that tend to limit the involvement of both patients and providers in influencing decisions that affect them: "gag rules" that inhibit providers from discussing selected treatment options with patients; "cram-down rules" that compel providers to participate in a state-mandated managed care program in order to receive benefits through other payor arrangements; selective or misleading plan marketing to potential enrollees; time constraints on patient-provider visits or failure to provide cultural competency training that could affect patient-provider communication; and adversarial or obstructionist consumer grievance and dispute resolution procedures. Though some of these practices or failures may have also been present in fee-for-service Medicaid provider arrangements, Medicaid eligibles' options are likely to be constrained as a function of mandated enrollment in what might be a limited number of competing managed care plans in a given area.

Though community or consumer participation has been an explicit component of health policy design, particularly in the context of public health–oriented community empowerment initiatives, it has not always been effectively realized in practice. Further, participation also has not been fully developed and considered as a criterion of the fairness of health policy or program design. The future directions for research in this area would be to extend the conceptual and methodological development of indicators of deliberative justice; to use them in evaluating the performance of policies and programs at the national, community, system, institutional, and patient levels; and to examine their import for ultimately influencing the health of the individuals and of the communities they were intended to serve.

In summary, the weight of the evidence regarding the extent to which equity has been achieved may be summarized as follows: not to a substantial extent. The evidence of the successes of the broad policy strategies for enhancing equity outlined earlier may be viewed at best as mixed, and at worst as falling far short of desired equity objectives. The bulk of the evidence regarding the goal of enhancing access to medical care is rooted in the distributive justice paradigm of individual rights to medical care. Though substantial investments in both the organization and financing of medical care services have been made at federal, state, and local levels, wide variations in access to care and coverage persist across regions and subgroups of the U.S. population, and both the costs and effectiveness of the care provided continue to present challenges to policymakers in deciding what rights should be assured, and at what cost to whom, within this framework.

The U.S. Public Health Service Year 2000 Objectives provide a template for examining the extent to which the social justice goals of minimizing health risks and health disparities have been achieved, based on indicators and evidence of subgroup variations in achieving desired health promotion, health protection, and preventive services goals. The data routinely gathered to monitor progress toward these objectives show progress on some, and persistent or widening disparities on many others.

Though there is emerging evidence of the importance of participation of affected parties in health policy and program design, the deliberative justice paradigm has been largely unexamined as a component of the fairness of the policy formulation and implementation process. The challenge to the public health and health services research community is to determine how best to conceptualize and measure norms of deliberative justice, so that both the presence and impact of this innovative benchmark of fairness can be more explicitly assessed.

The evidence available to date suggests that the major health policy strategies directed at achieving both procedural and substantive equity have, as a whole, fallen short of doing so. The next section examines the prospects for enhancing equity in the context of Medicaid managed care, with a particular focus on the norms of socially responsible managed care.

Criteria for Assessing Policy Alternatives in Terms of Equity

A number of innovations offer promise for transforming the disparate array of medical and non-medical programs and services into a comprehensive, coordinated system of healthcare directed toward improving the health of individuals and populations.

A historical Medicine and Public Health Initiative, sponsored by the AMA and the APHA, sought to explore the possibilities for fruitful collaboration between medicine and public health in education, research, and healthcare (Reiser 1996; The Medicine/Public Health Initiative 1997). The WHO has encouraged the promulgation of the Healthy Cities and Healthy Communities model for eliciting and inspiring interest across the array of diverse sectors within a community toward promoting the health of community residents (Ashton 1991). The concept of community empowerment perhaps most directly embodies a perspective and set of approaches mirroring the role that affected populations themselves play in promoting the health and well-being of the community. This perspective is manifest in the formulation and implementation of community-based health education and health promotion initiatives (Wallerstein 1992; Wallerstein and Bernstein 1994).

Community-oriented primary care (COPC) is a model focusing on the delivery of primary medical care in the context of identified community health needs. The COPC model has played a somewhat limited role in healthcare delivery in the United States, where medical care functions have tended to dominate over broader community and public health concerns. Further, the COPC model has not typically been successful in enhancing the efficient use of resources, which managed care alternatives have more often attempted to achieve (Lairson et al. 1997).

Evidence in more mature managed care–dominated markets suggests that MCOs are increasingly realizing that the entire community is their target population, as their penetration into these markets increases or as they experience a high degree of turnover in plan membership (Shortell, Gillies, and Anderson 1994; Shortell et al. 1996). As public health departments and community providers come to define and redefine their unique roles in these environments, the promise of a new form of medical care organization representing a partnership between managed care and public health interests—community-oriented managed care (COMC)—has emerged (Lairson et al. 1997; Starfield 1996).

COMC has its counterpart in Canada, which has traditionally emphasized community health over managed care through a comprehensive healthcare organization (CHO) in selected areas in the province of Ontario. These entities focus primarily on enhancing the health of the population or of the community as a whole with an integrated array of medical and non-medical programs and services. Another central component of healthcare reform in Canada is the involvement of affected individuals and subpopulations in the planning and management of the health system. The development of regional authorities is one of the main avenues used in various provinces to translate the principle of participation into practice (Mhatre and Deber 1992).

Managed care, and particularly for-profit managed care systems, are likely to increasingly dominate healthcare service provision in both the public and private sectors in the United States. Showstack et al. (1996) have delineated the dimensions of socially responsible managed care that reflect a set of normative yardsticks against which managed care plans can be evaluated in the contexts of the deliberative, distributive, and social justice underpinnings of equity developed in the previous chapter. Table 7.1 summarizes the indicators, drawn directly from Showstack et al. (1996), for evaluating health policy in terms of the equity criteria, and illustrates how the elements of socially responsible managed care might embody them. These criteria include the principles of participation within the deliberative justice paradigm; the distributive justice norms of freedom of choice and cost-effectiveness; social justice criteria related to need and the common good; and the similar treatment norm imbedded in both the distributive and social justice paradigms. (See Table 6.2 for a review of these criteria in general and Table 7.1 for how they might be interpreted and applied in assessing socially responsible managed care.)

An Application of Equity Criteria: Medicaid Managed Care

In the discussion that follows, the evidence on the extent to which Medicaid managed care manifests these elements of equity will be highlighted, based on health services research conducted in this area (Freund and Hurley 1995; Freund et al. 1989; Hurley, Freund, and Paul 1993; Mathematica 1997; The Robert Wood Johnson Foundation 1996; Rotwein et al. 1995; Rowland 1996; Rowland et al. 1995).

Table 7.1   Criteria for Assessing Health Policies in Terms of
Equity—An Application to Socially Responsible
Managed Care

Dimensions	Criteria	Indicators[1]
PROCEDURAL EQUITY		
Deliberative Justice		
Health Policy	Participation	Includes the community, broadly defined, in the governance and advisory structures of the managed care system.
Distributive Justice		
Delivery System	Freedom of choice	
• Availability		Participates actively in health
• Organization		professions education programs.
• Financing		Collaborates meaningfully with academic health centers, health departments, and other components of the public health infrastructure.
Realized Access	Cost-effectiveness	
• Utilization		Participates in community-wide data
• Satisfaction		networking and sharing. Publishes information regarding its financial performance and contributions to its community.
Distributive & Social Justice		
Population at Risk	Similar treatment	
• Predisposing		Enrolls a representative segment of the
• Enabling		general population living in the
• Need		system's geographic service area.
Social Justice		
Environment	Common good	
• Physical		Advocates publicly for community
• Social		health promotion and disease
• Economic		prevention.
Health Risks	Need	
• Environmental		
• Behavioral		
SUBSTANTIVE EQUITY		
Health	Need	
• Individuals		Identifies and acts on opportunities for
• Community		community health improvement.

[1]The indicators of socially responsible managed care were drawn directly from Showstack et al. (1996).
The classification of these elements according to the respective dimensions and criteria of equity was done
by the author. See the chapter text for further detail.

In terms of the deliberative justice norm of participation, socially responsible managed care would include viewpoints and representatives from a variety of sectors in the system's governance or advisory structures: plan enrollees and the population in the community in which the system operates, including underrepresented minorities; business and employee sectors; public health and social work professionals; and key community agencies such as school systems. Both consumer and provider participation in the design of Medicaid managed care plans has been limited in many states. In some states—Tennessee, for example—the transformation of the Medicaid program to managed care proceeded quite rapidly, in some instances with the explicit intent of avoiding direct opposition by affected stakeholders. The Oregon program has been quite visible and often criticized for adopting what has been deemed a "rationing" approach to providing services to Medicaid enrollees. That state was unique, however, in soliciting and using input from patients, providers, and other stakeholders gathered from surveys, community forums, and public hearings in developing this approach.

Socially responsible managed care systems would attempt to enhance the freedom of choice and the array of alternatives available to potential consumers and residents. This would include participating in the training of a broad array of health professionals and collaborating with academic health centers, health departments, and other components of the public health infrastructure in building a comprehensive, coordinated, prevention-oriented continuum of care (see Figure 1.1 in Chapter 1). Managed care, and the waivers granted to states to innovate managed care alternatives within Medicaid, are intentionally designed to limit "choices" on the part of both providers and patients. Enrolling Medicaid-eligible individuals in managed care plans was, however, intended to address a major access barrier under fee-for-service provision: the refusal of providers to accept Medicaid clients. Medicaid managed care patients may nonetheless come to find their choices constrained as academic health centers, teaching hospitals, and safety-net providers that have traditionally served Medicaid clients face severe cutbacks for medical education and are unable to compete with private for-profit providers for Medicaid contracts. Although more efficient models of care delivery may evolve over the long term, substantial disruptions in access and continuity are likely to result for Medicaid enrollees in the interim.

Participation in community-wide networking and sharing of data on enrollees' characteristics, health status, risk behaviors, healthcare utilization, satisfaction and outcomes, and on plan financial performance would provide a more complete picture of the extent to which cost-effective services are provided to enrollees across the array of providers in a community, and may indicate which programs or services need to be strengthened to assure their provision. States do, in fact, face major challenges in developing or adopting data systems for monitoring and tracking utilization and expenditures as the primary method of providing and paying for care shifts from fee-for-service to managed care practice arrangements. The health services research evidence regarding the cost and utilization impacts of Medicaid managed care were summarized in Chapter 5. In general, it suggests that the utilization of selected types of services (e.g., specialists and emergency rooms) is reduced under managed care. Cost savings vary by type of managed care model, and may be due in many cases to sharply constrained reimbursement to providers rather than to sustained reductions in more costly hospital and physician services overall. Patients seem satisfied, in general, with managed care arrangements. Those who are forced to switch providers at the time of enrollment remain the most dissatisfied.

The similar treatment standard compels a look at the extent to which the plan enrolls a representative segment of the general population living in the system's geographic service area, including socially and economically disadvantaged and vulnerable populations. Medicaid managed care policies have focused primarily on enrolling AFDC-eligibles—mostly low-income women and children. Many states are struggling to develop provider arrangements and incentives for accommodating elderly or disabled beneficiaries— groups that have traditionally not been sought out or served by managed care entities.

A socially responsible system of managed care would attempt to promote the common good of the community as a whole by advocating community health promotion and disease prevention, and by promoting personal, corporate, and civic responsibility for identifying and addressing the physical, social, and economic environmental risks to the health of populations and individuals within the community. Selected states (e.g., Minnesota) have attempted to forge partnerships with departments of public health and incorporate elements of population-oriented prevention efforts in the design of managed care–driven Medicaid reform. This is more likely to be the case in mature markets with a high penetration of HMOs or in those states for which there has been a history of involvement of not-for-profit HMOs in particular in such efforts. In such cases, broader population-oriented health promotion and disease prevention efforts are seen as ultimately benefiting the community residents that the plans directly serve.

And finally, the commitment of the system to substantive equity is evidenced by the extent to which it identifies and acts on opportunities for community health improvement by inventorying the *needs* of high-risk populations or neighborhoods through system-wide databases and data sharing, and by collaborating with other sectors and providers in enhancing the health and well-being of the community as a whole. The end points and associated assessments of Medicaid managed care have been focused primarily on access, cost, and quality performance issues within the distributive justice paradigm. The evolution of broader partnerships between managed care, public health, and other health-oriented sectors and a corollary concern with community-wide health impacts is an emerging reality in a few states, but is a far-distant or nonexistent vision in many others.

Summary and Conclusions

In summary, the goal of equity has not been achieved to a substantial extent. Significant health disparities persist between racial, ethnic, and socioeconomic groups. Vulnerable populations remain at risk of receiving less, or less than adequate, healthcare. Both public and private policymaking appears to eschew rather than elicit the views of affected stakeholders. A core argument of this book is that the ultimate measure of success of U.S. health policy is the level of improvement in the health of the population. This and the previous chapter have attempted to provide a new conceptual blueprint and methodological tools for designing health policy directed toward more effectively achieving this objective.

References

Aday, L. A. 1987. "The Ethical Implications of Prospective Payment and Corporate Medical Practice: A Research Agenda." *Social Justice Research* 1: 275–96.

——. 1992. "Indicators and Predictors of Health Services Utilization." In *Introduction to Health Services.* 4th ed. Edited by S. J. Williams and P. R. Torrens, 46–70. New York: John Wiley & Sons.

——. 1993. *At Risk in America: The Health and Health Care Needs of Vulnerable Populations in the United States.* San Francisco: Jossey-Bass.

Aday, L. A., R. Andersen, and G. Fleming. 1980. *Health Care in the U.S.: Equitable for Whom?* Beverly Hills: Sage Publications.

Andersen, R. M., L. A. Aday, C. S. Lyttle, L. J. Cornelius, and M. Chen. 1987. *Ambulatory Care and Insurance Coverage in an Era of Constraint.* Chicago: Pluribus Press, Inc.

Andersen, R. M., A. L. Giachello, and L. A. Aday. 1986. "Access of Hispanics to Health Care and Cuts in Services: A State of the Art Overview." *Public Health Reports* 101: 238–52.

Anderson, G. M., R. Brook, and A. Williams. 1991. "A Comparison of Cost-Sharing Versus Free Care in Children: Effects on the Demand for Office-Based Medical Care." *Medical Care* 29: 890–8.

Ashton, J. 1991. "The Healthy Cities Project: A Challenge for Health Education." *Health Education Quarterly* 18: 39–48.

Beauregard, K. M., S. K. Drilea, and J. P. Vistnes. 1997. *The Uninsured in America: 1996. Health Insurance Status of the U.S. Civilian Noninstitutionalized Population,* AHCPR Pub. No. 97-0025. Rockville, MD: Agency for Health Care Policy and Research.

Berk, M. L., C. L. Schur, and J. C. Cantor. 1995. "Ability to Obtain Health Care: Recent Estimates from the Robert Wood Johnson Foundation National Access to Care Survey." *Health Affairs* 14 (3): 139–46.

Billings, J., G. M. Anderson, and L. S. Newman. 1996. "Recent Findings on Preventable Hospitalizations." *Health Affairs* 15 (3): 239–49.

Billings, J., L. Zeitel, J. Lukomnik, T. S. Carey, A. E. Blank, and L. Newman. 1993. "Impact of Socioeconomic Status on Hospital Use in New York City." *Health Affairs* 12 (1): 162–73.

Bindman, A. B., K. Grumbach, D. Osmond, M. Komaromy, K. Vranizan, N. Lurie, J. Billings, and A. Stewart. 1995. "Preventable Hospitalizations and Access to Health Care." *Journal of the American Medical Association* 274: 305–11.

Blendon, R. J., J. Benson, K. Donelan, R. Leitman, H. Taylor, C. Koeck, and D. Gitterman. 1995. "Who Has the Best Health Care System? A Second Look." *Health Affairs* 14 (4): 220–30.

Blendon, R. J., A. C. Scheck, K. Donelan, C. A. Hill, M. Smith, D. Beatrice, and D. Altman. 1995. "How White and African Americans View Their Health and Social Problems: Different Expectations, Different Experiences." *Journal of the American Medical Association* 273: 341–46.

Bloom, B., G. Simpson, R. A. Cohen, and P. E. Parsons. 1997a. "Access to Health Care Part 1: Children." *National Center for Health Statistics. Vital and Health Statistics* 10 (196).

———. 1997b. "Access to Health Care Part 2: Working-Age Adults." *National Center for Health Statistics. Vital and Health Statistics* 10 (197).

Braveman, P., G. Oliva, M. G. Miller, R. Reiter, and S. Egerter. 1989. "Adverse Outcomes and Lack of Health Insurance among Newborns in an Eight-County Area of California, 1982 to 1986." *The New England Journal of Medicine* 321: 508–13.

Chiu, G. Y., L. A. Aday, and R. Andersen. 1981. "An Examination of the Association of 'Shortage' and 'Medical Access' Indicators." *Health Policy Quarterly* 1: 142–58.

Claxton, G., J. Feder, D. Shactman, and S. Altman. 1997. "Public Policy Issues in Nonprofit Conversions: An Overview." *Health Affairs* 16 (2): 9–28.

Davis, K. 1997. "Uninsured in an Era of Managed Care." *Health Services Research* 31: 641–49.

Davis, K., D. Rowland, D. Altman, K. S. Collins, and C. Morris. 1995. "Health Insurance: The Size and Shape of the Problem." *Inquiry* 32: 196–203.

Davis, K., and C. Schoen. 1997. *Managed Care, Choice, and Patient Satisfaction.* New York: The Commonwealth Fund.

Davis, K., C. Schoen, and D. R. Sandman. 1996. "The Culture of Managed Care: Implications for Patients." *Bulletin of the New York Academy of Medicine* 73 (Summer): 173–83.

Donelan, K., R. J. Blendon, J. Benson, R. Leitman, and H. Taylor. 1996. "All Payer, Single Payer, Managed Care, No Payer: Patients' Perspectives in Three Nations." *Health Affairs* 15 (2): 254–65.

Donelan, K., R. J. Blendon, C. A. Hill, C. Hoffman, D. Rowland, M. Frankel, and D. Altman. 1996. "Whatever Happened to the Health Insurance Crisis in the United States? Voices from a National Survey." *Journal of the American Medical Association* 276: 1346–50.

Ettner, S. L. 1996. "The Timing of Preventive Services for Women and Children: The Effect of Having a Usual Source of Care." *American Journal of Public Health* 86: 1748–54.

Farley, P. 1985. "Who Are the Underinsured?" *Milbank Memorial Fund Quarterly/Health and Society* 63: 476–503.

Franks, P., C. M. Clancy, and M. R. Gold. 1993. "Health Insurance and

Mortality: Evidence from a National Cohort." *Journal of the American Medical Association* 270: 737–41.

Freund, D. A., and R. E. Hurley. 1995. "Medicaid Managed Care: Contribution to Issues of Health Reform." *Annual Review of Public Health* 16: 473–95.

Freund, D. A., L. F. Rossiter, P. D. Fox, J. A. Meyer, R. E. Hurley, T. S. Carey, and J. E. Paul. 1989. "Evaluation of the Medicaid Competition Demonstrations." *Health Care Financing Review* 11 (2): 81–97.

Friedman, E. 1991. "The Uninsured: From Dilemma to Crisis." *Journal of the American Medical Association* 265: 2491–95.

———. 1994. "Money Isn't Everything: Nonfinancial Barriers to Access." *Journal of the American Medical Association* 271: 1535–38.

Gany, F., and H. T. de Bocanegra. 1996. "Overcoming Barriers to Improving the Health of Immigrant Women." *Journal of the American Medical Women's Association* 51: 155–60.

Ginzberg, E. 1991. "Access to Health Care for Hispanics." *Journal of the American Medical Association* 265: 238–41.

Gosfield, A. G. 1997. "Who Is Holding Whom Accountable for Quality?" *Health Affairs* 16 (3): 26–40.

Gray, B. H. 1986. *For Profit Enterprise in Health Care.* Washington, D.C.: National Academy Press.

———. 1997. "Conversion of HMOs and Hospitals: What's at Stake?" *Health Affairs* 16 (2): 29–47.

Grumbach, K., K. Vranizan, and A. B. Bindman. 1997. "Physician Supply and Access to Care in Urban Communities." *Health Affairs* 16 (1): 71–89.

Hacker, J. 1996. *The Road to Nowhere: The Genesis of President Clinton's Plan for Health Security.* Princeton, NJ: Princeton University Press.

Hadley, J., E. P. Steinberg, and J. Feder. 1991. "Comparison of Uninsured and Privately Insured Hospital Patients: Condition on Admission, Resource Use, and Outcome." *Journal of the American Medical Association* 265: 374–79.

Health Services Research. 1989. "Special Issue: A Rural Health Services Research Agenda." *Health Services Research* 23: 725–1083.

Hellander, I., J. Moloo, D. U. Himmelstein, S. Woolhandler, and S. M. Wolfe. 1995. "The Growing Epidemic of Uninsurance: New Data on the Health Insurance Coverage of Americans." *International Journal of Health Services* 25: 377–92.

Holahan, J., C. Winterbottom, and S. Rajan. 1995. "A Shifting Picture of Health Insurance Coverage." *Health Affairs* 14 (4): 253–64.

Hosek, S., M. S. Marquis, K. E. Wells, D. Garnick, and H. Luft. 1990. *The*

Study of Preferred Provider Organizations: Executive Summary, R-3798-HHS/NIMH. Santa Monica, CA: The Rand Corporation.

Hurley, R. E., D. A. Freund, and J. E. Paul. 1993. *Managed Care in Medicaid: Lessons for Policy and Program Design*. Chicago: Health Administration Press.

Institute of Medicine. 1988. *Prenatal Care: Reaching Mothers, Reaching Infants*. Washington, D.C.: National Academy Press.

———. 1989a. *Medical Professional Liability and the Delivery of Obstetrical Care: Volume I*. Washington, D.C.: National Academy Press.

———. 1989b. *Medical Professional Liability and the Delivery of Obstetrical Care: Volume II*. Washington, D.C.: National Academy Press.

———. 1993. *Access to Health Care in America*. Edited by M. Millman. Washington, D.C.: National Academy Press.

Israel, B. A., B. Checkoway, A. Schulz, and M. Zimmerman. 1994. "Health Education and Community Empowerment: Conceptualizing and Measuring Perceptions of Individual, Organizational, and Community Control." *Health Education Quarterly* 21: 149–70.

James, S. A. 1993. "Racial and Ethnic Differences in Infant Mortality and Low Birth Weight: A Psychosocial Critique." *Annals of Epidemiology* 3: 130–36.

Kleinman, J. C., and R. W. Wilson. 1977. "Are the 'Medically Underserved Areas' Medically Underserved?" *Health Services Research* 12: 147–62.

Komaromy, M., N. Lurie, and A. B. Bindman. 1995. "California Physicians' Willingness to Care for the Poor." *Western Journal of Medicine* 162: 127–32.

Kosecoff, J., K. L. Kahn, W. H. Rogers, E. J. Reinisch, M. J. Sherwood, L. V. Rubenstein, D. Draper, C. P. Roth, C. Chew, and R. H. Brook. 1990. "Prospective Payment System and Impairment at Discharge: The 'Quicker and Sicker' Story Revisited." *Journal of the American Medical Association* 264: 1980–83.

Krieger, N. 1992. "The Making of Public Health Data: Paradigms, Politics, and Policy."*Journal of Public Health Policy* 13: 412–27.

Kuder, J., and G. Levitz. 1985. "Visits to the Physician: An Evaluation of the Usual Source Effect." *Health Services Research* 20: 579–96.

Lairson, D. R., G. Schulmeier, C. E. Begley, L. A. Aday, Y. Coyle, and C. H. Slater. 1997. "Managed Care and Community-Oriented Care: Conflict Or Complement." *Journal of Health Care for the Poor and Underserved* 8: 36–55.

Lambrew, J. M., G. H. DeFriese, T. S. Carey, T. C. Ricketts, and A. K. Biddle. 1996. "The Effects of Having a Regular Doctor on Access to Primary Care." *Medical Care* 34: 138–51.

Langwell, K. M., and J. P. Hadley. 1989. "Evaluation of the Medicare

Competition Demonstrations." *Health Care Financing Review* 11 (2): 65–80.

LaVeist, T. A. 1994. "Beyond Dummy Variables and Sample Selection: What Health Services Researchers Ought to Know about Race as a Variable." *Health Services Research* 29: 1–16.

Levit, K. R., H. C. Lazenby, B. R. Braden, C. A. Cowan, P. A. McDonnell, L. Sivarajan, J. M. Stiller, D. K. Won, C. S. Donham, A. M. Long, and M. W. Stewart. 1996. "National Health Expenditures, 1995." *Health Care Financing Review* 18 (1): 175–214.

Lillie-Blanton, M., and A. Alfaro-Correa. 1995. In *The Nation's Interest: Equity in Access to Health Care*. Washington, D.C.: Joint Center for Political and Economic Studies.

Link, B. G., and J. Phelan. 1995. "Social Conditions as Fundamental Causes of Disease." *Journal of Health and Social Behavior* (Extra issue): 80–94.

Lipson, D. J., and N. Naierman. 1996. "Effects of Health System Changes on Safety-Net Providers." *Health Affairs* 15 (2): 33–48.

Lohr, K. N., R. H. Brook, C. J. Kamberg, G. A. Goldberg, A. Leibowitz, J. Kessey, D. Reboussin, and J. P. Newhouse. 1986. "Use of Medical Care in the Rand Health Insurance Experiment: Diagnosis and Service-Specific Analyses in a Randomized Controlled Trial." *Medical Care* 24 (Supplement): S1-S87.

Mark, T., and C. Mueller. 1996. "Access to Care in HMOs and Traditional Insurance Plans." *Health Affairs* 15 (4): 81–87.

Mathematica. 1997. Expanding Health Insurance Coverage for Low-Income People: Experiments in Five States [Online]. Available: http://www.mathematica-mpr.com/ [12/17/97].

McBeath, W. H. 1991. "Health for All: A Public Health Vision." *American Journal of Public Health* 81: 1560–65.

Mhatre, S. L., and R. B. Deber. 1992. "From Equal Access to Health Care to Equitable Access to Health: A Review of Canadian Provincial Health Commissions and Reports." *International Journal of Health Services* 22: 645–68.

Miles, S., and K. Parker. 1997. "Men, Women, and Health Insurance." *The New England Journal of Medicine* 336: 218–21.

Miller, R. H., and H. S. Luft. 1994. "Managed Care Plan Performance Since 1980: A Literature Analysis." *Journal of the American Medical Association* 271: 1512–19.

Mitchell, J. B. 1991. "Physician Participation in Medicaid Revisited." *Medical Care* 29: 645–53.

Moore, P., N. Fenlon, and J. T. Hepworth. 1996. "Indicators of Differences in Immunization Rates of Mexican American and White Non-Hispanic

Infants in a Medicaid Managed Care System." *Public Health Nursing* 13: 21–30.

Morrison, E. M., and H. S. Luft. 1990. "Health Maintenance Organization Environments in the 1980s and Beyond." *Health Care Financing Review* 12 (1): 81–90.

Muntaner, C., F. J. Nieto, and P. O'Campo. 1996. "The Bell Curve: On Race, Social Class, and Epidemiologic Research." *American Journal of Epidemiology* 144: 531–36.

National Center for Health Statistics. 1997. *Health, United States, 1996–97 and Injury Chartbook.* Hyattsville, MD: Public Health Service.

National Commission to Prevent Infant Mortality. 1988. *Malpractice and Liability: An Obstetrical Crisis.* Washington, D.C.: National Commission to Prevent Infant Mortality.

Nelson, L., R. Brown, M. Gold, A. Ciemnecki, and E. Docteur. 1997. "Access to Care in Medicare HMOs, 1996." *Health Affairs* 16 (2): 148–56.

Perloff, J. D., P. R. Kletke, J. W. Fossett, and S. Banks. 1997. "Medicaid Participation among Urban Primary Care Physicians." *Medical Care* 35: 142–57.

Perloff, J. D., and N. M. Morris. 1989. "Validating Reporting of Usual Sources of Health Care." In *Health Survey Research Methods.* Edited by F. J. Fowler, DHHS Publication No. PHS 89-3447, 59–64. Washington, D.C.: U.S. Government Printing Office.

Physician Payment Review Commission. 1997. *Annual Report to Congress, 1997.* Washington, D.C.: Physician Payment Review Commission.

Reiser, S. J. 1996. "Medicine and Public Health: Pursuing a Common Destiny." *Journal of the American Medical Association* 276: 1429–30.

Relman, A. 1980. "The New-Medical Industrial Complex." *The New England Journal of Medicine* 303: 963–70.

Robert Wood Johnson Foundation. 1996. The Robert Wood Johnson Foundation Changes in Health Care Financing and Organization (HCFO) Program Meeting Report. Research on and Evaluations of Medicaid Managed Care: What Do We Need to Know? [Online]. Available: http://www.ac.org/httpdocs/mmc1115.html [07/18/97].

Rosenbaum, S., R. Serrano, M. Magar, and G. Stern. 1997. "Civil Rights in a Changing Health Care System." *Health Affairs* 16 (1): 90–105.

Rosenbaum, S., P. Shin, A. Mauskopf, K. Fund, G. Stern, and A. Zuvekas. 1995. "Beyond the Freedom to Choose: Medicaid, Managed Care, and Family Planning." *Western Journal of Medicine* 163 (Supplement): 33–38.

Rotwein, S., M. Boulmetis, P. J. Boben, H. I. Fingold, J. P. Hadley, K. L. Rama, and D. Van Hoven. 1995. "Medicaid and State Health Care Reform:

Process, Programs, and Policy Options." *Health Care Financing Review* 16 (3): 105–20.

Rowland, D. 1996. "Medicaid Managed Care: State Experiences." *Bulletin of the New York Academy of Medicine* 73 (Winter Supplement 2): 496–505.

Rowland, D., B. Lyons, A. Salganicoff, and P. Long. 1994. "A Profile of the Uninsured in America." *Health Affairs* 13 (2): 283–87.

Rowland, D., S. Rosenbaum, L. Simon, and E. Chait. 1995. *Medicaid and Managed Care: Lessons from the Literature*. Kaiser Commission on the Future of Medicaid.

Schauffler, H. H., and J. Wolin. 1996. "Community Health Clinics Under Managed Competition: Navigating Uncharted Waters." *Journal of Health Politics, Policy and Law* 21: 461–88.

Short, P. F., and J. S. Banthin. 1995. "New Estimates of the Underinsured Younger than 65 Years." *Journal of the American Medical Association* 274: 1302–06.

Shortell, S. M., R. R. Gillies, and D. A. Anderson. 1994. "The New World of Managed Care: Creating Organized Delivery Systems." *Health Affairs* 13 (5): 46–64.

Shortell, S. M., R. R. Gillies, D. A. Anderson, K. M. Erickson, and J. B. Mitchell. 1996. *Remaking Health Care in America: Building Organized Delivery Systems*. San Francisco: Jossey-Bass.

Showstack, J., N. Lurie, S. Leatherman, E. Fisher, and T. Inui. 1996. "Health of the Public: The Private-Sector Challenge." *Journal of the American Medical Association* 276: 1071–74.

Silverstein, G., and B. Kirkman-Liff. 1995. "Physician Participation in Medicaid Managed Care." *Social Science and Medicine* 41: 355–63.

Skocpol, T. 1996. *Boomerang: Clinton's Health Security Effort and the Turn Against Government in U.S. Politics*. New York: W.W. Norton & Co.

Sloan, F. A., J. F. Blumstein, and J. M. Perrin. 1986. *Uncompensated Hospital Care: Rights and Responsibilities*. Baltimore, MD: The Johns Hopkins University Press.

Starfield, B. 1996. "Public Health and Primary Care: A Framework for Proposed Linkages." *American Journal of Public Health* 86: 1365–69.

The Medicine/Public Health Initiative. 1997. The Medicine/Public Health Initiative [Online]. Available: http://www.sph.uth.tmc.edu/mph/ [09/17/97].

Ullman, R., J. W. Hill, E. C. Scheye, and R. K. Spoeri. 1997. "Satisfaction and Choice: A View from the Plans." *Health Affairs* 16 (3): 209–17.

U.S. Department of Commerce. 1996. *Statistical Abstract of the United States, 1996*. 116th ed. Washington, D.C.: Bureau of the Census.

Wagner, E. H., and T. Bledsoe. 1990. "The Rand Health Insurance Experiment and HMOs." *Medical Care* 28: 191–200.

Wallerstein, N. 1992. "Powerlessness, Empowerment, and Health: Implications for Health Promotion Programs." *American Journal of Health Promotion* 6: 197–205.

Wallerstein, N., and E. Bernstein. 1994. "Introduction to Community Empowerment, Participatory Education, and Health." *Health Education Quarterly* 21: 141–48.

Ware, J. E., M. S. Bayliss, W. H. Rogers, M. Kosinski, and A. R. Tarlov. 1996. "Differences in 4-Year Health Outcomes for Elderly and Poor, Chronically Ill Patients Treated in HMO and Fee-For-Service Systems." *Journal of the American Medical Association* 276: 1039–47.

Ware, J. E., R. H. Brook, W. H. Rogers, E. B. Keeler, A. R. Davies, C. D. Sherbourne, G. A. Goldberg, P. Camp, and J. P. Newhouse. 1986. "Comparison of Health Outcomes at a Health Maintenance Organization with Those of Fee-For-Service Care." *The Lancet* 1: 1017–22.

Warner, D. C. 1991. "Health Issues at the U.S.–Mexican Border." *Journal of the American Medical Association* 265: 242–7.

Weiner, J. P., and G. de Lissovoy. 1993. "Razing a Tower of Babel: A Taxonomy for Managed Care and Health Insurance Plans." *Journal of Health Politics, Policy and Law* 18: 75–103.

Weisman, C. S. 1996. "Proceedings of Women's Health and Managed Care: Balancing Cost, Access, and Quality." *Women's Health Issues* 6: 1–38.

Weissman, J. S., C. Gatsonis, and A. M. Epstein. 1992. "Rates of Avoidable Hospitalization by Insurance Status in Massachusetts and Maryland." *Journal of the American Medical Association* 268: 2388–94.

Wenneker, M. B., A. M. Epstein, and J. S. Weissman. 1990. "The Association of Payer with Utilization of Cardiac Procedures in Massachusetts." *Journal of the American Medical Association* 264: 1255–60.

Wickizer, T. M., M. Von Korff, A. Cheadle, J. Maescr, E. H. Wagner, D. Pearson, W. Beery, and B. M. Psaty. 1993. "Activating Communities for Health Promotion: A Process Evaluation Method." *American Journal of Public Health* 83: 561–67.

Williams, D. R. 1994. "The Concept of Race in *Health Services Research*: 1966 to 1990." *Health Services Research* 29: 261–74.

Appendix 7.1 Highlights of Selected Indicators of Equity of Access to Healthcare

Potential Access

Delivery System
Availability: Distribution of providers (NCHS 1997; Perloff et al. 1997)
Active non-federal physicians per 10,000 civilian population (1995):
  U.S. = 24.2;   D.C. = 63.6;   Texas = 19.4;   Alaska = 15.7.

Registered nurses per 100,000 resident population (1994):
  U.S. = 785.1;   Northeast = 987.0;   Midwest = 856.3;   South = 703.0;   West = 657.4.

Percent of office-based, primary care physicians not participating in Medicaid:

	1993 and 1994
• Total primary care physicians	18.8%
• General practice/family practice	14.7
• General internal medicine	17.3
• Pediatrics	15.7
• Obstetrics/gynecology	29.0

Organization: Types of facilities (NCHS 1997)
Community hospital beds per 1,000 civilian population (U.S.):
  1940 = 3.2;   1950 = 3.3;   1960 = 3.6;   1970 = 4.3;   1980 = 4.5;   1990 = 3.7;
  1994 = 3.5.

Health maintenance organizations (all plans, U.S.):
  1976 = 174;   1980 = 235;   1987 = 647;   1990 = 572;   1991 = 553;   1992 = 555;
  1993 = 551;   1994 = 540;   1995 = 550;   1996 = 628.

Nursing home beds per 1,000 resident population 85 years of age and over (U.S.):
  1976 = 685.3;   1986 = 542.1;   1991 = 494.5.

Inpatient and residential treatment beds in mental health organizations per 100,000 civilian population (U.S.):
  1970 = 263.6;   1980 = 124.3;   1984 = 112.9;   1990 = 111.6;   1992 = 107.4.

Financing: Sources of payment (Levit et al. 1996)
Percent distribution of selected expenditures for health services and supplies (U.S.):

	1960	1970	1980	1985	1990	1995
Public						
Federal government	9.0%	23.0%	29.2%	29.6%	29.0%	34.5%
State & local government	12.6	12.2	10.9	9.7	10.6	10.1
Private						
Private health insurance	21.2	23.2	28.6	30.2	32.8	31.5
Other private funds	1.8	2.6	3.6	3.7	3.5	3.1
Out-of-pocket payments	55.3	39.0	27.8	26.7	24.1	20.8

Appendix 7.1 (*continued*)

Population at Risk
Enabling: Regular source of care (Bloom et al. 1997a, 1997b)
Percent distribution of regular care by race, income (1993):

	Race				Income		
	White	Black	Hispanic		<$20,000	$35,000+	
Children 0–17 years							
No regular source of care	4.7%	7.5%	12.9%		10.6%	2.5%	
				<$10,000	$10,000–$19,000	$35,000–$49,000	$50,000+
Those with location							
Private doctor	91.5%	66.9%	70.0%	62.5%	72.8%	93.8%	94.0%
Clinic	5.0	25.3	25.0	32.2	20.2	3.3	3.2
Emergency Room	0.6	4.7	1.8*	3.2	2.9	0.6*	0.2*
Adults 18–64 years							
No regular source of care	15.8%	16.9%	28.1%	25.6%	25.4%	12.5%	9.8%
Those with location							
Private doctor	89.7%	71.2%	76.5%	61.1%	75.6%	91.3%	92.5%
Clinic	5.8	19.9	18.4	29.9	15.5	4.8	4.3
Emergency Room	1.2	4.3	1.6*	3.7	3.7	0.8	0.6

(* Estimate does not meet NCHS standard of reliability or precision.)

Enabling: Insurance coverage (Hellander et al. 1995; NCHS 1997; Short and Banthin 1995)
Percent of U.S. population without insurance:
   1987 = 12.9%;   1990 = 13.9%;   1992 = 15.0%;   1993 = 15.3%;   1994 = 15.2%;
   1995 = 15.4% (40.6 million people).

Percent of privately insured U.S. population who are underinsured for catastrophic illness:

	1977	1994
Total	12.6%	18.5%
Type of insurance:		
Nongroup	51.6%	40.7%
Any group	8.6	16.0

Percent of uninsured by race/ethnicity, income (under 65, 1993):

Race			Income		
White	Black	Hispanic	$50,000+	$25,000–49,999	<$25,000
11.9%	20.5%	31.9%	5.9%	12.3%	22.5%

Appendix 7.1 (*continued*)

Actual Access

Utilization

Type of use: Use of selected services (NCHS 1997)
Percent having had procedure or contact by race/ethnicity:

	Race/Ethnicity			
	White	*Black*	*Hispanic*	*Native American*
Began prenatal care, 1st trimester (1995)	83.6%	70.4%	70.8%	66.7%
Vaccinations, children (19–35 months) (1995)				
• Measles-containing or MMR	90.9	86.6	88.0	87.8
• DTP (3+ doses)	95.7	92.3	92.6	96.8
• Polio	89.2	83.6	86.4	91.3
• Combined Series DTP, Polio, MMR	78.6	71.9	71.2	74.2
Saw dentist, past year (adults 25+ years, 1993)	64.0	47.3	46.2	—

Purpose of use: Use of services relative to need (NCHS 1997)
Physician visits relative to need by race, income (1994):

	Race		*Income*	
Need	*White*	*Black*	*$50,000+*	*$LT 14,000*
Percent in fair or poor health	8.6%	16.1%	3.9%	20.4%
Percent with limitation in usual activity due to chronic conditions	14.0	18.0	9.2	26.4
Use				
Percent saw doctor, past year	79.6	79.5	83.7	78.0
Mean doctor visits, past year	6.1	5.7	6.0	7.6

Unmet need (Berk, Schur, and Cantor 1995)
Percent of people unable to obtain care by race, health status, income, insurance status, usual source of care (1994):

Race:	White	14.5%
	Hispanic	17.5
	Black	24.3
Health:	Good/excellent	14.7
	Fair/poor	29.9
Income:	> $50,000	7.9
	$20,000 – $50,000	16.6
	< $20,000	24.4
Insurance:	Insured	13.6
	Uninsured	33.7
Source of Care:	Has usual source	15.1
	No usual source	22.1

Appendix 7.1 (*continued*)
Satisfaction

General: Public opinion (Blendon, Benson, Donelan, Leitman, Taylor, Koeck, and Gitterman 1995)

Public's overall view of healthcare system (1994):

	U.S.	Canada	West Germany
• On the whole the healthcare system works pretty well, and only minor changes are necessary to make it better.	18%	29%	30%
• There are some good things in our healthcare system, but fundamental changes are needed to make it work better.	53	59	55
• Our healthcare system has so much wrong with it that we need to completely rebuild it.	28	12	11
• Not sure.	2	*	4
		(* < 0.5%)	

Perceived problems with healthcare system (1994):

• Country is spending too little on healthcare	48%	38%	17%
• Treated unfairly by healthcare system	28	11	22
• Quality of healthcare in community is fair or poor	35	27	28
• Had problem paying doctor and hospital bills last year	20	6	3
• Couldn't get needed medical care last year	12	8	6

Visit-specific: Patient opinion (Donelan, Blendon, Benson et al. 1996)
Consumers' views on general, specialist, and preventive care (1995):

	U.S.	Canada	West Germany
Access to care:			
• Not able to see a specialist	15%	14%	9%
• Not able to get diagnostic tests	18	19	12
• Not able to get needed medical care	12	8	6
Cost of medical care:			
• Out-of-pocket expenditures last year	$993	$302	$328
• Serious problem having enough money to pay doctor or hospital bills	20%	6%	3%

Chapter 8

Integrating Health Services Research and Policy Analysis

Health services researchers are routinely involved in producing information relevant to public policy debates. To further an understanding of suppliers and users of policy-relevant information, this chapter examines the role of health services research in policy analysis. The first section provides a brief overview of objectives and methods in policy analysis. The objectives of policy analysis are discussed in the context of the policymaking process, and different types of analysis are related to different stages of policymaking. Next, the application of health services research in policy analysis is explored. Aspects of effectiveness, efficiency, and equity research are related to policy-analytic tasks such as defining policy problems, predicting the potential consequences of proposed policies, and explaining the results of past policies. The final section reviews the limitations of health services research as a resource for policy analysis.

Concepts and Methods in Policy Analysis

Objectives of Policy Analysis

Whether public policies take the form of laws, programs, rules and regulations, or judicial decisions, they are made through a process of decisions or choices about the objectives of government and the means of achieving them.[1] This general characterization of policymaking applies to any level of government—federal, state, and local—and to any policy area, including education, defense, welfare, and health. The focus of policy analysis is on the decision-making process and the associated need for both descriptive and prescriptive information to facilitate public debate.

Descriptive information is factual material that documents social conditions (e.g., an increase in the number of uninsured people, or a decrease in health status variations among populations), or analyzes the potential or actual consequences of different policy alternatives (e.g., the number of people uninsured who would be covered under a national health insurance option, or an improvement in birth outcomes of women covered under Medicaid). The types of questions that descriptive information addresses are: Does a particular social condition exist? What are the consequences of a given policy? What are the potential consequences of a future policy?

Prescriptive information, on the other hand, goes beyond factual analysis to develop normative recommendations about whether a particular problem deserves the attention of policymakers, or whether a particular policy should be adopted. For example, after providing factual information about the populations that would be covered under various universal health insurance proposals, the analyst may recommend a proposal based on its potential for achieving a particular equity objective (e.g., an appropriate utilization pattern based on need). The goal of prescriptive analysis is to combine factual information about problem situations and policy consequences with normative information about the goals and objectives of policy to influence, redirect, or affirm a policymaker's attitudes, preferences, or beliefs. The assumption is that the analyst understands the policymaker's values, goals, and objectives and that the policymaker expects, or will at least consider, a recommendation. Prescriptive analysis is controversial in the policy analysis field because of its normative nature.

Recognizing these informational needs, the objectives of policy analysis are to contribute to the policymaking process by (1) producing or interpreting descriptive information about problems and the consequences of past or future options; and (2) developing prescriptive arguments or claims translating such information into recommendations for defining problems and formulating solutions (Dunn 1994; Patton and Sawicki 1993). The first objective involves conducting or interpreting analyses related to understanding the nature and causes of problems, and the effects of past or future policies on individual, institutional, system, or population behavior. The findings become the information used to develop or influence the arguments that support a specific policy recommendation. The second objective involves creating and critically assessing policy arguments by examining the values, logic, and underlying assumptions used by the analyst to translate the information into a policy claim.

The dual objectives of policy analysis suggest criteria for judging an analysis: *relevance, validity,* and *reasonableness.* Relevance refers to the extent to which the analyst addresses important policy questions, that is, those that are directly related to the decisions faced by the policymaker. For example, does the information respond to the specific and detailed questions that arise over a bill before Congress or over a legislative proposal being considered in the governor's office? It also refers to the extent that the analysis incorporates the policy context. Does the analysis reflect the appropriate degree of uncertainty about the nature of the problem, the state of existing programs, budgetary or administrative limitations, and appropriate time frames?

The information that is produced for the analysis must be valid. Validity in policy analysis is the same as for traditional science. Validity refers to the degree of accuracy of the information that is being used to identify actual causes of problems or to determine the consequences of policy alternatives. Unfortunately, causal statements about the effects of policy options cannot be verified in most instances short of the actual implementation of the policy. Therefore, although validity is an important criterion, establishing validity is problematic in policy analysis because decisions have to be made prior to policies being implemented. Conceptual frameworks, theories, and logical deduction, however, do provide guidance regarding the likely outcomes of a given policy and illuminate the assumptions underlying it.

The importance of reasonableness arises from recognizing the degree of uncertainty in policy analysis. The same facts (e.g., data showing that disparities in health status are growing among socioeconomic groups) often lead different analysts to different definitions of policy problems or to different recommended solutions (e.g., reforms in healthcare financing versus investments in social infrastructure). Such conflicts often focus on ideological or value differences that are typical in the policy process, such as different views of the basic role and responsibility of government in health. Sometimes the differences result from alternative frames of reference taken by the analyst, such as economic analysis versus political feasibility, as the basis for decision making. They may also rest on the underlying assumptions used by the analyst regarding human or institutional behavior. Recognizing that the same information may be interpreted in different ways leads to the realization that all policy analysis is to some extent subjective. Therefore, the reasonableness of a policy claim is used as a standard in lieu of the scientific standard of empirical verification. Reasonableness is defined as the extent to which a policy claim or argument meets certain criteria of logical structure and completeness. The goal of reasonableness is assessed through examining a policy argument's factual base, its underlying assumptions, and the logical structure supporting its conclusions (Bobrow and Dryzek 1987; Dunn 1994).

Dunn (1994) has specified that the key elements of a reasonable policy argument are

1. policy-relevant information leading to a recommendation;
2. warrants or assumptions that provide reasons why the information supports the recommendation;
3. backing to support further the warrants and recommendation, particularly under conditions of high uncertainty or controversy;
4. any special qualifiers to the recommendation; and
5. consideration of possible rebuttals to the argument.

A recommendation that the federal government contract with HMOs to serve the Medicare population illustrates the nature of each element. The basis of the argument is the information that HMOs are more efficient than traditional fee-for-service group or solo practices. A warrant explains why this information leads to the recommendation. In this case, the warrant might refer to the impact of healthcare costs on the federal budget or to the prospect of the Medicare system becoming insolvent. Further assumptions, arguments, or principles for the recommendation may be needed.

Additional backing for the HMO investment might include evidence that other cost-control strategies, such as physician fee controls, are less effective or have disadvantages compared to the HMO alternative. In the rebuttal, the analyst considers the information, reasons, assumptions, or qualifications under which the original claim would be false. The rebuttal in the HMO case might challenge the healthcare cost impact on the budget, the projected insolvency of Medicare, or the efficiency claim of HMO supporters.

Models of Policy Analysis

Different models of policy analysis exist, each with different views of the role of analysis and the type of analysis thought to be most useful to policymakers. The models are based on different views of the policy process and the nature of social problem solving. A broader comprehension of policy analysis in relation to these models facilitates a deeper understanding of the possible contribution of health services research.

The *rational-comprehensive model* of analysis, which dates back to the philosophical writings of John Dewey (1927) and other American pragmatists, depicts the policymaking process as a series of logical, well-defined stages of problem solving:

1. define the problem;
2. identify a range of alternatives with the potential to resolve the problem;
3. evaluate and select the alternative that best addresses the problem;
4. describe and evaluate the consequences of the selected alternative after it has been implemented; and
5. evaluate and modify the alternative in light of its consequences.

This model idealizes the policymaker as an objective well-informed individual whose primary purpose is to serve the public interest by selecting policies that maximize community welfare. The model, as applied by one of the founders of modern policy analysis (Lasswell 1951), suggests a process of relevant analyses for resolving problems in a logical and orderly manner. It implies a major role for policy analysis as a "meta-discipline," providing information and clarifying values needed to pursue logical solutions to substantive problems through multidisciplinary research. The objectives of such analysis are to consider all possible definitions of a problem in arriving at the correct definition; to express policy goals clearly and specifically so that policymakers can reach agreement; to conduct a thorough examination of all possible consequences of the variety of potential alternatives in developing a resolution; and to undertake an exhaustive assessment of all possible effects in evaluating the performance of the adopted policy and related actions. With this information, policy formulation becomes a straightforward, logical exercise in social problem solving.

Recognizing that information needed for policymaking is often limited and difficult to interpret, and that policymakers bring conflicting objectives to the policymaking process, leads to an alternative view of policy analysis referred to as the *incremental* or *satisficing model* (Hayes 1992; Lindblom 1959; Simon 1982). The policymaker's goal, according to the incremental model, is less ambitious: to find policies that are acceptable to a reasonable number of people and that alleviate some of the shortcomings in past policies. Whereas the rational-comprehensive model looks to correctly define the problem and select the optimal course of action to solve the problem, the incremental model selects the first choice that is minimally acceptable and through a process of feedback or successive experimentation strives to improve on the original choice. In this model, prospective policy analysis, which involves the production and analysis of information before policy actions are initiated and implemented, is less important than retrospective analysis, which provides feedback after policy actions have been taken.

For example, the rational-comprehensive approach to selecting a Medicaid managed care enrollment policy for clients might involve an extensive review of existing theory and empirical research on the effectiveness of different models of marketing and education. The policy selected would be that which seemed to best meet the objectives of the state. The incremental model would draw upon research to some extent, but would take into account the limits of research and the problem of getting policymakers to agree, arriving at an approach similar to the current approach and letting the results determine future policy. Proponents of this model of decision making believe that the process of successive incremental changes leads to the clarification of problems, objectives, and consequences of various alternatives, and eventually leads to better policy design. The major roles of analysis are to supply feedback through empirical testing of policies and to translate that information into policy modification.

The *mixed-scanning model* (Etzioni 1967) proposes that rationality in policymaking may be best served by applying aspects of both the comprehensive and incremental models at different times in policy development. Etzioni proposes that the strategic decisions that set basic policy directions—typically questions about the overall purpose of government and the priorities set for a program— be approached with detailed comprehensive analysis focused on goal attainment and identification of optimal strategies. However, for operational choices (e.g., budgeting, finance, and acquisition questions) incremental analysis and observation is perhaps more rational, because these policies are made in narrower and more discrete areas in which incremental actions are likely to be optimal.

The three rationalistic models—comprehensive, incremental, and mixed-scanning—have all been criticized for their failure to recognize the political nature of the policy process. As an alternative, a *political model* of policy analysis has been proposed that emphasizes the institutions and processes that are involved in policymaking, the multiplicity of stakeholders, the complex and sometimes overlapping systems of responsibility, and the conflicting motives and interests of policymakers (Longest 1994). This model challenges the characterization of policymaking as a rational process and the assumption that policymakers are motivated primarily to provide solutions to social problems or that policymaking institutions, such as Congress or state legislatures, are structured to facilitate such problem solving (Jones 1976; Peterson 1995). The political model portrays policymaking as a messy, fragmented, and often illogical process of conflict resolution and consensus building among self-interested groups (Stone 1988). Problems and solutions are addressed in this process only to the extent that they reflect the individual goals of powerful interest groups, not as a result of a cooperative process of problem solvers attempting to make the best possible decisions for the general public. Outcomes of the policy process depend more on the ability of affected groups to organize and to participate in the political process than on the extent to which a policy achieves a given performance standard.

The question for policy analysis, therefore, is how best to aggregate and reconcile the conflicting preferences to produce decisions. The symbolic analogy of the garbage can is used to depict the political model's view of policymaking as irrational and nonsystematic (March and Olsen 1976). The mix of garbage in the can depends on the garbage being produced at the moment, the number of cans available, and the speed with which garbage is collected and removed from the scene. This model suggests a role for analysis aimed primarily at predicting the potential winners and losers among stakeholders participating in the policymaking process.

The associated *radical planning model* for policy analysis also argues against the relevance of the rational model, and in its place offers a political process that encourages reasonable discourse among affected populations as a policymaking standard (Dryzek 1993). Habermas (1989) is a contributor to this model. It relies on participatory modes of inquiry (e.g., focus groups or other group processes) and the pursuit of reasonable debate in policy design (Fischer and Forester 1993; Forester 1993; Friedmann 1987). The emphasis on reasonable discourse shifts attention to important issues of political process and consensus formation largely ignored by the rational models. A particular group's success in mobilizing and the variations in involvement of one group or another become as important as the quality of the analysis and evidence that is used in the debate.

Textbooks on policy analysis continue to adhere to the rational model as a framework for analysts to follow in relating research to the policy process, despite the limitations of the model in describing the actual policy process (Dunn 1994; Patton and Sawicki 1993; Stokey and Zeckhauser 1978; Weimer and Vining 1989). It is widely recognized, however, that actual analysis may not follow the sequence of steps suggested by the model, may not be as thorough or rigorous as the model implies, and is much more politicized than the model suggests. The implication is that the execution of policy analysis should generally follow the rational model (i.e., attempt to clarify problems, systematically search for alternatives, and comprehensively evaluate alternatives) but that the analyst should also be aware of and influenced by the political process and, to the extent possible, be involved in ensuring that affected parties are included in the policymaking process.

The stages specified in the rational model do not imply a sequential strategy of carrying out the analysis relevant to a stage, completing that stage, moving to the next stage, and so forth. In order to assess new policies under realistic political and administrative conditions, it is necessary to produce information from each phase of policy analysis: problem structuring, forecasting policy consequences, and monitoring and evaluating past policies. Both prospective and retrospective analyses are required, making policy analysis truly interdisciplinary. Retrospective analysis typically draws on the disciplines of political science, sociology, and law, which have placed primary emphasis on providing information about the consequences of policies after they have been implemented. Prospective analysis typically builds on disciplines such as economics, information processing, and operations research, that have specialized tools for modeling and forecasting.

The limits of information and the political nature of the process in a given context must be considered in determining the type of analysis appropriate to a given question. Analyses should not be viewed as a substitute for the judgment, insight, and creativity of the policymaker. It is suggested, however, that more systematic analysis at different stages of the policy process will enhance policymakers' decisions. Finally, the analyst should seek greater involvement in the process of analysis of the groups and individuals to be affected by the policy, should encourage an open and visible process of decision making, should emphasize negotiation, and should recognize the role that values play in the entire policy process.

In the remainder of this chapter the types of analysis that are associated with different stages of the policymaking process are described and discussed.

Policymaking and Policy Analysis

The policy analyst works with a variety of research frameworks and methods to address policy questions. The appropriateness of a particular approach depends on the kind of question being asked and on the current stage of the policy process. In broad terms, one might include among the analyst's duties the collection and organization of data, the application of appropriate analytical techniques, the clarification of the issues involved, and the formulation of alternatives for resolution of a problem, perhaps with a recommendation on the best policy to adopt. This section describes in greater detail the types of analysis that are typically needed in different stages. Table 8.1 provides a summary list of policy decisions associated with each stage, the relevant information at each stage, and the various types of research and analysis that are appropriate.

Define problems

The objective in this stage is to clarify what the problem is about, why it exists, who it affects, and possible solutions. Analysis is necessary because most problems typically appear to the policymaker as the vaguely defined concerns of some interest group. There are two fundamentally different tasks involved in analysis. One is to determine what the policy goals ought to be. This is a values question that in the broadest terms is subject to differing views of the nature of health, the role of medical care and of non-medical factors in producing health, and the responsibility of government for health. Prescriptive arguments that assess the importance of various policy objectives (i.e., effectiveness, efficiency, and equity) and relate prevailing policy conditions to a more ideal mix of objectives or to a

Table 8.1   Stages of Policymaking, Relevant Information, and Type of Research

Stages of Policymaking	Relevant Information	Type of Research
1. Define problems	Scope, severity, causes, importance of the problem	Conceptual analyses or descriptive studies of the problems and causes
2. Identify alternatives	Forecasts of likely consequences of alternatives	Conceptual or empirical projections of the consequences of alternatives
3. Evaluate alternatives	Normative evaluations prior to action	Applications of normative frameworks for prescription
4. Describe consequences	Implementation and impact of policies and programs	Descriptive studies of program and policy effects
5. Evaluate consequences	Normative evaluation of consequences	Normative studies of program and policy effects

higher level of each are relevant to this task. The second is to suggest measures and techniques for clarifying the scope and magnitude of the problem and determining possible causes. Conceptual and empirical information that describes the scope and magnitude of the problem, explains the causes of existing conditions, and suggests possible solutions is relevant to the second task.

The first task involves clarifying the norms for judging whether a situation is problematic; a problem exists only when a perceived discrepancy between what ought to be and what is becomes a policy issue. To clarify the values at stake, policy objectives—including general goals and more detailed objectives and criteria—must be specified. Although there may be general concern about a situation, stakeholders often disagree on a precise standard to use in defining the seriousness of the problem, necessitating this first task.

To obtain information on policy objectives, one can conduct population surveys, consult experts or stakeholders, or review reports from public hearings or focus groups. One can ask the relevant policymaking body or affected populations, or rely on some kind of observational analysis of past decisions, legislation, testimony, or other written material to infer what the norms might be (Nagel 1988; Patton and Sawicki 1993). Sometimes expert panels can provide a standard. For instance, the AHCPR clinical guidelines described in Chapter 3 offer a standard for identifying a problem in the existing Medicare benefits policy: lack of coverage of mammography screening, an effective preventive procedure. There are occasions when government officials have defined a normative standard in specific terms, such as the Hill-Burton standard for the ratio of hospital beds to population (Blumstein 1986), or the Healthy People 2000 Health Objectives of the U.S. Public Health Service (NCHS 1996).

The second task is to describe the scope and magnitude of an undesirable situation. Usually, vague and often conflicting perceptions of an undesirable situation initially exist. The objective is to delineate the boundaries of the problem: the geographic location, the time the problem has existed, the historical events that have shaped it, the number of people it has affected, etc. For example, to address concerns about the high cost of medical care, the analyst might try to locate data showing the growth in costs; the relationship between the growth in medical service costs and other economic indicators, such as wages or price inflation; and the distribution of the cost burden on third-party payors and patients.

Different theoretical models or frames of reference are applied to classify problems and analyze possible causes (i.e., to explain the relationships between different dimensions or elements of a problem). For example, there are a variety of views on the nature and causes of problems represented by rapidly rising healthcare costs, by the uneven distribution of physicians between urban and rural areas, and by the general surplus of hospital beds. Much of the disagreement is based on the different theoretical frames of reference used by analysts to define the problem. Studies of the effects of health insurance coverage on hospital use and costs, research on factors affecting physicians' choices of practice locations, and inquiries about the social and behavioral determinants of health are the types of research to help define and clarify the nature and causes of a problem.

Successful completion of the two tasks involved in problem definition provides necessary information for moving to the next stage of policymaking—suggesting solutions through an understanding of the problem and of the policy objectives at stake. For example, critics of traditional fee-for-service Medicaid cite the following deficiencies in the program: inappropriate expensive services are often provided (e.g., primary care is obtained in hospital emergency rooms); no accountability for outcomes exists (e.g., information is rarely collected at the provider level on measures such as childhood immunization rates or pregnancy outcomes); and there is a lack of access to care (e.g., many providers do not accept Medicaid reimbursement). Many states are attempting to remedy these shortcomings by implementing managed care in their Medicaid programs.

Identify alternatives

In this stage, the analyst seeks to identify policy alternatives that have the potential to correct, compensate for, or counteract the causes of the problem. The generation of alternative policy options for consideration by policymakers combines methods for searching among existing strategies and conceiving, or creating, entirely new ideas (Alexander 1982). The identification phase may involve efforts designed to facilitate creativity, to carry out a systematic search, or both. Facilitating the creation of new solutions involves a variety of techniques ranging from group processes that strive to be non-judgmental or to enhance participants' ability to retrieve unrelated ideas or information from memory, to methods for an analyst to develop new solutions by modifying existing solutions in light of a given problem. A variety of more-or-less systematic search techniques may be employed to identify alternatives ranging from in-depth research and experimentation to quick surveys and literature reviews. The best approach will vary with the policy context and the resource and time limitations of the analysis.

Forecasting the potential consequences of alternatives provides useful information to policymakers in this phase of formulation. Statistical models and simulation techniques may aid the analyst in generating projections of policy consequences. For example, the PPRC compared baseline projections of physician payments under the Medicare RBRVS fee schedule prior to its actual implementation with payments under the customary, prevailing, and reasonable charge methodology (Colby 1992). During the 1992–94 national health reform debate, U.S. Congressional Budget Office forecasts of the budget effects of the Clinton Health Security Act and of other reform plans played a particularly important role (Peterson 1995). More commonly, the analyst must rely on theoretical inference or subjective opinion to project consequences.

Chapters 4 and 5 illustrate the use of economic reasoning and empirical evidence in the debate over the allocation of health resources through market incentives or through government regulations. Economic theory is often used to suggest that certain market conditions will lead to allocative efficiency or inefficiency. Such projections are based upon the validity of assumptions about the behavioral responses of providers and consumers to certain market conditions. A more subjective approach is to base forecasts on the opinions of others who have expertise or insight in a policy area. This may be done through personal interviews or literature reviews. The assessment of the validity of a subjective forecast depends solely on the recognized authority of the source.

In reforming Medicaid, many states considered incremental tactics other than managed care that had been used in the past to address the program's cost problems, such as shifting funds from

other state budgetary items, reducing benefit coverage for beneficiaries, or tightening eligibility requirements. In many instances,
these options were rejected because of their inconsistency with other
goals of the program. In other cases, they became options that were
seriously considered for evaluation.

Evaluate alternatives

In this stage of analysis, the projected consequences of policy alternatives are evaluated in terms of defined values and objectives.
Analytical tasks are the identification of the mix of goals and objectives that are to be used to evaluate different alternatives; the
translation of these goals and objectives into specific quantitative or
qualitative criteria; and their application to the projected effects of
alternatives (Weimer and Vining 1989). For example, to evaluate
alternative proposals for emergency transportation services, the
analyst may define the average rush-hour delay for vehicles as the
criterion related to the goal of improving access to urban trauma
centers. Changes in the cost of private ambulances may be another
criterion derived from the goal of economic efficiency. The analyst
applies these criteria to policy alternatives in order to clarify the
performance trade-offs represented by each alternative.

Practical difficulty arises when multiple goals must be balanced
to develop an overall assessment of alternatives. Various decision
models are available to assist the analyst with this problem. Some
of the more rigorous techniques include CBA, multiattribute utility
analysis, threshold analysis, optimum-mix analysis, and multigoal
analysis (McKenna 1980; Nagel 1988; Stokey and Zeckhauser 1978).
Unfortunately, these models require quantitative data and a level of
precision that is often not available to policy analysts. In practice, the
analyst's role is typically limited to clarifying how each alternative
meets each objective, leaving their prioritization to the policymaker.
In addition, qualitative methods such as focus groups and informal
polling are increasingly being used by analysts to assist the policymaker when conflicting goals are at stake (Friedmann 1987).

Again using Medicaid managed care as an illustration, a variety
of evaluation criteria must be considered in determining the consequences of such design issues as eligibility and enrollment, service
coverage, provider enrollment and selection, payment systems and

rate setting, and program administration issues (Freund and Hurley 1995). Criteria such as cost savings, administrative difficulty, political feasibility, impact on quality of care, and impact on access to care must be operationalized and applied to each design option in the context of a particular state. Summaries of the evaluation results, such as a table showing the results of the evaluations of each option in terms of each criterion, may be developed to guide decision making.

Describe consequences

A shift in focus occurs from prospective, or ex ante, analysis to retrospective analysis once the policy has been enacted. The analytic objectives in this stage are twofold: to determine the degree to which a policy or program was implemented as intended, and to measure anticipated and unanticipated effects. When monitoring implementation, the analyst asks if certain standards are being followed or if the policy or program reflects the intended use of resources. Specific indicators often used in monitoring policies and programs include measures of inputs (e.g., personnel, facilities, equipment, and supplies), processes (e.g., administrative, organizational, clinical, behavioral, political, and attitudinal), and outputs (i.e., the goods and services provided).

In measuring effects, the analyst attempts to determine whether a policy has brought about change, for example, in the behavior, attitudes, or health status of targeted individuals, groups, organizations, or communities. Quantitative methods for determining effects range from social systems accounting, in which the analyst monitors overall changes in health or other social status indicators (i.e., infant mortality rates) over time and attempts to relate the changes logically to past policies (prenatal care access interventions), to experimental and quasi-experimental evaluations of specific programs designed explicitly to isolate the effects of the programs from other factors (overall downward trends in infant mortality) (Dunn 1994).

As indicated in previous chapters, a substantial amount of research is being done to determine the consequences of state implementation of Medicaid managed care. This includes the examination of a variety of implementation issues, surveys of client and provider reaction, claims data analyses to determine changes in utilization and costs, as well as efforts to document any effects on the quality of care received by Medicaid recipients. Both qualitative and quantitative methods are being used in this research.

Evaluate consequences

This stage involves collecting and analyzing performance information to help policymakers decide to continue, to modify, or to terminate existing policies. In some cases, this stage leads to a redefinition of the original problem. To assess performance, the consequences of a policy are evaluated normatively in light of designated objectives and criteria. The menu of analytic tasks and methods used in the ex ante evaluation of alternatives is also relevant to this stage, but the focus is on evaluating actual rather than potential consequences. To evaluate performance, the analyst must define policy objectives, transform them into specific criteria that can be used in evaluation, and evaluate the consequences of a policy or program in terms of the criteria. As discussed earlier, the identification and use of norms in policy analysis is plagued with difficulties. Policymakers may not be able to determine from their various constituencies the appropriate goals in a particular context, they rarely are able to make explicit trade-offs between these goals, and they may have to consider implicit goals or hidden agendas that are not made explicit in the policy process. For example, evaluations indicating the cost-savings potential of Medicaid managed care are praised by those policymakers most concerned with the fiscal solvency of the program but are a concern for those who worry about the financial solvency of academic medical centers that are dependent on Medicaid revenues (Meyer and Blumenthal 1996).

The Role of Health Services Research in Policy Analysis

As described in the previous chapters, health services research seeks to clarify the goals and performance of the healthcare system in terms of the effectiveness, efficiency, and equity of service delivery. Theoretical frameworks, conceptual definitions and measures, methods and procedures, and data sources that have been developed in this research can be applied in policy analysis. The field has much to offer the policymaker interested in knowing the degree to which health policy goals are being realized and in identifying what alternatives improve the performance of the health system. The discussion that follows describes the health services research tools that are relevant in defining policy problems, identifying and evaluating alternatives, and monitoring and evaluating the consequences of past decisions.

Define Problems

The health services research field offers concepts and measures that can be used to clarify the standards of effectiveness, efficiency, and equity for use in defining problems. It has a variety of methods for describing the scope and magnitude of problems, and it offers both theory and method for examining causes of problems.

Effectiveness

As indicated in Chapter 2, the health services research literature suggests two possible ways of defining the goal of effectiveness in health policy analysis: the population perspective, focusing broadly on the importance of social, behavioral, and medical care factors to the health of the population; and the clinical perspective, focusing more narrowly on the clinical effectiveness of medical care for the individual patient. From the population perspective, effectiveness is defined in terms of the proportion of the population with a health problem who are benefited by treatment or by changes in social or behavioral circumstances. Policy analysis aimed at improving effectiveness in this way would compare the relative contributions of medical care and other population-oriented factors to the quality and quantity of life. The health problems associated with poverty, inadequate housing, smoking, or drug abuse might be contrasted with those resulting from poor access to medical care. Explicit analyses of the health effects of patient behavior and environmental conditions as well as the quality of medical care are relevant in this perspective.

The clinical perspective on effectiveness focuses more narrowly on the benefits achieved by patients receiving medical care under conditions of actual practice. Although often confused with the population perspective, this perspective is relevant when the policy question is limited to the performance of the medical care system as opposed to improving the health of the population as a whole. The evaluation standard might be stated in terms of actual benefits in medical practice compared to maximum achievable benefits—that is, in terms of efficacy. As noted previously the framework for defining problems of clinical effectiveness may involve the system, institution, or patient level (see Table 2.2).

Efficiency

The policy goal of efficiency in healthcare may also be approached in two ways: at the macrolevel, by encouraging the right mix of medical and non-medical health-related investments to maximize social welfare (i.e., allocative efficiency); or at the microlevel, by encouraging the right mix of inputs and production methods to maximize the productivity of the investments made (i.e., production efficiency). Criteria for analysis in both cases include production and cost standards deduced from microeconomic theory, and measures derived from applying the cost-effectiveness or cost-benefit frameworks.

The microeconomic model of the healthcare provider shows the relationship between different levels and mixes of inputs, input prices, and technology that minimizes the cost of services. It can be used in policy analysis when the concern is the production of a specific service or mix of services. For example, each setting for healthcare—such as a community health center, hospital, or nursing home—uses a particular combination of health personnel, supported by other inputs, to produce services. The microeconomic model suggests criteria that can be used to empirically identify the most efficient combination of personnel, supplies, and other inputs to support a particular level of health service.

The cost-effectiveness framework, on the other hand, may be used when the concern is the comparison of the relative efficiency of policies or programs that try to improve health through alternative methods of production. A cost-effectiveness ratio (e.g., cost per encounter, per case found, or per quality-adjusted life year) is computed for each alternative and compared to ratios for other alternatives. It is important to note that production efficiency also requires that services be effective. Efficiency analysis must be preceded by the technical appraisal of effectiveness. Once a policy or program is shown to be effective, either in clinical or population-oriented terms, cost-effectiveness analysis compares its relative effectiveness and costs to other options.

The broader goal of allocative efficiency is assessed using the cost-benefit framework. The analyst calculates and compares the costs and benefits of a policy, program, or service to determine if it adds to social welfare—that is, if the social benefits exceed the social costs. All relevant social costs—including cost-savings that may be associated with prevention services—and benefits must be identified and measured in dollars, if possible, so that comparisons of costs versus benefits can be made across all possible actions. Future costs and benefits must be discounted to reflect their present value. Subtracting costs from benefits yields net benefits, the criterion indicating increased social welfare. Allocative inefficiencies are indicated when the aggregate costs of a policy or program exceed its aggregate benefits.

Equity

As discussed in Chapter 6, equity goals of healthcare policy have traditionally derived from ethical principles of distributive justice involving the fair distribution of the benefits and burdens of medical care. Public health policy has been primarily governed by the social justice notion of promoting the health of the community as a whole. The deliberative justice paradigm is proposed as a policy formulation guide, bridging competing values by suggesting a process for policymaking in which affected parties participate and contribute. While debate continues over which norms should serve as the basis for defining equity in healthcare delivery and policy, specific goals and criteria can be derived that embody aspects of a number of alternative theories of equity (Table 6.2). Each can, in turn, be translated into quantitative or qualitative indicators, as explained in Chapters 6 and 7, to evaluate the extent to which equity has been achieved.

Equity criteria related to the healthcare delivery system are based on the characteristics of the delivery system (e.g., the availability and distribution of services), the characteristics of the population (e.g., ethnicity, gender, insurance coverage, and the availability of a regular source of care), the use of services, and satisfaction with services (Table 6.2). Equity-of-access objectives may be evaluated at the institutional, system, or community level by applying these criteria. Equity analysis in the context of the social justice paradigm may be applied to the distribution of health and health risks, and the relationship of health risks to the physical, social, and economic environment. Deliberative justice norms would assay the extent to which individuals and groups affected by policies at the micro or macrolevel participate in the formulation and implementation of these policies.

Identify and Evaluate Alternatives

In addition to defining and clarifying problems, health services research is helpful to policymakers in determining strategies for solving problems. Theoretical models may be adopted as the rational foundation for new proposals. In other instances, both theory and empirical studies may be referenced to depict the potential success of a strategy.

Effectiveness

The structure-process-outcomes framework developed by Donabedian (1966) as the conceptual guide for effectiveness research is useful in the policy-analytic task of a priori identification and evaluation of policy alternatives. This framework may be applied at the population level, with medical care and non-medical care strategies evaluated in terms of their contribution to the health of the population. It can also be applied at the system, institution, or patient level to evaluate possible ways to improve the effectiveness of medical care through manipulation of structure and process variables. The framework suggests the kind of data needed to identify possible solutions to an effectiveness problem. Evidence linking the elements of the framework to outcomes suggests targets for interventions. For example, in clarifying a policymaker's concern about the quality of care in nursing homes, the structure-process-outcomes framework suggests that the quality of nursing home care is influenced by structural factors such as the quantity of staff and their qualifications.

Quality, in turn, has an influence on outcomes, including mortality, morbidity, functional status, and client satisfaction. The framework indicates the structure and process factors that are subject to policy manipulation to improve the effectiveness of care.

From the population perspective, the evidence on the limited effectiveness of medical care in reducing mortality can be presented to suggest the need for investment in non-medical interventions. For example, in the case of certain forms of cancer mortality, it may be more effective to alter the physical environment—a structural intervention—in such a way that exposure to harmful pollutants is reduced—a process result. This reduced exposure should show reduced mortality from certain cancers over time as the outcome. Ultimately, this could prove a more cost-effective intervention than continued investment in medical care to treat cancer, the causes of which continue unabated.

Efficiency

Research concerned with allocative and production efficiency informs policymakers about what alternatives tend to result in the provision of effective services that are relatively inexpensive to deliver. Numerous empirical studies, for example, document that physicians and hospitals generally could use nonphysician inputs more efficiently (Reinhardt 1975), that HMO patients' use of hospitals is much less than that of fee-for-service patients with no corresponding reduction in the effectiveness of care (Miller and Luft 1994), and that cost sharing results in lower use and lower cost of medical care with little or no decline in health status for the average patient (Manning et al. 1987). Researchers are attempting to provide better information on the efficiency of a variety of specific medical care services aimed at common medical problems and on the resources, organizational arrangements, and financing mechanisms involved in their provision.

Solutions to efficiency problems may also be identified and evaluated through analysis of medical care market conditions (see Chapter 4). Microeconomic theory identifies market conditions that lead to inefficiencies in production or allocation if not corrected. Many of these conditions have been shown to be present in medical care markets. For example, the uncertain consequences of some types of medical care make it difficult for patients to judge what care is in their best interest. The gap in knowledge between patients and providers leaves patients vulnerable to inappropriate care, or care they would not choose for themselves if they were well informed. The external benefits and costs of some types of medical care (e.g., immunization to prevent infectious disease, which benefits populations as well as individuals), as well as investments in education, housing, and the environment, may not be appropriately valued by private markets, leading to inefficient allocation. Documenting the presence of such adverse conditions is another method used by analysts to suggest government interventions designed to improve efficiency.

It should be noted that applying the competitive economic model to enhance efficiency in healthcare assumes that maximizing satisfaction of consumer preferences is an appropriate policy goal. This is a value judgment that should be clearly stated when applying the model. An alternative model that emphasizes maximizing the population's health status, or meeting healthcare needs, is a substitute for consumer satisfaction in efficiency analysis. Both models are discussed in Chapter 4. Criteria for judging the determinants of allocative efficiency in the needs-based model are not as well developed as those in the competitive economic model.

Equity

The three primary policy strategies for enhancing equity, lodged in the distributive, social, and deliberative justice paradigms, were identified as (1) enhancing access to medical care; (2) reducing health disparities; and (3) assuring affected parties' participation in policy and program design. Empirical analyses of the relative importance of various factors presumed to influence whether or not people receive care, experience social and behavioral risk factors and poor health, and participate in the health policy process point to possible points of intervention for health policy to enhance equity. Potential access indicators discussed earlier may be used to identify potential solutions to an equity problem by examining the correlation of these indicators with realized access measures—utilization and satisfaction. Those factors that most directly influence access to needed services, such as insurance coverage or a regular source of medical care, then become the focus of the design and implementation of programs and services to enhance access.

Like efficiency analysis, equity research is ultimately concerned with those medical and non-medical services that are effective in the clinical or population sense—that is, in improving health and reducing health disparities. Equity criteria incorporating norms regarding those conditions that medical care can help to ameliorate (e.g., sentinel events, avoidable hospitalizations, or ambulatory care-sensitive conditions) embody the clinical effectiveness perspective (Weissman, Gatsonis, and Epstein 1992). Criteria incorporating norms regarding the health and health risks related to medical and non-medical (e.g., social-structural, cultural, and environmental) factors embody the population effectiveness perspective. The extent to which norms of democratic participation are involved in policy formulation or implementation is a criterion of equity based on the deliberative justice paradigm.

Describe and Evaluate Consequences

One of the major contributions made by health services researchers is informing policymakers about what does and does not work. The health system performance perspective of much of this research provides evidence that analysts can use to show the effects of past policies.

Effectiveness

Effectiveness research supplies a conceptual framework, methods, and evidence to describe and evaluate the technical effectiveness of health policies. Research linking structural factors—the quantity and efficacy of medical and non-medical inputs—to health outcomes can be conducted to assess the impact of a particular intervention on desired policy outcomes. In the same way, studies on the effects of process—the quantity, quality, and appropriateness of services delivered or of investments made—on health outcomes guide us in evaluating the success of options in changing the process of medical and social service delivery. Analysts use this information in measuring the consequences (e.g., lessening health disparities) of any given solution (investments in public housing), that can then be related to desired policy objectives (to improve the health of the population). Other examples of alternative interventions aimed at the policy objective of improving the health of the population include lifestyle modification through health promotion programs such as anti-smoking campaigns, or fluoridation of an entire community's water supply to reduce the incidence of dental caries.

Efficiency

The concepts, definitions, and methods health economists have developed to examine the allocative and production efficiency of healthcare are important resources for describing and assessing the consequences of policy actions. There are numerous studies of production efficiency, as outlined in Chapters 4 and 5, to guide evaluations of the organization and production of health services. The RAND Health Insurance Experiment discussed in prior chapters is a good example of this kind of research carried out with a rigorous, large-scale, experimental design. Findings indicated the costs and effects of alternative insurance strategies ranging from first-dollar coverage to catastrophic plans. Estimates were made of the excess spending that occurred under first-dollar coverage given the low marginal value of the added medical care services consumed. Studies of the efficiency of prepaid group practice are another important example. Many well-conducted cost-effectiveness studies have provided useful information on the relative efficiency of alternative services and technologies (see Chapter 5).

Equity

Both analytic research and evaluative research are relevant to the task of describing and evaluating the equity consequences of health policy and programs. Analytic research suggests causes of equity problems that are likely to be altered by private or government interventions. Empirical measurement of the effects of specific factors (e.g., social support available to high-risk mothers) form the primary basis for evaluating the equity consequences (prenatal care utilization rates) of alternative service delivery options (case management services). Evaluative research on access (reviewed in Chapter 6) is useful in actually informing policy analysts of the success of specific programs or policies (e.g., Healthy Cities and Community-Oriented Primary Care, aimed at community health) in enhancing procedural and substantive equity.

Difficulties in Linking Health Services Research to Policy

To the extent that the conceptual theories and empirical studies from effectiveness, efficiency, and equity research are neither well developed nor clear, the research is limited as a source of information and argument in policy analysis. The prior sections reviewed the potential contributions of health services research to policy analysis, while the discussion that follows highlights some of the limitations.

Effectiveness

No policy or professional consensus exists on whether the population or clinical perspective is more appropriate for defining effectiveness in healthcare delivery. The clinical perspective leaves out important factors that contribute to the health of the population. The population perspective requires that health policy address factors beyond the medical care system (e.g., housing and jobs). As indicated in Chapter 2, the clinical perspective has become more prominent of late in the United States in giving emphasis to research evaluating the outcomes of specific clinical practices. Related to the debate over perspectives is the question of defining health. From the population perspective, community health indicators are important. From the clinical perspective, individual patient health status is emphasized.

The imprecision of measures of effective medical practice is a critical weakness in applying effectiveness analysis at the clinical and population levels. Only rough estimates can be made of the direction and strength of the relationships between structure and outcomes and between processes and outcomes of care. Studies of variations in practice indicate that there is an extremely wide range of acceptable practice patterns (Chassin et al. 1986; Eisenberg and Nicklin 1981; Roos 1984; Schroeder et al. 1973; Wennberg and Gittelsohn 1982). However, the efforts by the federal government to invest in this type of research notwithstanding, it is difficult to determine precisely how much of the variation can be attributed to the provision of ineffective services.

Another limitation is that the extensive research on the medical and non-medical determinants of health has not often been well linked across the levels of analysis defined in Chapter 2. Approaches that appear to be beneficial at one level may not be effective at the next level of analysis. For example, improving the quality of care of individual patients may not be effective at the community level because of the limited potency of medical care interventions. When policymakers decide how they will invest societal resources in improving the health of the population, they must take into account not only what works for the individual patient, but how these resources are best utilized. Without information across all levels of analysis, ineffective decisions can and will be made.

Efficiency

Efficiency research provides useful but limited information on the optimal allocation of resources and on optimal production methods. We are only beginning to understand the effects of healthcare and other important medical and non-medical investments on health and well-being. Without this information, the social value of resource-allocation decisions cannot be determined with precision. The relative efficiency of different organizational models and resource mixes for producing medical care are not clear, despite the extensive research in some areas—for example, comparing managed care and non-managed care models of physician care, and comparing hospital inpatient and outpatient settings for the provision of various procedures and services. A conceptual difficulty in applying allocative efficiency criteria to the evaluation of policy alternatives is that the distributional consequences of alternatives (i.e., some win and some lose as a result of each alternative) cannot be assessed. Pareto optimum criteria that the beneficiaries compensate the payors can be used (Chapter 4), but this may not be ethically acceptable if there are no mechanisms for ensuring that winners compensate losers.

Another important limitation is that different methods are applied by researchers doing efficiency research (e.g., cost-effectiveness, cost-benefit, cost-utility, and cost-of-illness), limiting the ability to make comparisons across projects. Guidelines have been developed, however, for researchers to follow (Gold et al. 1996). There are also limitations associated with macrointernational comparisons of efficiency—the lack of standard definitions of health services, the differences in national accounting practices, and difficulties in adjusting for currency differences.

Equity

The focus of equity research would be enhanced if there were greater clarity and consensus on equity objectives. Chapter 6 proposes multiple paradigms that provide the basis for alternative principles and indicators of equity. Some of the frameworks potentially conflict, making it difficult to apply the criteria in policy analysis. In addition, each framework has multiple criteria. An expanded conceptual framework of equity (Figure 6.1) has been presented that integrates these criteria, considering procedural and substantive equity and their interrelationship. The causal relationships between procedural and substantive indicators of equity have not been thoroughly and uniformly documented. The challenge to health services research and policy analysis is to more accurately and fully document the contribution of medical and non-medical factors to reducing health inequalities—the ultimate criterion of substantive equity—across social and economic groups.

Summary and Conclusions

This chapter describes competing models of the policy process and their implications for policy analysis. The rational model is described as a guide that policy analysts and health services researchers can use to identify the types of research most relevant to specific health policy questions. This model identifies the sequential stages of the policymaking process, the relevant policy analysis that is most appropriate, and the information and types of research needed to guide decision making at each stage. The stages of the rational model of policy analysis, however, have been augmented by adding an awareness of, and attempting to take into account, the critiques of this model offered by the political and radical models. Health services research that meets the standards of scientific integrity, and is concerned broadly with both medical and non-medical determinants of health, provides a rich resource for the policymaking process.

Note

1. Our discussion focuses on public policymaking. However, the concepts, terms, and methods presented are generally applicable to the private sector as well.

References

Alexander, E. R. 1982. "Design in the Decision-Making Process." *Policy Sciences* 14: 279–92.

Blumstein, J. F. 1986. "Providing Hospital Care to Indigent Patients: Hill-Burton as a Case Study and a Paradigm." In *Uncompensated Hospital Care: Rights and Responsibilities*. Edited by F. A. Sloan, J. F. Blumstein, and J. M. Perrin, 94–107. Baltimore, MD: The Johns Hopkins University Press.

Bobrow, D. B. and J. S. Dryzek. 1987. *Policy Analysis by Design*. Pittsburgh, PA: University of Pittsburgh Press.

Chassin, M. R., R. H. Brook, R. E. Park, J. Keesey, A. Fink, J. Kosecoff, K. Kahn, N. Merrick, and D. H. Solomon. 1986. "Variations in the Use of Medical and Surgical Services by the Medicare Population." *The New England Journal of Medicine* 314: 285–90.

Colby, D. 1992. "Impact of the Medicare Physician Fee Schedule." *Health Affairs* 11 (3): 216–26.

Dewey, J. 1927. *The Public and Its Problems*. New York: H. Holt.

Donabedian, A. 1966. "Evaluating the Quality of Medical Care." *Milbank Memorial Fund Quarterly* 44 (Part 2): 166–206.

Dryzek, J. S. 1993. "Policy Analysis and Planning: From Science to Argument." In *The Argumentative Turn in Policy Analysis and Planning*. Edited by F. Fischer and J. Forester, 213–32. Durham, NC: Duke University Press.

Dunn, W. N. 1994. *Public Policy Analysis: An Introduction*. 2nd ed. Englewood Cliffs, NJ: Prentice Hall.

Eisenberg, J. and D. Nicklin. 1981. "Use of Diagnostic Services by Physicians in Community Practice." *Medical Care* 19: 297–309.

Etzioni, A. 1967. "Mixed Scanning: A Third Approach to Decision Making." *Public Administration Review* 27: 385–92.

Fischer, F. and J. Forester. 1993. *The Argumentative Turn in Policy Analysis and Planning*. Durham, NC: Duke University Press.

Forester, J. 1993. *Critical Theory, Public Policy and Planning Practice: Toward a Critical Pragmatism*. Albany, NY: State University of New York Press.

Friedmann, J. 1987. *Planning in the Public Domain: From Knowledge to Action*. Princeton, NJ: Princeton University Press.

Freund, D. A. and R. E. Hurley. 1995. "Medicaid Managed Care: Contribution to Issues of Health Reform." *Annual Review of Public Health* 16: 473–95.

Gold, M. R. J. E. Siegel, L. B. Russell, and M. C. Weinstein. 1996. *Cost-Effectiveness in Health and Medicine*. New York: Oxford University Press.

Habermas, J. 1989. *The Structural Transformation of the Public Sphere: An Inquiry Into a Category of Bourgeois Society*. Translated by T. Burger. Cambridge, MA: MIT Press.

Hayes, M. T. 1992. *Incrementalism and Public Policy*. New York: Longman.

Jones, C. 1976. "Why Congress Can't Do Policy Analysis (Or Words to that Effect)." *Policy Analysis* 2: 251–64.

Lasswell, H. D. 1951. "The Policy Orientation." In *The Policy Sciences: Recent Developments in Scope and Methods*. Edited by D. Lerner and H. D. Lasswell, 3–15. Stanford, CA: Stanford University Press.

Lindblom, C. 1959. "The Science of Muddling Through." *Public Administration Review* 19: 79–88.

Longest, B. B. Jr. 1994. *Health Policymaking in the United States*. Chicago: AUPHA Press/Health Administration Press.

Manning, W. G., J. P. Newhouse, N. Duan, E. B. Keeler, A. Leibowitz, and M. S. Marquis. 1987. "Health Insurance and the Demand For Medical Care: Evidence from a Randomized Experiment." *American Economic Review* 77 (3): 251–77.

March, J. and J. Olsen. 1979. *Ambiguity and Choice in Organizations*. 2nd ed. Bergen: Universitetsforlaget.

McKenna, C. K. 1980. *Quantitative Methods For Public Decision Making*. New York: McGraw-Hill.

Meyer, G. S. and D. Blumenthal. 1996. "TennCare and Academic Medial Centers: The Lessons from Tennessee." *Journal of the American Medical Association* 276: 672–76.

Miller, R. H. and H. S. Luft. 1994. "Managed Care Plan Performance Since 1980: A Literature Analysis." *Journal of the American Medical Association* 271: 1512–19.

Nagel, S. 1988. *Policy Studies: Integration and Evaluation*. New York: Greenwood Press.

National Center For Health Statistics. 1996. *Healthy People 2000 Review, 1995–96.* Hyattsville, MD: Public Health Service.

Patton, C. V. and D. S. Sawicki. 1993. *Basic Methods of Policy Analysis and Planning.* 2nd ed. Englewood Cliffs, NJ: Prentice Hall.

Peterson, M. A. 1995. "How Health Policy Information Is Used in Congress." In *Intensive Care: How Congress Shapes Health Policy.* Edited by T. E. Mann and N. J. Ornstein, 79–125. Washington, D.C.: American Enterprise Institute, The Brookings Institution.

Reinhardt, U. E. 1975. *Physician Productivity and the Demand For Health Manpower: An Economic Analysis.* Cambridge, MA: Ballinger Publishing Company.

Roos, N. P. 1984. "Hysterectomy: Variations in Rates Across Small Areas and Across Physicians' Practices." *American Journal of Public Health* 74: 327–35.

Schroeder, S. A., K. Kenders, J. K. Cooper, and T. E. Piemme. 1973. "Use of Laboratory Tests and Pharmaceuticals: Variation among Physicians and Effect of Cost Audit on Subsequent Use." *Journal of the American Medical Association* 225: 969–73.

Simon, H. A. 1982. *Models of Bounded Rationality.* Cambridge, MA: MIT Press.

Stokey, E. and R. Zeckhauser. 1978. *A Primer For Policy Analysis.* New York: W.W. Norton.

Stone, D. A. 1988. *Policy Paradox and Political Reason.* Glenview, IL: Scott, Foresman and Co.

Weimer, D. L. and A. R. Vining. 1989. *Policy Analysis: Concepts and Practice.* Englewood Cliffs, NJ: Prentice Hall.

Weissman, J. S., C. Gatsonis, and A. M. Epstein. 1992. "Rates of Avoidable Hospitalization by Insurance Status in Massachusetts and Maryland." *Journal of the American Medical Association* 268: 2388–94.

Wennberg, J. E. and A. Gittelsohn. 1982. "Variations in Medical Care among Small Areas." *Scientific American* 246 (4): 120–34.

Chapter 9

Applying Health Services Research to Policy Analysis

This chapter concludes the book by applying the effectiveness, efficiency, and equity objectives to a policy analysis of state health reform. Seven state models that represent a broad range of strategies for expanding coverage, controlling costs, and improving the quality of healthcare are described and analyzed. The analysis is patterned after prospective policy analyses that have appeared in the health services research literature comparing and evaluating major reform initiatives at the national or state level (Aday et al. 1993; Brown 1988; Feldstein 1988; Somers and Somers 1977; Thorne et al. 1995).

First, the state plans are described in terms of five key dimensions related to the inclusiveness and comprehensiveness of public coverage, methods for expanding private coverage, and strategies for containing costs and assuring the quality of care. Each state's plan is then classified on continua for each dimension locating the state's strategy along the spectrum of possible strategies for each dimension. The likely effectiveness, efficiency, and equity of strategies on particular points of the continua are assessed. Explicit criteria are developed for each objective and applied to the respective dimensions to determine if, and how, a particular strategy is likely to perform within a given dimension with respect to the criteria. Evidence for the evaluation is conceptual and descriptive, based on a review of health services research literature.

The purpose of the analysis is to illustrate the application of health services research in helping policymakers choose among state reform options. The evaluation builds upon descriptive comparisons of state reforms that have appeared in the literature (Gold, Sparer, and Chu 1996; Holahan et al. 1995; Moon and Holahan 1992). These analyses are helpful in comparing different strategies, but they stop short of analyzing the strengths and weaknesses of different approaches. In an attempt to be more analytical, the likeliness of reforms to affect the effectiveness of care, equity of access, and efficiency of service delivery is assessed. A normative framework is proposed for evaluating alternative plans, and the framework is used to suggest a set of criteria that might guide policy decisions.

The analysis focuses on a realistic range of policy options that are being considered or implemented as the responsibility for healthcare reform shifts to the states. It should be noted that state health reform is a moving target, changing as political and economic circumstances change (Crittenden 1995; McDonough, Hager, and Rosman 1997; Sparer 1995). This analysis is based on formulated or, in some cases, implemented policies in particular states as of 1995–1996. The strategies represented by the state plans will undoubtedly evolve in the future as they have in the recent past. Nevertheless, the issues that have generated the reforms are not likely to disappear and the strategies examined here illustrate options that are likely to be considered in the future as well.

The analysis is limited to the theoretical potential of the plans. Clearly, states face numerous political and administrative challenges in effectively implementing reforms and a comprehensive analysis should include an examination of the prospects for successful implementation as well (Moon and Holahan 1992; Sparer 1995). The evaluation also does not explicitly address the role that the healthcare environment plays in determining a strategy's success in a particular state. For example, reliance on a pro-market strategy to achieve cost containment may be more likely to succeed in a state with a large and relatively mature managed care system. On the other hand, a regulatory or market-minimizing approach is more likely to succeed in a state with a history of regulatory policies and practices upon which to build. The analysis also does not consider other criteria besides health system performance for judging policy options. Obviously, the impact of health reform on labor markets and the economy, their consistency with current financing and organizational structures, and their political feasibility are important factors that policymakers must consider.

Dimensions of State Health Reform

Many states have been making changes in their health systems since the late 1980s and early 1990s. Several states were pursuing broad-based reform in the direction of controlling costs, increasing access and coverage, and improving healthcare performance for all. The options considered by states ranged from mandates that employers provide health coverage to their workers (e.g., Massachusetts, Oregon, and Washington), to serious consideration of a "Canadian-style" single payor system (e.g., Vermont) to an intermediate tax-financed managed competition system (e.g., Colorado). Proponents argued that comprehensive reform was needed for effective cost control and significant coverage expansion. Due to the demise of national reform in 1992–93 in some cases and to a simple change in local political support in others, the comprehensive reform efforts were short-lived. Currently, incremental strategies for reform have gained center stage with moderate, but steady, progress by several states in this regard.

Table 9.1 classifies the seven selected state plans in terms of continua for five dimensions: (1) inclusiveness of public coverage; (2) comprehensiveness of public benefits; (3) regulatory versus voluntary methods for expanding private coverage; (4) regulatory versus pro-market methods to contain costs; and (5) regulatory versus pro-market methods to ensure quality of care. The state plans are similar in some respects; for example, all states are encouraging publicly and privately covered populations to enroll in managed care plans. Diversity is present in the varying degrees of reliance on private mechanisms—in market-maximized plans—versus government interventions—market-minimized plans—to achieve goals of improved health system performance. (See Chapter 5 for a discussion of market-maximizing versus market-minimizing policy strategies.)

Inclusiveness of Public Coverage

The first continuum, which concerns the inclusiveness of public coverage, groups states according to the extent to which the state is attempting to provide coverage for all citizens who have not obtained coverage in the private sector through a single public program. States following an inclusive strategy are attempting to cover

Table 9.1   Dimensions of State Health Reform

States	Calif.	Florida	Hawaii	Maryland	Minn.	Oregon	Tenn.
1. Inclusiveness of public coverage							
Universal							
↑ All uninsured in single program		X	X		X	X	X
Medicaid expansion for child and family				X			
Independent program for ↓ child and family	X	X					
Narrowly targeted							
2. Comprehensiveness of public benefits							
Comprehensive							
↑ Broad package with few limits or copays					X		X
Basic package with limits or copays		X	X			X	
↓ Limited package	X			X			
Limited							
3. Regulatory vs. voluntary methods to expand private coverage							
Regulatory							
↑ Employer mandates			X				
Systemwide regulatory reform				X			
Systemwide market reform	X	X			X		
Small group insurance ↓ reform	X	X	X	X	X	X	X
Voluntary							
4. Regulatory vs. pro-market methods to contain costs							
Regulatory							
↑ Price and budget controls				X	X	X	X
Managed competition	X	X			X		
↓ Managed care	X	X	X	X	X	X	X
Pro-market							
5. Regulatory vs. pro-market methods to ensure quality							
Regulatory							
↑ Specific mandates		X		X		X	
Collection/dissemination of performance data	X			X	X		X
↓ Licensing			X				
Pro-market							

all uninsured populations through statewide Medicaid expansions (e.g., a Medicaid waiver program enrolling low-income adults not categorically eligible for Medicaid as well as populations typically eligible for Medicaid, such as pregnant women and children). These extensive public programs are funded through a variety of federal, state, and local taxes. They differ in terms of the maximum level of income allowed for eligibility, with the highest level at 400 percent and the lowest at 100 percent of the federal poverty level (FPL), and in the extent to which the coverage is subsidized.

In the middle of the continuum is a more common strategy being followed by states in which Medicaid is extended to certain groups categorically eligible for the program. This strategy focuses on expanding coverage for optional groups allowed by Medicaid law, for example, "near-poor" children and pregnant women. The goal of these state initiatives is to make public coverage broader and more consistent across age groups. This more incremental strategy became a national policy with the Children's Health Insurance Program, the five-year $24 billion federal initiative to expand coverage of low-income children passed as part of the 1997 Federal Budget Agreement. The strategy leads to much larger Medicaid programs. However, it is significantly less inclusive than the universal strategy, leaving major responsibility for coverage of uninsured populations who do not fit the categorical requirements for Medicaid—mainly non-disabled adults without children—to other levels of government or to the private sector.

At the targeted end of the continuum are the independent coverage programs being adopted in some states in which Medicaid expansions have proved politically or administratively unworkable. Most states are financing coverage for children through such programs, but a few states have developed programs to subsidize coverage for families—adults and children—without the benefit of federal Medicaid funds.

Comprehensiveness of Public Benefits

The second dimension—comprehensiveness of public benefits—refers to the types of services and copayment provisions of the public insurance programs. On one end of the continuum are states covering a set of services equal to or greater than that included in state Medicaid programs with few restrictions or copayments. Medicaid benefit packages typically are more comprehensive than commercial insurance plans, and include such services as inpatient and outpatient care; mental health and substance abuse treatment; vision; hearing; dental care; nursing home care; and an enhanced set of primary care and preventive benefits, such as well-child screening, home visits, nutrition counseling, childbirth education, and parenting classes. Medicaid coverage has no copays and deductibles unless specifically granted by federal waiver.

In the middle of the benefits continuum are expansion programs that attempt to provide coverage for a "basic" benefit package. These states typically design a public benefit package that is roughly similar to that available in the private insurance market with additional exclusions, such as preventive care services, or with restrictions or caps on the use of services. They also may have significant copays and deductibles.

On the other end of the continuum are state initiatives that provide coverage for only a limited set of basic services, such as inpatient care only or primary and preventive care only. This strategy is designed to improve access to important services but it also further segments and distinguishes the coverage available to different groups, creating administrative and political issues related to eligibility determination and to continuity and coordination of care.

Expanding Private Coverage

The third dimension is concerned with strategies for expanding private coverage. The main benefit of these strategies is that the government can pursue the goal of additional private coverage while avoiding the political risks of raising taxes to fund public programs. These strategies also have the advantage of building on the current system of employment-based coverage. The strategies range from employer mandates that require employers to finance health insurance for their employees to small group insurance reforms designed to make coverage more attractive to employers and employees in small businesses. Government-imposed mandates requiring employers to offer employee health insurance have been proposed in several states but implemented only in Hawaii, and represent the most regulatory strategy being used to expand private coverage.

Several states are following voluntary coverage strategies that involve price and budget controls or market reforms to reduce costs and make private coverage more available and more attractive. These strategies are voluntary in the sense that they rely on voluntary coverage expansions as employers and individuals respond to improved conditions in the market achieved either through systemwide regulatory reform or through such market reform strategies as competitive bidding, purchasing pools, and the provision of better information for providers and consumers.

The least interventionist voluntary strategy is reflected in small business and individual insurance reforms designed to encourage private coverage. This strategy is being followed by all seven states, and is the most voluntary because it requires insurers serving only a particular part of the market to include or to offer certain benefits in their health policies and prohibit certain restrictive underwriting practices. These reform laws attempt to expand coverage by making insurance more available and less costly for small businesses.

Cost Containment

Cost-containment strategies also are highly variable, ranging from regulatory efforts with government-imposed price and budget controls, to a mix of regulatory and market-enhancing interventions promoting managed competition, to reliance on the current market shift to managed care. Regulatory states are attempting to contain costs through strategies aimed at controlling the organization or supply of healthcare resources, the prices charged by providers or their operating or capital budgets, or the premiums or capitation rates charged by insurance companies and HMOs. Managed competition states are attempting to control costs through publicly sponsored health financing reforms designed to enhance price competition among health plans and providers. This strategy includes the development of purchasing pools and other state-sponsored provisions of managed competition. The extreme pro-market strategy relies solely on the expansion of managed care to increase effectiveness and efficiency, without any market enhancing or regulatory efforts by the state. States following this strategy are relying on the increasingly competitive market forces to produce change in healthcare delivery and financing.

Improving Quality

The final dimension of state reform concerns the efforts to ensure accountability for high quality care. The range of strategies within this dimension include those focusing on specific mandates for consumer or provider protection, those encouraging self-regulation through the collection and dissemination of performance data, or, in some states, strategies relying on licensing and the industry's motivation to voluntarily self-regulate. The growth of managed care is shaping these policies. Concerns about arbitrary treatment of providers and consumers have prompted government enactment of "any willing provider" and "freedom-of-choice" laws mandating certain procedures and practices among managed care plans. Safeguards include guidelines to regulate the use of participating provider lists as marketing tools and procedures that plans must use when terminating provider agreements. Several states have passed laws requiring managed care companies to contract with any physician who agrees to the terms and conditions of a health plan, and have also passed laws requiring insurers and MCOs to provide enrollees with descriptions of their benefit contracts. These actions reflect the policy strategy of mandating protections for consumers or providers (Mariner 1996; Tannenbaum 1996). State laws requiring health insurance and managed care plans to pay for minimum postnatal hospital stays are another illustration of this approach.

Rather than mandates, some states are pursuing a more indirect educational and informational strategy. Assuming that the problem of poor quality is associated with the lack of performance data, many states are actively involved in the collection and dissemination of data aimed at improved decision making by consumers, purchasers, and policymakers (Tanenbaum 1996). A number of states are developing standardized encounter data to analyze utilization and treatment patterns, consumer report cards that rate plans, and comprehensive health plan quality indicators.

At the other extreme of this dimension is the strategy of relying on the industry to weed out poor quality plans and providers. Under this strategy, the state's role in ensuring quality is limited to its licensing function.

Description of State Plans

The following provides a brief characterization of the major features of selected state's reform efforts. The descriptive material is based on a variety of sources describing and comparing different state reforms (Alpha Center 1995; Beatrice 1996; Boles and Hicks 1996; Casey, Wellever, and Moscovice 1997; Coughlin et al. 1994; Crittenden 1995; Gold, Sparer, and Chu 1996; Holahan et al. 1995; Iglehart 1994; Intergovernmental Health Policy Project 1995; Lipson and Schrodel 1996; McManus and Thai 1996; Moon and Holahan 1992; National Institute for Health Care Management 1994; Riley 1995; Shriber 1997; Stearns et al. 1997; Thorne et al. 1995; Vladeck 1995). In addition, a number of sources specifically concerned with a given state's plan were incorporated for California (Sparer 1995), Florida (Gold, Aizer, and Salganicoff 1997; Mitchell and Norton 1996; Vogel and Miller 1995), Hawaii (Gardner and Neubauer 1995), Minnesota (Blewett 1994; Kralewski et al. 1995; Wascoe 1995), Oregon (Fleck 1994; Gates 1995; Gold, Chu, and Lyons 1995; Tengs 1996), and Tennessee (Gold, Frazer, and Schoen 1995; Meyer and Blumenthal 1996; Mirvis et al. 1995).

Inclusiveness of Public Coverage

Table 9.2 summarizes the strategies of the state plans for expanding public coverage. Inclusive strategies covering all low-income uninsured in one program are represented by Florida, Hawaii, Minnesota, Oregon, and Tennessee—states that are attempting to cover all uninsured families and individuals in single state and federal sponsored Medicaid plans. Florida created the Health Security Plan, a government-subsidized, low-premium basic benefit health plan for people below 250 percent of the federal poverty level (FPL) who have been uninsured for 12 months. The plan received an 1115 federal waiver allowing the state to use federal Medicaid funds for the expansion. In order to meet the required federal budget neutrality provision, Florida sought to accomplish the expansion

Table 9.2 Inclusiveness of Public Coverage

State	Universal ← All Uninsured in Single Program	Medicaid Expansion for Children & Families	→ Narrowly Targeted Independent Program for Children & Families
California			Children up to 100% of poverty who are ineligible for Medicaid
Florida	All citizens up to 250% FPL with persons above 100% FPL required to pay percent of premium		School children who qualify for school lunch program
Hawaii	All citizens up to 300% FPL with persons above 100% required to pay percent of premium		
Maryland		Children up to age 5 between 133–185% FPL, and from age 6–13 between 100–185% FPL	
Minnesota	All children and families with children up to 275% FPL, single adults and couples without children up to 125% FPL, with persons above 100% required to pay percent of premium		
Oregon	All persons up to 100% FPL		
Tennessee	All citizens up to 400% FPL with persons above 100% FPL required to pay percent of premium		

by requiring all Medicaid recipients to receive care from managed care plans that would compete for enrollees through regional purchasing alliances. However, the waiver to implement the program has not been approved by the legislature. It would have guaranteed coverage in private plans with an amount subsidized by the state.

Hawaii Health QUEST, created in 1993, integrates Medicaid, the State Health Insurance Program, and the state's general assistance program into a single purchasing pool to provide a standard package of benefits for all uninsured individuals with incomes up to 300 percent of the FPL. The program began in the summer of 1994 and all beneficiaries are enrolled in managed care plans. Faced with growing costs, the program has had to restrict eligibility and introduce additional copayments. Under the current plan, people between 100 and 133 percent of the poverty level are required to pay a portion of the premium; self-employed people must pay at least half of their premiums; people who are unemployed are not eligible; and college students under age 21 must have their parents' income taken into account when applying for coverage.

Like Health Quest and the Health Security Plan, MinnesotaCare, the Oregon Health Plan, and TennCare are comprehensive statewide programs that reflect the government's commitment to provide coverage to all low-income uninsured persons. Originally passed in 1992, MinnesotaCare will be the primary source of coverage for uninsured families and individuals. Currently, the program provides comprehensive coverage for those not on Medicaid who have been uninsured for at least four months and have not had access to employer-subsidized coverage for at least 18 months. Subsidized coverage is available on a sliding scale to single adults and childless couples with incomes up to 125 percent of the FPL. MinnesotaCare covers children and families with children with incomes up to 275 percent of the FPL. Over time, the state plans to apply for waivers to incorporate Medicaid and other indigent care programs in the state into MinnesotaCare.

Oregon is taking responsibility for providing publicly subsidized coverage of all persons below poverty who are uninsured. The expansion is broad in that coverage is being extended to adults not normally covered by Medicaid. The state has obtained a waiver of statutory Medicaid requirements to extend federally assisted Medicaid coverage to adults and children below poverty. It also includes simplifying the eligibility criteria and the eligibility process to eliminate barriers that might otherwise keep people from applying. In the inclusive approach, the role of private insurance companies in selling insurance to low-income populations is minimized for services provided under the government plans.

TennCare is designed to cover all Medicaid enrollees, including categorically eligible families with children and the chronically disabled and frail elderly groups, citizens who are uninsurable because of current or prior medical conditions, and persons not eligible for an employer-sponsored or government-sponsored health plan. TennCare provides fully subsidized coverage for those with incomes below poverty. Those with incomes between 100 and 199 percent of the FPL pay a premium of up to 20 percent of the capitation rate and copayments of up to 10 percent of costs. Those with incomes of 200 percent or higher of the FPL are expected to pay a premium of up to as much as the full capitation rate, with copayments of 10 percent of costs. Maximum deductibles are set at $250 for an individual and $500 for a family per year.

In the middle of the continuum are states like Maryland that are extending coverage to more broadly defined Medicaid-eligible groups (e.g., women, children, and the disabled), but these strategies do not include additional subsidies to attract all low-income uninsured. Maryland is extending coverage of primary care and preventive care only for children up to age 5 with incomes between 133 and 185 percent of the FPL, and from ages 6 to 13 with incomes between 100 and 185 percent of the FPL. This model builds on the existing commitment that the states have to cover traditional Medicaid groups and they continue to rely on the private sector or other local government sources for coverage of many low-income and non-poor uninsured populations.

On the narrowly targeted end of the continuum are several states that have created special programs that focus on populations ineligible for Medicaid and at risk of being uninsured, often using state funds or encouraging the private sector to expand coverage to narrowly targeted populations. California created a program to extend outpatient coverage to children who are ineligible for Medicaid. The program builds on an existing state-funded screening initiative, improving access to more sophisticated follow-up diagnostic procedures and primary care.

Florida created the Healthy Kids Program to provide school-based health insurance coverage for uninsured children at several sites. This program covers low-income uninsured children, grouping them by school districts and then obtaining affordable coverage rates with managed care plans through competitive bids. The program provides subsidized premiums ranging from $5 to $57 a month per child, using the guidelines of the National School Lunch Program to determine the family's ability to pay. About half the program's cost is paid by the state, 35 percent by family contributions, and 16 percent by a mix of local sources, including school districts, hospitals, children's services councils, and other groups.

Comprehensiveness of Public Benefits

In their expansion programs, Minnesota and Tennessee provide comprehensive benefit packages similar to Medicaid (Table 9.3). A broad set of services is typically covered in Medicaid programs and there are very few restrictions or caps on those services. Traditional medical services include inpatient and outpatient hospital services, physician services, laboratory and x-ray, dental services, home health services, physical therapy, prescription drugs, and several other acute care services. Preventive services typically include family planning, early periodic screening and diagnostic testing (EPSDT), and genetic services. Most states also cover long-term care, adult day health care, hospice, primary home care, and medical transportation. There are no copays or deductibles in the Medicaid benefit package.

Because of budget constraints, many states' public insurance expansion programs provide benefit packages that are less comprehensive than Medicaid. They may cover most traditional medical services but may have substantial restrictions and copayments. The Florida Health Security Plan, for example, will provide a government-subsidized, low-premium health program that covers traditional medical services but includes many restrictions and copayment provisions. Hawaii QUEST offers a choice between two low-cost insurance plans that meet state standards. The insurance stresses primary care and preventive services. It covers only five days of inpatient hospital care, with hospitals agreeing to continue care for those who need longer stays.

Table 9.3   Comprehensiveness of Public Benefits

| | Comprehensive ← | → Limited | |
State	Broad Package with Few Limits or Copays	Basic Package with Limits or Copays	Limited Package
California			Outpatient services
Florida		Basic benefit package with restrictions and copays	
Hawaii		Basic benefit package plus coverage of clinical preventive services	
Maryland			Primary and preventive services
Minnesota	Full Medicaid package		
Oregon		Prioritized list of services*	
Tennessee	Medicaid package including the entire EPSDT service package for children		

*Varies with fiscal conditions of the state.

Oregon's plan is unique in proposing that eligibility and payments to providers should remain stable while the benefits available to covered populations vary based on the availability of funds. To accomplish this, the traditional package of Medicaid benefits was exchanged for one based on a prioritized list of services. Each year after reviewing the list, the Oregon legislature determines how far down the prioritized list of health services funding will reach. The list is based on combinations of conditions and treatments (i.e., treatments may be covered or not covered depending on the condition for which they are used). The funded services then define the benefit package and payments to the plans are based on the estimated reasonable cost of providing the covered services.

Funding limitations have constrained many states to offer a more limited package of benefits. California and Maryland's recent expansions illustrate this approach. California's expansion covers outpatient services only for indigent children who do not qualify for Medicaid. Maryland's proposed Medicaid expansion covers primary and preventive care only for children.

Expanding Private Coverage

Hawaii's employer mandate, passed in 1974, illustrates the most interventionist strategy being used to expand private coverage (Table 9.4). The mandate requires all employers in the state to offer their full-time employees health insurance with either indemnity plans or HMOs. The employer must cover at least half of the costs of the insurance and the employee must not have to pay more than 1.5 percent of his or her wages as a premium share. The mandate does not extend to dependents, but many employers do offer such coverage. Both Florida and Oregon's legislatures adopted "play-or-pay" plans that would have required all employers to either provide basic coverage to their workers or pay into a state insurance pool. Both states subsequently have repealed their employer mandates, however.

At the other end of the continuum are states that have implemented small group and individual insurance reform, including such provisions as guaranteed renewal and issue, preexisting condition limits, portability, modified community rating, and standardized benefit plans. These reform laws seek to achieve expanded coverage by making insurance more available and less costly for high-risk individuals. The specific provisions are designed to ensure that groups who are older and sicker are offered coverage on an equal basis as the young and healthy. For example, under modified community rating, rate differences are compressed so that everyone can obtain coverage under the same plan, regardless of health status or other risk factors. When such rate regulation is coupled with open enrollment or guaranteed issue (i.e., the requirement that carriers offer coverage to all comers), these laws are designed to give everyone an equal chance to buy insurance at a similar price. While these reforms are designed to spread risk more broadly, they are not expected to make insurance more affordable for low-income individuals and families.

Table 9.4   Regulatory versus Voluntary Methods to Expand Private Coverage

| | Regulatory ⟵ | | ⟶ Voluntary | |
State	Employer Mandates	Systemwide Regulatory Reform	Systemwide Market Reform	Small Group Insurance Reform
California			Purchasing pools, standardized benefits, and central administration	Guaranteed issue and renewal, portability, basic benefit plan
Florida			Purchasing pools, standardized benefits, and central administration	Guaranteed issue and renewal, portability, community rating, basic benefit plan
Hawaii	Employers required to offer coverage to full-time employees			Guaranteed issue and renewal, portability, basic benefit plan
Maryland		Rate restrictions		Guaranteed issue and renewal, portability, pre-existing conditions limits, basic benefit plan
Minnesota			Purchasing pools, standardized benefits, and central administration	Guaranteed issue and renewal, portability, basic benefit plan
Oregon				Guaranteed issue and renewal, portability, community rating, basic benefit plan
Tennessee				Guaranteed issue and renewal, portability, basic benefit plan

Maryland has gone beyond most states in making private coverage more affordable by enacting several unique provisions such as limiting the premium cost of the standard benefit plan and extending its hospital rate setting to other health services. California, Florida, and Minnesota are also going beyond most states in attempting to increase private coverage. However, rather than a regulatory approach to systemwide reform, they are pursuing a strategy of managed competition. This approach incorporates a purchasing pool, standardized benefits and out-of-pocket requirements, and centralized administration and data collection in order to make coverage less costly and more accessible. These strategies are discussed in more detail in the next section, which addresses cost containment.

Cost Containment

Table 9.5 summarizes the state plans with respect to their strategies for cost containment. Maryland is continuing its regulatory approach by extending its hospital rate regulation program to other services (e.g., controlling insurance premiums and limiting payments to practitioners and for diagnostic tests). It has also established a statewide program of medical practice parameters. Maryland created the Health Care Access and Cost Commission to establish a statewide healthcare database on all healthcare practitioners, to compare and analyze fees charged by healthcare practitioners, to develop a payment system for office-based health services, to compare quality of care among practitioners and establish medical practice parameters, and to develop a comprehensive benefit package. In addition, Maryland is the only state to include limits on the premium cost of health benefit plans offered to small employer groups. The average community-rated premium is limited to 12 percent of the average annual wage in the state. If the average community rate exceeds 12 percent, the commission must alter the standard benefit package.

To contain physician costs, Maryland has a voluntary arrangement between the state and physicians to implement a new payment methodology based on a fee comparison system. If the state determines that providers of a particular specialty service have excessively high charges, the state can work with the group to bring them into compliance or can establish mandatory rates. Similarly, if charges for certain medical services exceed the commission's cost-containment goals, the commission is authorized to establish mandatory rates.

Table 9.5   Regulatory versus Pro-Market Methods to Contain Costs

	Regulatory ←		→ Pro-Market
State	Price and Budget Controls	Managed Competition	Managed Care
California		Purchasing pools for state and local employees and small business	Medicaid managed care in urban areas
Florida		Regional purchasing pools for low-income and small business	Statewide Medicaid managed care
Hawaii			Managed care plans compete to bid for Health Quest contracts
Maryland	State may exclude or limit benefits if community rated plans exceed percent of wages		Statewide Medicaid managed care
Minnesota	Providers encouraged to form integrated networks; state sets rates and total revenue caps for the networks	Purchasing pools for small business, state employees	Medicaid managed care expanded to 14 counties
Oregon	State determines services covered based on budget		Oregon Health Plan enrollees select managed care plan
Tennessee	State capitation for TennCare based on budget limits		TennCare enrollees select managed care plan

Minnesota is pursuing a strategy with a substantial degree of regulation to assure that healthcare spending goals are met. The regulatory component includes provider rate setting for payors and providers not in managed care networks, aggregate premium or spending limits for providers in networks, and oversight authority based on the monitoring of statewide healthcare spending limits. Minnesota also has specified annual growth limits on health insurance expenditures and provider revenues. The objective is to reduce the annual growth rate for all health spending by 10 percent per year over a five-year period.

Tennessee introduced global budgeting in its financing for TennCare. A budget for the program was determined, forming the basis for determining an annual capitation rate. The capitation rate was then discounted by the anticipated continuing charity care, local government contributions, and average copayments by beneficiaries.

California, Florida, and Minnesota exemplify the managed competition strategy of cost containment. The major provision of this strategy, as implemented in these states, is state-sponsored purchasing pools offering a menu of competing plans; standardized benefits and out-of-pocket requirements; and incentives for individuals to purchase the lowest-cost plans. The pools negotiate with the plans in order to obtain the best rates for the members. California has two programs: (1) the California Public Employees Retirement System (CalPERS), a health insurance plan for state and local workers which, since its inception in the late 1960s, has grown to cover over 1 million employees; and (2) the Health Insurance Plan of California (HIPC), a publicly administered purchasing pool for small businesses and individuals. Both programs group employees together to offer them a choice of health plans. In both cases, the sponsor negotiates with health plans to obtain the best rates for its members.

Florida's 1993 law provided the authority to create eleven regionalized purchasing alliances to manage competition among accountable health partnerships (AHPs) (i.e., indemnity and HMO health plans offered through the alliances). The alliances are to function as collective purchasing agents for insurance on behalf of small employers and individuals. Health Security Plan enrollees, Medicaid beneficiaries, and employees of small businesses would be enrolled in AHPs through the purchasing alliances. Within a geographic area, individuals choose between two standard benefit plans—each with a PPO and HMO option. Only plans formally designated as AHPs are allowed to compete. To qualify, the plan must offer the complete array of services to all potential enrollees and use modified community rating to establish its premiums. While the alliances will assist small employers and individuals in the acquisition of healthcare coverage, the small employers are not required to offer employee coverage. Large business participation with the alliances is limited to obtaining information on the AHPs. Thus, the plan seeks to achieve cost containment through voluntary activities by employers, education of healthcare consumers, insurance reform, and improved state administration.

Minnesota has created state-sponsored purchasing pools for employees of small businesses, state employees, and MinnesotaCare enrollees. The state is also encouraging the development of voluntary purchasing pools open to private employers. The state has adopted a number of reforms focused on restructuring the delivery system so that providers will form integrated service networks. These small plans are being encouraged because of the concern that market consolidation in Minnesota may have gone too far, and that the system may become monopolistic rather than competitive.

Hawaii and Oregon illustrate state plans that are relying primarily on managed care to improve performance. In Hawaii, cost control is pursued through what the state calls a "managed cooperative" approach, in which managed care plans compete against one another to bid for Hawaii QUEST contracts. The state also relies on prevention to try to hold down healthcare costs, and when it instituted its employer mandate it required community ratings from insurers. Oregon's efforts to have all care delivered to publicly covered enrollees by fully capitated healthcare plans, combined with its unique process of prioritizing services, is the state's major cost-containment strategy.

All states are pursuing managed care as a cost-containment strategy to some extent. They already have developed, or are in the process of developing, managed care infrastructures serving commercial and Medicare populations. Medicaid managed care is not far behind as states are rapidly enrolling their Medicaid and other public insurance program recipients into managed care plans.

Improving Quality

As cost-containment strategies have been intensified in both the public and private sectors, policymakers have been prompted to consider a variety of options for ensuring that patients receive high-quality care. Table 9.6 summarizes the state plans in terms of their strategies for ensuring quality of care. Florida has "any willing provider" legislation to improve the treatment of providers by HMOs and prepaid health plans and to protect consumers against certain marketing practices. Oregon also enacted a Patient Protection Act, which—albeit without requiring the insurance department to develop standards for managed care plans—nevertheless includes protections for providers and a point-of-service coverage option. Maryland was one of the first states to enact provisions mandating coverage for 48-hour, doctor-recommended hospital stays following childbirth. Maryland also has a Patient Protection Act, which established a range of criteria to be followed by health plans in provider selection, participation, and financial incentives. One provision of the Act requires HMOs to offer point-of-service plans, allowing enrollees to see providers outside their plan's panel of providers.

Table 9.6   Regulatory versus Pro-Market Methods to Ensure Quality

| | Regulatory ←——————————————————————→ Pro-Market | | |
State	Specific Mandates	Collection and Dissemination of Performance Data	Licensing
California		Outcomes analyses of managed care plans	
Florida	Any-willing-provider law and marketing protections		
Hawaii			Relies on the market
Maryland	Coverage mandates for childbirth; criteria for provider selection, participation and financial incentives	Report cards for comparisons among HMOs	
Minnesota		Data collection and dissemination; quality report cards	
Oregon	Provider protections		
Tennessee		Data collection and dissemination	

In California, lawmakers enacted a measure calling for comprehensive outcomes analyses in order to provide consumers with objective reports on successful treatment records of managed care plans. Minnesota passed several laws related to collecting and sharing information, including establishing an office of consumer information to act as a resource for plan enrollees, disseminating information on health plan performance and on hospital and health plan quality. Results of consumer satisfaction surveys are to be included in quality report cards that will be developed annually according to standards defined by the state. A Health Data Institute was created to provide information on all health plans and to provide consumer information on obtaining coverage, covered options, purchasing pools, and other consumer data. Tennessee authorized its Community Health Management Information System to collect and analyze data from providers.

Hawaii is an example of a state with neither a regulatory nor informational strategy to improve quality. The state relies on the market, its comprehensive coverage policy, and its requirements for licensure of managed care plans to improve the quality of care.

Evaluation of State Plans

The principal questions to be addressed in assessing the performance of healthcare policies and programs with respect to effectiveness, efficiency, and equity are summarized in Table 9.7. At the microlevel (i.e., system, institution, and patient), the focus is on the performance of the health care system, and at the macrolevel (i.e., community), the focus is on the health of the population at which programs and services are directed. The general criteria to be used in assessing the extent to which these goals of effectiveness, efficiency, and equity are likely to be achieved were elaborated in the preceding chapters. They will be applied here in assessing the state healthcare reform models that are viewed as policy options for states to consider. The various strategies within each reform dimension are placed on a scale of high, medium, or low potential for satisfying criteria from each perspective. A summary evaluation table (Table 9.8) is developed that provides the results of the evaluation in terms of the scale scores and their justification. The remainder of this section discusses the evaluation criteria, evidence, and results from each perspective.

Effectiveness

The criteria for assessing the effectiveness of healthcare programs and policies were delineated in Chapter 3 (Table 3.3). Two of the criteria relate to the population perspective, as defined in Chapter 2: (1) policy design guided by community or population needs assessment; and (2) plan inclusion of options contributing to comprehensiveness through integration of services across the entire continuum of health services (see Figure 1.1 in Chapter 1). Two other criteria relate to the clinical perspective, as defined in Chapter 2, and concern professional performance: (1) improved precision through advance specification of expected guidelines for professional performance; and (2) performance monitoring of process and outcome indicators for selected conditions to assure clinical accountability. Both sets of the effectiveness criteria are derived from Shortell, Gillies, and Devers' (1995) scheme for a community healthcare management system described in Chapter 3.

Implicit in these criteria is a value judgment about whether the population or the clinical perspective guides the evaluation.

Table 9.7 Summary of Effectiveness, Efficiency, and Equity Performance Criteria

Level	Performance Criteria		
	Effectiveness	Efficiency	Equity
Microlevel	Clinical effectiveness: Does healthcare contribute to improving the health of individuals?	Production efficiency: Is healthcare being produced at the lowest cost?	Procedural equity: Are the procedures for allocating healthcare fair?
Macrolevel	Population effectiveness: Is the health of the population improved?	Allocative efficiency: What mix of investments produces improvements in the population's health?	Substantive equity: Are subgroup disparities in health within the population minimized?

The assumption underlying the criteria and critique presented here is that the population perspective—whether the intervention contributes to an improvement in the health of the population—should be the basis for judging any health policy option, and therefore any aspect of state health reform. In most arenas, and in state healthcare reform in particular, however, the clinical perspective—whether the intervention yields positive benefits for patients—is the basis on which policies are likely to be formulated and judged.

From the clinical perspective and in terms of structural elements, several states have provisions relating to provider selection and participation that appear to be directed more at equity than at effectiveness issues. Some use cost controls to regulate the supply and organization of medical care resources. These structural interventions may represent the neglect of accountability for professional performance in the processes of medical care.

In the discussion that follows, the effectiveness criteria will be applied to an evaluation of the state health reform options presented in the previous sections of this chapter.

Need-based

There is no evidence that population needs assessments form the basis for these reforms; in fact, they appear to be based largely on the overwhelming need to control the costs of medical care to the state while assuring or enhancing access. There is a certain rationale, mentioned in Chapter 3, for using medical care as the means to improve the health of the most vulnerable population groups in a state: while the point of diminishing returns for medical care may have been reached for the population overall, its basic benefits have not yet been fully realized for many vulnerable population groups. To the degree that an attempt is made to include all uninsured in a single program and to mandate the expansion of private coverage, there may be a chance of improving the health of the population by bringing the benefits of medical care to all, including those most at risk. These judgments are reflected in the medium effectiveness rating on these poles in the inclusiveness of public coverage and in the regulatory versus voluntary methods to expand private coverage dimensions in Table 9.8. The medium rating recognizes the benefits of medical care, but also recognizes the limits of a policy focus that fails to take into account the non-medical determinants of health.

Comprehensiveness

These reforms reflect modest attention to the full continuum of healthcare services. Most state healthcare reform efforts, using the broad Medicaid package, offer or guarantee a comprehensive set of medical care benefits. These range from preventive care through acute and long-term care on the continuum of services portrayed in Figure 1.1 in Chapter 1. This judgment is reflected in the medium rating assigned to the broad package in the comprehensiveness of public benefits category in Table 9.8. Broad benefits packages may contribute to this comprehensiveness, but they still focus largely on medical care.

Precision

Improving the precision of medicine is a key purpose of AHCPR and the related development of clinical practice guidelines. An example of such a process intervention is Maryland's use of information on performance to develop medical practice parameters, or practice guidelines. From a clinical perspective, practice parameters offer some evidence of their possible impact on the health of beneficiaries. Managed care and managed competition, combined with the need to achieve greater cost-effectiveness, may enhance clinical performance through the specification of guidelines. This rationale is the basis for the medium rating associated with both of these strategies in the regulatory versus pro-market methods to contain costs portion of Table 9.8.

It is also the basis for the high rating given to the specific mandates of regulation versus pro-market methods for ensuring quality. Practice guidelines, however, are specific mandates and should not be confused with the proliferation of specific legislative acts related to the processes of medical care, such as the legislation of minimal postnatal hospital stays. This represents legislative micromanagement of medical care triggered by publicity of flagrant abuses by some MCOs, and contributes little to ensuring the overall quality of medical care.

Table 9.8 Evaluation of State Health Reform Options

OPTIONS FOR STATE HEALTH REFORM	CRITERIA		
	Effectiveness	Efficiency	Equity
1. Inclusiveness of public coverage			
Universal			
↑ All uninsured in single program	Medium	High	High
Medicaid expansion for child & family	Low	Low	Medium
↓ Independent program for child & family	Low	Low	Low
Narrowly targeted			
	Single program contributes to improving population health	Single program contributes to administrative production efficiency and cost containment	Single program provides universal coverage. Contributes to minimizing disparities between different types of public coverage. Minimizes constraints on choice of provider for more people.
2. Comprehensiveness of public benefits			
Comprehensive			
↑ Broad package with few limits or copays	Medium	Medium	High
Basic package with limits or copays	Low	Low	Medium
↓ Limited package	Low	Low	Low
Limited			
	Broad package contributes to integration of medical services across continuum	Broad package contributes to allocative efficiency	Broad package minimizes constraints on consumer choice of providers. Contributes to similar treatment. Meets greater needs of low-income population.
3. Regulatory vs. voluntary methods to expand private coverage			
Universal			
↑ Employer mandates	Medium	High	High
Systemwide regulatory reform	Low	Low	Low
Systemwide market reform	Low	Low	Low
↓ Small group insurance reforms	Low	Low	Low
Voluntary			
	Mandated coverage contributes to improving population health	Mandates only proven method to expand private coverage to low-income employees and their dependents	Mandates extend more universal coverage. Contributes to minimizing disparities between public and private coverage.

Table 9.8 (*continued*)

OPTIONS FOR STATE HEALTH REFORM	CRITERIA		
	Effectiveness	Efficiency	Equity
4. Regulatory vs. pro-market methods to contain costs			
Regulatory			
↑ Price and budget controls	Low	Medium	Low
│ Managed competition	Medium	Medium	High
↓ Managed care	Medium	Low	Medium
Pro-market	Managed competition may enhance clinical performance	Managed competition contributes to allocative efficiency and cost control. Budget and price controls may contain costs, but are likely to have limited impact when applied only to the public sector	Managed competition prioritizes benefits, based on costs and outcomes
5. Regulatory vs. pro-market methods to ensure quality			
Regulatory			
↑ Specific mandates	High	Low	High
│ Collection/dissemination of performance data	Medium	Medium	Medium
↓ Licensing	Low	Low	Low
Pro-market	Practice guidelines with process and outcome monitoring improves precision and performance	Performance regulation will contribute to competition on basis of price and quality, thereby providing better value for money to consumers	Specific mandates and performance monitoring attempt to directly mitigate adverse health consequences

Performance monitoring

Performance monitoring and reporting, to the degree that it addresses outcomes and not just processes, has the potential to yield positive benefits. Specifically, by providing information on performance to patients and purchasers, it may affect choices, and in the long run may improve clinical accountability. The dissemination of information, however, is not a strongly deterministic strategy, and so the collection and dissemination of performance data, such as that being accomplished through HEDIS, is judged only a medium contributor to effectiveness in the regulatory versus voluntary methods for ensuring quality portion of Table 9.8. The usefulness of this information is enhanced when it is used to evaluate care and to derive practice guidelines, as is being done in Maryland.

Summary

Not surprisingly, state health reform options do not contribute greatly to improving effectiveness, especially not when assessed from the population perspective. They were not designed to do so; they have been adopted to enhance access to care while containing costs. Effectiveness benefits tend to be secondary, such as improvements in health due to better access to medical care for the most vulnerable and cost containment due to improvements in the precision of medical care.

Efficiency

The criteria for assessing the efficiency of healthcare programs and policies were summarized and applied to the evaluation of Medicaid managed care in Chapter 5 (see Table 5.5). These criteria address the issues of macro–cost control, allocative efficiency, production efficiency, and dynamic efficiency. Judgments about the likely effects of state healthcare reforms on certain indicators in each of these areas reflect the extent to which these reforms would achieve these broad goals. Efficiency criteria are often conflicting. For example, regulation may contain costs at the macrolevel, but may reduce allocative and dynamic efficiency. In general, when there is conflict between these criteria, greater weight will be given to allocative efficiency because it addresses the attainment of the highest level of population health from the available resources.

Macro–cost control

All states are concerned about budget deficits incurred due to expansion of healthcare and other entitlement programs. Deficits may violate state law and result in unpopular tax increases. Expanding health spending may curtail opportunities to invest in other programs that may have a greater effect on population health, resulting in resource misallocation. Defining an appropriate fraction of gross state product for healthcare has served to operationalize this issue in European countries. However, states use various approaches, including a growth target for state health spending (e.g., Minnesota) and limits on premiums of health benefits offered to small employers tied to a percent of the average annual wage (e.g., Maryland).

Assuming that the political will to control cost is strong, international evidence (see Chapter 5) suggests that the market-minimized regulatory approach to macro–cost control has the best chance of controlling health spending. States with global budgets or fee and volume controls are more likely to realize their cost-containment goal than states that rely solely on competition among managed care plans, for example. An important caveat is that states do not control all health spending within their borders and this fact limits the degree to which state regulation can contain healthcare costs within the United States. Finally, regulation may slow innovation in healthcare delivery and cause resource misallocation. Regulators may misjudge patient needs and demands and budget limits and artificial prices may result in perverse economic incentives for providers (e.g., incentives to keep patients hospitalized when the same outcome could be achieved at lower cost within an outpatient setting).

These findings are reflected in the medium efficiency ratings given to both price and budget controls and to managed competition in the cost-containment dimension in Table 9.8. A medium, rather than high, rating is assigned to these options to reflect the limitations of price and budget controls in containing costs at the state level, and to reflect the fact that while managed competition has some advantage in terms of allocative efficiency, it too may have a limited ability to contain overall state healthcare costs.

Allocative efficiency

The goal of allocative efficiency is extremely difficult to operational-ize given the paucity of evidence on ways to improve population health. As much of the national and international evidence suggests that the marginal expansion of curative medicine may yield very little improvement in population health, new spending should be heavily directed toward selective preventive medicine and those investments that enhance the social and physical environments in which people live. Within curative medicine, spending should first go toward those services that consumers value most highly per dollar of investment. Thus, programs that simply fund medical treatments without explicit rationing between prevention, treat-ment, and alternative treatments are unlikely to enhance allocative efficiency. Because state reforms focus on medical care services, the prospects for large allocative efficiency improvements are quite small. A potential exists for states that constrain growth in medical care spending to allocate more funds to improving the quality of the social and physical environment, but this is generally not an explicit part of any state's plan. Within the confines of the medical care budget, states that explicitly consider the value per dollar of investment while allocating limited state dollars may improve the allocative efficiency of the healthcare sector. This market-minimized approach is being applied to low-income populations in Oregon.

Managed competition offers the possibility for consumers and payors to constrain the growth in spending and to shape health-care resource allocation to meet their health needs. These ends are achieved through selective contracting, competitive bidding, and consumer choice within a regulated market. The flexibility of this approach compared to direct regulation of prices and budgets offers the opportunity for the reallocation of resources toward cost-effective prevention and treatment, cost-effective input substitution, and rapid innovation in the production and delivery of health ser-vices. This approach is most effective when private sector payors also pursue a managed competition strategy, yielding a large active market of managed care providers who compete on both quality and price.

These assessments are reflected in the medium ratings assigned to a broad package of comprehensive public benefits and managed competition as a method for containing costs in Table 9.8. The rationale for the rating assigned managed competition was reviewed in the macro–cost control section. Broad coverage opens financial access to preventive services, and prior studies showed that the health status of the poor suffered under policies with high copayments (Manning et al., 1987). This likely impact is reflected in the low rating assigned more restrictive policies, based on the allocative efficiency criterion.

Production efficiency

For program administration, evidence suggests that having a multiplicity of programs increases administrative costs (e.g., programs for the poor in the United States), while a single insurance program (e.g., health insurance in Canada and Medicare in the United States) results in lower administrative costs. This is reflected in the high efficiency rating assigned to all uninsured in a single program in the inclusiveness of public coverage category in Table 9.8. Similarly, if the objective is to expand private coverage for the uninsured, the method that is proven to yield the largest gains is the employer mandate. This is likely to be the most efficient method to achieve this goal, and is therefore assigned a high rating in the expanding private coverage category in Table 9.8.

Comparing providers and health plans to national performance benchmarks operationalizes production efficiency. Policies that support managed care in a competitive market context are most likely to achieve this goal. Faced with competitive pressure to serve health plan enrollees at competitive levels of quality, amenity, and cost, managed care plans search for the least costly ways to provide care. Managed care plans are criticized for skimping on care and or service, but these problems have not been demonstrated to impact population health or the ability of these plans to grow and increase their market share to date. As more and better information on outcomes and on quality of care becomes available, there will be further pressure to maintain high quality while increasing the productivity of healthcare providers. Thus, collection and dissemination of performance data is given a medium efficiency rating for the methods for ensuring quality in Table 9.8

Dynamic efficiency

Achievement of the goal of dynamic efficiency is indicated by the degree to which the health system is induced to research and develop new health services and better ways to organize and deliver health services. Health policies that encourage competition based on quality and price are more likely to lead to innovations in the healthcare system. Thus, a higher efficiency rating is given for a broad benefits package, managed competition, and collection and dissemination of performance data in Table 9.8 in dimensions 2, 4, and 5, respectively. One caveat is that price competition reduces the ability of teaching hospitals to cost shift patient care funds to basic and clinical research. This may be partially offset by providers who choose to invest in clinical research to enhance their reputation for excellence. Eventually research and education investment should be transparent and centrally funded as public goods in the public domain.

Summary

State health reform options do not directly address allocative efficiency. Their main objective is to achieve access to a "good" standard of care and to contain healthcare costs. Their ability to achieve this latter goal is limited at the state level. The most promising approach appears to be a combination of coverage mandates and explicit controls on the state healthcare budget coupled with a healthcare delivery system based on managed competition.

Equity

The criteria for assessing the equity of healthcare programs and policies in terms of the respective paradigms of justice were summarized in Chapter 6 (Table 6.2) and applied to delineating socially responsible managed care in Chapter 7 (Table 7.1). These criteria include the norm of participation derived from the deliberative justice paradigm; the principles of freedom of choice and cost-effectiveness within the distributive paradigm; the standards of need and the common good lodged in the social justice perspective; and the ideal of similar treatment, which has roots in both the distributive and social justice paradigms.

State healthcare reform is a policy strategy fitting primarily within the distributive justice paradigm and its emphasis on improving access to medical care. (See a discussion of the alternative policy strategies defined by the respective paradigms in Chapter 7.) The criteria of the common good, based in the social justice paradigm, as well as community participation, rooted in the deliberative justice paradigm, have not tended to shape the formulation and implementation of state healthcare reform.

The policy formulation process undertaken in Oregon in the 1980s to reform its Medicaid program represents the most fully developed effort to assure the involvement of affected parties through a variety of participatory policy formation devices—community forums, population surveys, and public hearings (Garland 1992). The Tennessee state healthcare reform initiative in the mid–1990s represents another pole along the participatory/nonparticipatory policymaking continuum (Gold, Frazer, and Schoen 1995). In that case, no, or minimal, input was sought from providers and patients as an explicit strategy to assure swift enactment of the proposed reform measures. Both approaches stirred considerable controversy. Experience in Oregon suggests that the program has, in large measure, been accepted and adopted by providers and patients (Kitzhaber 1996). Assessments of the early experience of the Tennessee program suggest considerable disruption and disaffection on the part of physicians, patients, and safety-net providers affected by these changes (Gold, Frazer, and Schoen 1997). The respective approaches in these two states provide a natural experiment for assessing the evolution and success of the models of reform grounded in sharply contrasting expressions of the deliberative norm of participation in the policy formulation and implementation process.

Similarly, state healthcare reform efforts have not been primarily directed toward the community-wide health improvements demanded by the common good criterion. The relevance of the need criterion in the formulation of the alternative reform efforts was addressed in the effectiveness evaluation. The critique of the state healthcare reform initiatives with respect to equity will therefore focus primarily on the freedom of choice, similar treatment, and cost-effectiveness norms, which may be viewed as the principal criteria of equity—grounded in the distributive justice paradigm— implicitly or explicitly shaping these reform efforts.

Freedom of choice

The freedom-of-choice norm, as applied to an evaluation of the equity consequences of state healthcare proposals, may be used to judge the limits on consumers' choice of care required by a proposal. Implicit in this norm is the enhancement of availability of care. Those proposals that enhance the availability of services and minimize constraints on consumers' choices would be the fairest, according to this criterion.

The vast majority of the uninsured are employed workers or their dependents, which argues most definitively for the full involvement of employers in forging such expansions (Rowland et al. 1994). Employer mandates would entail an assessment of the extent to which the federal Employee Retirement Income Security Act (ERISA) provisions limit states' abilities to enact these reforms, and of the possible avenues for shared public and private responsibility for funding such initiatives (Chollet 1996).

The primary objective underlying the expansion and the extension of both public and private coverage is the enhancement of the overall availability of services by providing some form of coverage to those who currently have none. Those market-minimized reforms that attempt to cover all of the insured through expanded public programs or employer mandates and to provide comprehensive, rather than limited, public benefits offer the greatest promise for enhancing both the choice and availability of services to the uninsured. These assessments are mirrored in the high ratings assigned to the more expansive options for expanding public and private coverage and benefits in Table 9.8.

Strategies for expanding insurance coverage do not, however, explicitly address the extent to which the choices of consumers are limited by the restrictions encompassed in the reforms themselves or by other means. A key foundation for enacting Medicaid reform in the public sector is the federal approval of waivers that permit certain limitations—including the freedom to select providers—required for mandated enrollment of Medicaid-eligible individuals in selected managed care alternatives. These and related Medicaid reform provisions were enacted, however, with the intent of mitigating the major restrictions on choice that resulted from providers' unwillingness to serve Medicaid clients under the fee-for-service system.

The main discretion consumers can exercise over the care they ultimately receive is a function of the choice of provider they have. The more doors that are closed to consumers—because of the unavailability of providers in an area; closings of traditional safety net institutions; selected marketing to low-risk individuals or selected de-marketing to high-risk individuals; the limited number of plans or of providers offered to potential enrollees; or the lack of an informed knowledge basis for choosing among them—the fewer effective choices that are available to them. State healthcare reforms are unlikely to be successful in enhancing access without consideration of these organizational and delivery system issues.

Similar treatment

According to the similar treatment norm, those options that cover everyone in a similar fashion are deemed the fairest because they minimize the disparities in the type and extent of coverage and in the associated access differentials that have been widely documented to exist—particularly between the publicly and privately insured. In addition, the promulgation of coverage methods that are more universal would reduce the increasing tendency of the private health insurance market to exclude or limit coverage for high-risk individuals who are likely to need it the most.

An associated effect of disparate public and private means of financing medical care has been the evolution of disparate and distinct systems of providing care for those with public or no coverage and for the privately insured. An underlying intent of the national universal healthcare reform efforts in the early 1990s, as well as of more recent state reforms, was to assure more equal treatment and wider availability of services. However, initiatives that are primarily limited to expanding coverage for traditionally Medicaid-eligible individuals or to incremental, voluntaristic small-business reforms are unlikely to effectively reduce access and availability gaps between groups based on the type—or absence—of coverage. Reinhardt (1996) and others (Priester 1992) have argued that these gaps may widen and harden in the absence of more universal health-care reform—particularly in the context of managed care–driven healthcare system changes.

In summary, market-minimized state healthcare reform strategies that attempt to cover all of the insured, provide comprehensive public benefits, and mandate more extensive involvement of employers in providing private coverage appear to offer the most promise in realizing the similar treatment norm, reflected in the high ratings assigned these options (Table 9.8).

Cost-effectiveness

The cost-effectiveness criterion—grounded in the distributive justice paradigm of equity—is concerned with weighing the relative benefits, or outcomes, and burdens, or costs, of care provision. Approaches that place primary emphasis on containing costs without attendant considerations of likely health consequences would not fare well on this criterion. Price and budget controls may be successful in containing the overall growth in costs in specific sectors or throughout the system if they are broadly applied and enforced. However, they may also stifle technological innovations that enhance the quality of care provision and may ration effective, as well as ineffective, services. Managed care, to the extent that it is concerned with covering and providing preventive care services and promoting the use of effective but less costly ambulatory care or outpatient services, offers promise of delivering more cost-effective care. An array of abuses, however, have been identified in unfettered managed care environments (e.g., hasty discharges for normal deliveries or breast cancer surgery) and have led to charges that the quality and effectiveness of care may be compromised in the interest of cost containment.

The highest cost-effectiveness rating is assigned to a managed competition cost-containment strategy (Table 9.8). As discussed earlier in the context of the efficiency criterion, managed competition offers greater theoretical promise for overseeing both the costs and outcomes of care and for monitoring and prioritizing benefits based on outcomes, through the development of statewide standardized benefits packages and provider participation and bidding arrangements. The empirical reality of the impact of managed competition in selected markets within the United States has yet to be fully documented, however.

Those policy options that entail specific mandates for ensuring quality or entail the collection and dissemination of performance data would fare better—earning high and medium ratings, respectively—in terms of the cost-effectiveness criterion than strategies that rely on broad licensing requirements alone, which earn a low rating, because the former options focus more directly on mitigating adverse health consequences.

Summary

Overall, those state reform strategies that seek to extend more universal public and private coverage and more comprehensive public benefits fare best in terms of both the freedom-of-choice and similar treatment norms of equity. Cost-containment strategies that consider quality and health impacts and quality assurance approaches that focus most directly on health consequences receive the highest rating in terms of the cost-effectiveness criterion of fairness.

Summary and Conclusions

The analyses point out both the convergence and conflicts among the goals of effectiveness, efficiency, and equity that are suggested by the respective state reform proposals. Four of the proposed strategies have been judged to consistently optimize all three goals: universal coverage of the uninsured provided in a single public program; a comprehensive benefit package with few caps or copays offered in the public coverage plan; mandated employer coverage to expand private coverage; and managed competition to contain costs. A regulatory strategy for ensuring quality in the managed care environment ranked highest for effectiveness and equity, but a strategy collecting and disseminating performance data was preferable from the efficiency perspective. No state is implementing all four of the preferred strategies. Minnesota's plan includes three of the four—all except employer mandates—and Hawaii and Tennessee are both attempting to provide universal coverage: Hawaii supports employer mandates and Tennessee a broad package of benefits.

The results also reveal the number of criteria that are not addressed by state reform. Most notable from an effectiveness perspective is the lack of consideration of behavioral and environmental determinants of health. State reform aimed at improving health must incorporate a broader set of concerns than that reflected by the current focus on medical care and the healthcare system. In the instance of the equity norm, the analysis indicates that the criteria of participation and the common good that relate more broadly to community-level health protection interventions are not addressed in a significant way by the reform strategies.

Finally, the analysis also reveals the difficulties encountered in bringing health services research to bear on evaluations of policy options due to gaps in knowledge of the consequences of selected provisions that must be addressed to make effective judgments of their probable impact. Nevertheless, health policy design decisions that fail to take potential consequences into account often rely on political expediency. The uncertainties presented pose challenges to the health services research community to further document the performance of the U.S. healthcare system with respect to the effectiveness, efficiency, and equity criteria. Health services research can assist in framing current and future state and national policy debates by clarifying the goals, trade-offs, and assumptions of alternative proposals based on the valued system-performance criteria of effectiveness, efficiency, and equity.

In summary, the discussion in this and previous chapters examines the conceptual and normative blueprints of the major healthcare system goals of effectiveness, efficiency, and equity. It analyzes the balances and trade-offs that influence policies and programs designed to realize these objectives. It reviews the methods used to measure the extent to which each of these goals has actually been achieved. And it encourages dialogue among health services researchers, policy analysts, policymakers, and administrators who study, recommend, formulate, and implement health policy. Designing a healthcare system that optimizes the policy ideals of effectiveness, efficiency, and equity requires critical inquiry into the meaning of these goals and how best to achieve them. This book invites such inquiry.

References

Aday, L. A, C. E. Begley, D. R. Lairson, and C. H. Slater. 1993. *Evaluating the Medical Care System: Effectiveness, Efficiency, and Equity.* 1st ed. Chicago: Health Administration Press.

Alpha Center. 1995. *More for Less? Increasing Insurance Coverage Through Medicaid Waiver Programs.* Washington, D.C.: Alpha Center.

Beatrice, D. F. 1996. "States and Health Care Reform: The Importance of Program Implementation." In *Strategic Choices for a Changing Health Care System.* Edited by S. H. Altman and U. E. Reinhardt, 183–206. Chicago: Health Administration Press.

Blewett, L. A. 1994. "Reforms in Minnesota: Forging the Path." *Health Affairs* 13 (3): 200–209.

Boles, K. E., and L. L. Hicks. 1996. "A Compilation of State Activities in Legislatively Mandated Reporting of Health Services Data." *Journal of Health and Human Services Administration* 19: 133–62.

Brown, E. 1988. "Principles for a National Health Program: A Framework for Analysis and Development." *Milbank Quarterly* 66: 573–617.

Casey, M. M., A. Wellever, and I. Moscovice. 1997. "Rural Health Network Development: Public Policy Issues and State Initiatives." *Journal of Health Politics, Policy and Law* 22: 23–47.

Chollet, D. J. 1996. "Redefining Private Insurance in a Changing Market Structure." In *Strategic Choices for a Changing Health Care System.* Edited by S. H. Altman and U. E. Reinhardt, 33–62. Chicago: Health Administration Press.

Coughlin, T. A., L. Ku, J. Holahan, D. Heslam, and C. Winterbottom. 1994. "State Responses to the Medicaid Spending Crisis: 1988 to 1992." *Journal of Health Politics, Policy and Law* 19: 837–64.

Crittenden, R. A. 1995. "Rolling Back Reform in the Pacific Northwest." *Health Affairs* 14 (2): 302–5.

Feldstein, P. 1988. *Health Care Economics.* 3rd ed. New York: John Wiley & Sons.

Fleck, L. M. 1994. "Just Caring: Oregon, Health Care Rationing, and Informed Democratic Deliberation." *Journal of Medicine and Philosophy* 19: 367–88.

Gardner, A., and D. Neubauer. 1995. "Hawaii's Health QUEST." *Health Affairs* 14 (1): 300–303.

Garland, M. J. 1992. "Justice, Politics and Community: Expanding Access and Rationing Health Services in Oregon." *Law, Medicine, and Health Care* 20: 67–81.

Gates, V. 1995. *Employer Based Insurance and the Employer Mandate.* Salem, OR: Office of Health Plan Administrator.

Gold, M., A. Aizer, and A. Salganicoff. 1997. *Managed Care and Low-Income Populations: A Case Study of Managed Care in Florida*. Washington, D.C.: Kaiser Family Foundation and The Commonwealth Fund.

Gold, M., K. Chu, and B. Lyons. 1995. *Managed Care and Low-Income Populations: A Case Study of Managed Care in Oregon*. Washington, D.C.: Kaiser Family Foundation and The Commonwealth Fund.

Gold, M., H. Frazer, and C. Schoen. 1995. *Managed Care and Low-Income Populations: A Case Study of Managed Care in Tennessee*. Washington, D.C.: Kaiser Family Foundation and The Commonwealth Fund.

————. 1997. *Managed Care and Low-Income Populations: A Case Study of Managed Care in Tennessee. 1996 Update*. Washington, D.C.: Kaiser Family Foundation and The Commonwealth Fund.

Gold, M., M. Sparer, and K. Chu. 1996. "Medicaid Managed Care: Lessons from Five States." *Health Affairs* 15 (3): 153–66.

Holahan, J., T. Coughlin, L. Ku, D. J. Lipson, and S. Rajan. 1995. "Insuring the Poor Through Section 1115 Medicaid Waivers." *Health Affairs* 14 (1): 199–216.

Iglehart, J K. 1994. "Health Care Reform: The States." *The New England Journal of Medicine* 330: 75–79.

Intergovernmental Health Policy Project. 1995. *Fifty State Profiles: Health Care Reform, 1995*. Washington, D.C.: Intergovernmental Health Policy Project at George Washington University.

Kitzhaber, J A. 1996. "The Governor of Oregon on Medicaid Managed Care." *Health Affairs* 15 (3): 167–69.

Kralewski, J. E., A. De Vries, B. Dowd, and S. Potthoff. 1995. "The Development of Integrated Service Networks in Minnesota." *Health Care Management Review* 20 (4): 42–56.

Lipson, D. J., and S. P. Schrodel. 1996. *"State-Subsidized Insurance Programs for Low-Income People."* Washington, D.C.: Alpha Center.

Manning, W. C., J. P. Newhouse, N. Duan, E. B. Keeler, A. Leibowitz, and M. S. Marquis. 1987. "Health Insurance and the Demand for Medical Care: Evidence from a Randomized Experiment." *American Economic Review* 77: 257–77.

Mariner, W. K. 1996. "State Regulation of Managed Care and the Employee Retirement Income Security Act." *The New England Journal of Medicine* 335: 1986–90.

McDonough, J. E., C. L. Hager, and B. Rosman. 1997. "Health Care Reform Stages a Comeback in Massachusetts." *The New England Journal of Medicine* 336: 148–51.

McManus, S. M., and K. V. Thai. 1996. "Coping with the Health Care Crisis: State Government Responses." *Journal of Health and Human Services Administration* 19: 206–31.

Meyer, G. S., and D. Blumenthal. 1996. "TennCare and Academic Medial Centers: The Lessons from Tennessee." *Journal of the American Medical Association* 276: 672–76.

Mirvis, D. M., C. F. Chang, C. J. Hall, G. T. Zaar, and W. B. Applegate. 1995. "TennCare: Health System Reform for Tennessee." *Journal of the American Medical Association* 274: 1235–41.

Mitchell, J. M., and S. A. Norton. 1996. "Provider Assessments, the Uninsured, and Uncompensated Care: Florida's Public Medical Assistance Trust Fund." *Milbank Quarterly* 74: 545–69.

Moon, M., and J. Holahan. 1992. "Can States Take the Lead in Health Care Reform?" *Journal of the American Medical Association* 268: 1588–94.

National Institute for Health Care Management. 1994. *Health Care Problems: Variation Across States.* Prepared by Lewin-VHI, Inc. Report No. 94FMS230. Washington, D.C.: The National Institute for Health Care Management.

Priester, R. 1992. "A Values Framework for Health System Reform." *Health Affairs* 11 (1): 84–107.

Reinhardt, U. E. 1996. "A Social Contract for the 21st Century Health Care: Three-Tier Health Care with Bounty Hunting." *Health Economics* 5: 479–99.

Riley, T. 1995. "Medicaid: The Role of the States." *Journal of the American Medical Association* 274: 267–70.

Rowland, D., B. Lyons, A. Salganicoff, and P. Long. 1994. "A Profile of the Uninsured in America." *Health Affairs* 13 (2): 283–87.

Shortell, S. M., R. R. Gillies, and K. J. Devers. 1995. "Reinventing the American Hospital." *Milbank Quarterly* 73 (2): 131–60.

Shriber, D. 1997. "State Experience in Regulating a Changing Health Care System." *Health Affairs* 16 (2): 48–68.

Somers, A., and H. Somers. 1977. "A Proposed Framework for Health and Health Care Policies." *Inquiry* 14: 115–70.

Sparer, M. 1995. "Great Expectations: The Limits of State Health Care Reform." *Health Affairs* 14 (4): 191–202.

Stearns, S. C., R. T. Slifkin, K. E. Thorpe, and T. A. Mroz. 1997. "The Structure and Experience of State Risk Pools: 1988–1994." *Medical Care Research and Review* 54: 223–38.

Tanenbaum, S. J. 1996. "'Medical Effectiveness' in Canadian and U.S. Health Policy: The Comparative Politics of Inferential Ambiguity." *Health Services Research* 31: 517–32.

Tengs, T. O. 1996. "An Evaluation of Oregon's Medicaid Rationing Algorithms." *Health Economics* 5: 171–81.

Thorne, J. I., B. Bianchi, G. Bonnyman, C. Greene, and T. Leddy. 1995. "State

Perspectives On Health Care Reform: Oregon, Hawaii, Tennessee, and Rhode Island." *Health Care Financing Review* 16 (3): 121–38.

Vladeck, B. C. 1995. "Medicaid 1115 Demonstrations: Progress Through Partnership." *Health Affairs* 14 (1): 217–20.

Vogel, W. B., and M. K. Miller. 1995. "Florida's Managed Competition Approach to Health Care Reform." *Advances in Health Economics and Health Research* 15: 185–208.

Wascoe, D. 1995. "A State of Flux: Minnesota." *Business and Health* 13 (2): 43–52.

Index

Access: actual, 244–45; equity,
185–95; framework, 178–84;
geographic rate variations,
30–31, 46; issues, x, 14, 33–34;
policy strategies, 78; potential,
214, 215–16, 218–19, 242–43;
realized, 180, 189–90, 214–15,
217–18, 219, 222–25; utilization
issues, 222–25
Accountability, ix
Accountable health partnership,
295–96
Acute Physiological and Chronic
Health Evaluation. See APACHE
scale
Administrative costs, 148–49
Agency for Health Care Policy and
Research. See AHCPR
AHA, 15, 197
AHCPR: funding, 16; practice
guidelines, 79–80, 257; purpose,
301; research teams, 122; surveys,
196
AHP, 295–96
AHSR, 16
Alcohol, 41
Allocative efficiency, 2; assessment,
119–23; criteria, 111–14;
definition, 107; evidence,

138–48, 164; focus, 11; market-
maximized model, 132–34;
market-minimized model,
134–35; Medicaid managed care,
159–60; policy, 108–10, 156–58,
265; problems, 108; qualitative
analysis, 132–33; state health
reform, 304–6
AMA, 15, 197, 228
American Hospital Association, 15,
197
American Medical Association. See
AMA
American Public Health
Association. See APHA
American Public Welfare
Association. See APWA
Analytic research, 199–200
Andersen, Ronald, 177–78
Anderson, D.W., 131
Anderson, J.P., 122
Any willing provider laws, 284, 297
APACHE scale, 57, 58, 65–66
APHA, 15, 228
Appropriateness, 51, 52
APWA, 15
Arnstein, S., 188
Arrow, K.J., 112
Asklepios, 73

Association for Health Services Research. *See* AHSR
Attitudinal scales, 225–26

Barer, M.L.: health determinants, 9, 48, 81, 83; social/economic hierarchies, 19, 46
Bed blocker phenomenon, 142
Behavioral risk, 21, 76, 180
Bentham, Jeremy, 190
Bernstein, E., 184
Biomedical research, 77–78, 85
Blue Cross/Blue Shield, 30, 63
Blum, H.L., 83
Blumenthal, D.S., 90
British National Health Services, 88, 134
Brock, R., 47
Brown, D.M., 149
Bunker, J.P., 85, 151
Burt, V.L., 47–48
Business Census of Hospitals, 15

CABG, 31
California Medicaid initiative, 285–312
California Public Employees Retirement System, 295
Cancer: death rates, 43; environmental cause, 83; progress, 42; race/gender factors, 24; screening, 23
CBA, 119–23, 124, 190, 265
CCMC, 14–15
CEA, 119–23, 124, 190
Centers for Disease Control and Prevention, 62, 85
Center for Studying Health System Change, 197
Charles, C., 188
Children's Health Insurance Program, 281

CHO, 228–29
Claims data, 62
Clinical effectiveness, 2; assessment, 52, 54–66; components, 50–52; criteria, 94, 269; evidence, 90–91, 92; focus, 11, 46–48, 271–72; framework, 48–50, 53; policy strategies, 75, 79–80; problem definition, 263–64; research, 208
Clinical evaluation science, 47
Clinical guidelines. *See* Practice guidelines
Clinical indicators, 79
Clinical outcomes, 50
Clinical practice guidelines. *See* Practice guidelines
Clinical trials, 59–60
Clinton, Bill, 133
CMCC, 15–16
Cochrane, A.L., 86
Cochrane Collaboration, 60–61
Colby, D.C., 182
COMC, 228–29
Commission on Chronic Illness, 15
Commission on Financing, 15
Commission on the Health Care Needs of the Nation, 15
Commission on Hospital Care, 15
Committee on the Costs of Medical Care. *See* CCMC
Committee on Monitoring Access to Personal Health Care Services, 190
Common good, 192–93, 232–33, 308
Commonwealth Fund, 16
Communication, 185, 187
Communitarian theory, 175–77, 192–93
Community: collaboration, *x*; empowerment, 225–26, 228; health improvements, 11;

influence, *xiv*; information system, 298; needs assessment, 93;outcome studies, 14

Community Health Care Management System, 93

Community-level analysis, 12–14, 49; cross-sectional study, 61; data, 62, 195–96; effectiveness study, 64; framework, 53; outcome measures, 54; risk adjustment, 57; social justice, 180

Community-oriented managed care, 228–29

Community-oriented primary care, 228

Community Tracking Stucy, 197

Competitive bidding, 145

Competitive market: assumptions, 114–16; conditions, 117; healthcare, 116–18; Pareto optimum, 112–13

Comprehensive healthcare organization, 228–29

Comprehensive health planning, 77, 78

Congressional Budget Office, 150

Conrad, D., 153

Consensus Development Program, 77, 78, 91

Consensus statement guidelines, 79

Consumer: choice, 216; demand, 113–14, 116–18; preference, 268

Contractarian theory, 193, 194

Copayment, 140–41, 219–20, 282

COPC, 228

Coronary artery bypass graft. *See* CABG

Cost-benefit analysis. *See* CBA

Cost-containment strategies, 106, 163–64, 283–84, 293–96

Cost-effectiveness: analysis. *See* CEA; criteria, 189–90; indicators,

190; managed care, 229, 232; problem definition, 264–65; ratio, 264; state health reform, 311–12

Cost function, 119

Cost-utility analysis. *See* CUA

Cram-down rules, 226

Cream-skimming, 146

Cross-sectional study, 61–62, 64, 85–87

CUA, 119–23, 124, 190

Culyer, A.J., 107

DALY, 54

Daniels, Norman, 187, 193, 194

Data: collection, 15–16, 57–58; descriptive, 12; effectiveness research, 62–63; sources, 53, 65–66, 195–99; system, *xiv*, 42

Database, 63, 80

Death rate: age-adjusted, 43

Decision analysis, 60–61, 260

Deliberative justice: analysis, 266; criteria, 186–91, 229–31; evidence, 209–10, 225–27; indicators, 186–93; paradigm, 177–81, 183–84, 201; policy, 208–9, 265

Delivery system: access indicators, 242; availability, 25, 213–15; characteristics, 49; community influence, *xiv*; corporatization, 215–18; equity, 188–89, 265–66; financing, 28–30, 218–20; impact, 47; integrated, 78; organization, 26–28, 215–18; performance evaluation, *xiv*; study design, 60

DeMaio, S., 188

Demand, 113–14, 116–18, 180

Demand curve, 114, 115, 116

Dental health, 22, 28, 42

Descriptive analysis, 199

Descriptive information, 248
Dewey, John, 251
DHEW, 15
Diabetes, 23, 24, 42, 43
Disability-adjusted life year. *See* DALY
Discharge data, 63
Discourse theory, 184, 185, 187
Distributive justice, 174; criteria, 229, 230; evidence, 209–10, 213–25, 226–27; paradigm, 175, 178–83, 201; policy, 207–8, 265
Docteur, E.R., 182
Donabedian, A., 47, 48–49, 266
Donabedian's triad, *xiv-xv*
Dowd, B., 154
DRG, 219
Dunn, W.N., 250
Dynamic efficiency: criteria, 157, 158; evidence, 164–65; managed care, 162; state health reform, 306–7

Economies of scale, 110, 149–51
Education, 24, 108
Effectiveness: assessment, 52–66; clinical perspective. *See* Clinical effectiveness; criteria, 94–98; data sources, 62–63; definition, 1, 2, 51, 52; dimensions, 50–52; evidence, 80–93; framework, 53; health services research, 271–72; issues, *x*; outcome measures, 53, 54–56; policy, 74–80, 93–94, 263–64, 266–67, 269–70; population perspective. *See* Population effectiveness; questionnaire, 56; research levels, 47–52; risk adjustment, 53, 56–59; role, 11–12; state health reform, 299–303; study design, 53, 59–66; trade-offs, 2–3

Efficacy: assessment, 59–60; definition, 50, 51, 52
Efficiency: allocative. *See* Allocative efficiency; assessment, 118–24; criteria, 156–62; definition, 1, 2; dynamic. *See* Dynamic efficiency; evidence, 138–55; framework, 107–18; health services research, 272–73; international comparisons, 123–24; issues, *x*; limitations, 272–73; overview, 105–7; payment arrangements, 135–37; policy, 131–38, 264–65, 267–68, 270; production. *See* Production efficiency; program evaluation, 7; trade-offs, 2–3; utilization management, 137–38
Egalitarian theory, 191
Elderly population, 216, 219
Emergency transportation services, 260
Employer, 30, 154
Employer Retirement Income Security Act, 309
Encounter data, 284–85
Enthoven, A.C., 133, 151
Environment: equity issues, 192–93; health status relationship, 41, 211–13; influence, 46; physical, 19; policy strategies, 76; risks, 19–22, 83, 180, 212–13; role, 9
Environmental indicators, 193, 195–96
Equity: access issues, *x*, 33–34; assessment, 181–200; criteria, 185–95, 227–33, 265–66; data sources, 195–99; definition, 1, 2; evidence, 209–27; framework, 174–81; goals, 233; health services research, 273; indicators, 185–95, 242–45; overview, 173–74;

policy, 207–9, 265–66, 268–71; procedural. *See* Procedural equity; study design, 199–200; substantive. *See* Substantive equity; test, 185; trade-offs, 2–3
ERISA, 309
Etzioni, A., 253
Evaluative research, 200
Evans, R.G., 93, 106; health determinants, 9, 48, 81, 83; social/economic hierarchies, 19, 46
Evidence-based practice initiative, 80
Exercise, 21, 41
Expert panels, 257
Externalities, 117

FAACT, *ix*
Family planning, 28, 41
Feasibility, 54
Fee-for-service arrangements, 28–29, 96, 136, 225
Feldstein, Paul, 132–33, 151, 154
Fielding, J.E., 84
Flexner report, 14
Florida Medicaid initiative. *See* Health Security Plan
Focus groups, 198
Folland, S., 139
Food and Drug Administration, 122
Food safety, 22, 42
Foundation for Accountability, *ix*
Foundations, 16
Frazier, H.S., 85
Freedom-of-choice: equity criteria, 188–89; laws, 284; managed care, 229, 231; state health reform, 308–10
Freire, Paulo, 187
Friedlander, L.J., 86

Fund holding, 146

Gag rule, 187, 226
GDP, 30, 105–6, 146–47, 156
Gender, 24
General practitioner, 146
Gifford, G., 154
Glanz, K., 84
Global budget, 135–37, 143, 145, 295
Glover, J.A., 31
Gold, M., 182
Golladay, F.L., 149
Goodman, A.C., 139
Gordis, L., 87
Government: healthcare expenditures, 30; policy role, 17–19; programs, 17 18
GP, 146
Greenberg, B.G., 48
Greenfield, S., 65
Greenlick, M.R., 109
Grimshaw, J.M., 91
Gross domestic product. *See* GDP
Group Health of Puget Sound, 151
Group-model HMO, 25, 109, 216

Habermas, Jürgen: deliberative democracy, 177; discourse theory, 184, 185, 187; radical planning model, 254
Hannan, E.L., 151
Hansen, K.K., 151
Harvard study, 139
Hawaii Medicaid initiative. *See* Health QUEST
HCFA, 16, 63, 79; data, 197; demonstration projects, 159–60, 217
HCIA-MERCER project, 157–58
Health: determinants, 47, 48, 75–76, 81, 83; disparities, 81, 208, 210–13; education, 28; epidemiology,

46; expenditures, 109, 143, 145;
goals, 123–24; improvement,
2, 11, 45–46, 48; information
system, 75, 76; planning, 78,
87; program evaluation, 7, 8;
promotion, 21, 41, 76, 84–85;
protection, 22, 41–42, 76, 192–93;
risks, 19–21, 193–95; status, 82
Healthcare: alternatives, 108,
138–39; categorization, 49–
50; delivery system. *See*
Delivery system; developed
countries, 105–6; disease-
specific interventions, 86;
disparities, 45–46; ecology,
47, 48–49; effectiveness,
85–90; epidemiology, 47;
geographic variations, 46;
market assumptions, 116–18;
program evaluation, 122;
rationing, 106, 231; reform, 45,
208, 225; resources, 77–78, 86–87,
92
Health Care Access and Cost
Commission, 293
Healthcare expenditures, 29–
30, 31, 105–7; international
comparisons, 146, 147; per
capita, 143, 145; trends, 152–53
Health Care Financing
Administration. *See* HCFA
Healthcare services: continuum, 4–
5, 93; definition, *xiii*; geographic
rate variations, 32
Healthcare system: analysis levels,
12–14; descriptive data, 12;
objectives, 1–3; outcomes, 10, 11;
process, 10, 11; structure, 10–11
Health, Education, and Welfare,
U.S. Department of. *See* DHEW
Health employer data and
information system. *See* HEDIS

Health and Human Services, U.S.
Department of, 20, 109
Health Insurance Association of
America, 197
Health Insurance Plan of California,
295
Health insuring organization, 33
Health maintenance organization.
See HMO
Health plans: cost-sharing
provisions, 219–20; efficiency
evidence, 152–55
Health policy. *See* Policy
Health Professions Educational
Assistance Act, 77, 78
Health QUEST, 285–312
Health-related quality of life, 57
Health Resources and Services
Administration, 197
Health Security Act, 259
Health Security Plan, 285–312
Health services research: analysis
levels, 12–14; comparisons, 8;
components, 10–12; criticisms,
8–9; data, 12; definition, 3–5;
equity considerations, 201,
208; focus, 5; framework, *xiv*;
goals, 1, 6; managed care,
155; motivations, 9–10; policy
role, 6–7, 14–16, 262–73; topic
classification framework, 9–12
Health: United States, 25
Healthy Cities and Healthy
Communities model, 195, 208,
227
Healthy Kids Program, 289, 291
Healthy People 1990, 76
Healthy People Report, 75
Healthy People Review (1995–96),
81
Healthy People Year 2000, 11–12,
76, 257; health promotion, 21;

health protection, 22; indicators, 81; preventive services, 22–23; progress, 41–42

Heart disease, 22, 24, 42, 43, 85

HEDIS, *ix*, 63, 91; database, 90, 198; performance information, 158

HHS, 20, 109

Hill-Burton Act, 15, 77, 78, 257

Hillman, Alan, 122

HIO, 33

HIPC, 295

HIV, 23, 24, 28, 42, 43

HMO, 35; enrollee satisfaction, 155, 217; growth, 26; impact, 161; market penetration, 153–54; Medicaid, 33–34; Medicare, 26; outcome studies, 88; preventive services, 109

Homicide, 21, 24, 41, 43

Horizontal integration, 27

Hospital: admission rates, 141; alliances, 27; care, 15; construction program, 15; cost-containment, 152; data, 63; expenditures, 153–54; industry changes, 25; inpatient days, 142, 144; international comparisons, 142–46; payment arrangements, 29, 133, 136, 151–52; risk adjustment measures, 58; services, 150–52; tax-status, 27; utilization rates, 219

HRQOL, 57

Hume, David, 190

Hurley, Robert, 160

Hygeia, 73, 74

Hypertension, 23, 48

Indicators: access, 242; clinical, 79; cost-effectiveness, 190; deliberative justice, 186–93; demand, 180; environmental, 193, 195–96; equity, 185–95, 242–45; health; status, 82; need, 194–95; procedural equity, 185–95; quality, 47, 49; satisfaction, 244–45; social justice, 186–93; social status, 261; substantive equity, 186, 193–95; utilization, 243–44

Iezzoni, L.I., 57, 58, 59

Immunization, 23, 27, 42

Income tax, 17

Incremental model, 252–53

Individual practice association, 216

Inefficiency, 110

Injury, 22, 24, 41, 118–19

Input, 264

Institute of Medicine, 3–4, 76, 190

Institution-level analysis, 12–14, 49; cross-sectional study, 61; data, 198; effectiveness study, 65–66; framework, 53; outcome measures, 55; risk adjustment, 57

Instrumentalities, 49

Insurance, 30, 224

Integrated delivery systems, 78

Intermediate outcomes, 10, 11

Internal market, 134, 145

International comparisons, 105–6, 131–32; administrative costs, 148–49; allocative efficiency, 142–48; healthcare expenditures, 143, 145–47; hospitals, 142–46; inpatient days, 142, 144; market-minimized models, 134–35; payment arrangements, 136–37; public coverage, 140–41, 143; satisfaction, 224–25; utilization, 146

Interpersonal characteristics, 50

Interventions: costs, 139–40; effectiveness, 266–67; efficiency, 139–40, 268

Invisible hand, 188
IPA, 216

JCAHO, *ix*, 63, 80
Johnson (Robert Wood)
    Foundation, 16, 196, 197
Joint Commission on Accreditation
    of Healthcare Organizations. *See*
    JCAHO
Justice paradigm, 174–84, 201, 207

Kaiser Family Foundation, 16, 151
Kaplan, R.M., 122
Key clinical findings, 58
Kindig, D.A., 149
Kosecoff, J., 91

Lalonde, M., 74–75, 83
Lead hazards, 22
Lewis, F.M., 84
Libertarian theory, 175–77, 188
Life expectancy, 84
Life-saving interventions, 139
Lifestyle, 14, 21, 76, 108
Lohr, K., 47, 90
Lomas, J., 79, 91
Luft, H.S.: economies of scale, 151;
    HMO impact study, 88, 109,
    154–55

McGlynn, E.A., 90
McKeown, T., 84
McKinlay, J.B., 84, 86
McKinlay, S.M., 84, 86
Managed care, 25, 26; distributive
    justice, 182–83; dynamic
    efficiency, 162; employer
    expenditures, 154; enrollee
    satisfaction, 225; enrollment
    data, 196; health expenditure
    trends, 152–53; hospital
    expenditures, 153–54; Medicaid

programs, 32–34, 94–98, 133,
    158–62, 229–33; organization. *See*
    MCO; participation indicators,
    188; physician services, 149;
    social justice, 183; socially
    responsible, 229, 231–32;
    utilization management, 137–38,
    154–55
Managed competition, 305
Manning, W.G., 141
Marine Hospital Service, 17, 76, 77
Market: demand, 114; incentives,
    133; internal, 134, 145; supply,
    115
Market-maximization model, 131,
    162–65; allocative efficiency,
    132–34; payment arrangements,
    135–39; public sector insurance,
    142–43; utilization management,
    137–38
Market-minimization model, 131–
    32, 162–63; allocative efficiency,
    134–35; payment arrangements,
    135–37; public sector insurance,
    142–43; utilization management,
    137–38
Marmor, T.R.: health determinants,
    9, 48, 81, 83; social/economic
    hierarchies, 19, 46
Martini, C.J.M., 86
Maryland Medicaid initiative,
    285–312
MCO: accountability, 218; cross-
    subsidies, 216; enrollees,
    217; limitations, 226; market
    penetration, 228; restriction
    consequences, 218
Measles, 23
*Measuring Health—A Guide to
    Rating Scales and Questionnaires,*
    55
Medicaid, 16, 18; allocative

efficiency, 159–60; demonstration projects, 95–97, 159–60; economic problems, 32–33; enrollment growth, 222; expenditures, 32, 158–59, 218–19; HMO arrangements, 33–34; managed care arrangements, 32–34, 94–98, 133, 158–62, 229–33; production efficiency, 160–61; provider involvement, 32–33; reform, 259–60; state initiatives, 281–82, 285–312; utilization rates, 223

Medical care. *See* Healthcare

Medical education, 14, 17, 25

Medical Illness Severity Grouping System, 57, 58

Medical indigency programs, 17

Medical-industrial complex, 216

Medical necessity guidelines. *See* Practice guidelines

Medical Outcomes Study, 16, 89, 218

Medical Outcomes Study Short Form, 55–56, 65

Medicare, 16, 18, 133; enrollee satisfaction, 217–18; expenditures, 150, 218–19; HMO enrollment, 26; payment arrangements, 25, 29, 135; PPS, 29, 133, 136; utilization rates, 223

Medicare Provider Analysis and Review, 63

MedisGroups, 57, 58

MEDPAR, 63

Melnick, G.A., 152, 153

Mental health, 41, 216

Meta-analysis, 60–61

Milio, N., 46

Mill, John Stuart, 190

Miller, M., 149

Minkler, M., 184

MinnesotaCare, 285–312

Mixed-scanning model, 253

Moore, F., 86

Mortality and Morbidity Weekly Report, 62

Mosteller, F., 85

National Ambulatory Medical Care Survey, 62

National Cancer Institute, 62

National Center for Health Services Research and Development, 16

National Center for Health Statistics. *See* NCHS

National Committee for Quality Assurance. *See* NCQA

National healthcare expenditures, 29

National Health Interview Survey. *See* NHIS

National Health and Nutrition Examination Survey, 47–48

National Heart Institute, 77

National Hospital Discharge Survey, 62

National Institute of Aging, 16

National Institute of Mental Health, 16

National Long-Term Care Survey, 62

National Medical Care Expenditure Survey, 196

National Program to Conquer Heart Disease, Cancer and Stroke, 77

National School Lunch Program, 289

NCHS, 25; data, 47, 62, 197; surveys, 196

NCHSRD, 16

NCQA, *ix*, 63, 80, 198

Need, 113, 180; assessment, 222,

233, 300–301; criteria, 193–94, 229; indicators, 194–95
Newhouse, J.P., 86, 149
NHANES, 47–48
NHE, 29
NHIS, 15, 54, 62
NIH, 77, 78
Normal species functioning, 193
Nozick, R., 188
Nutrition, 41

OBRA, 33
Observational study, 61–62, 65, 88
Occupational health, 22, 41
OECD, 62, 123, 124, 142
Office of Health Promotion and Disease Prevention, 75–76
Omnibus Budget Reconciliation Act, 33
Oregon Medicaid initiative, 285–312
Organization for Economic Cooperation and Development. *See* OECD
Organized delivery systems, 78
Outcomes, 10, 11; analysis, 12–14, 298; clinical, 50; community studies, 14; definition, 50; effectiveness, 89, 91, 266–67; measures, 51, 53, 54–56, 62; observation timeframe, 57; policy process, 253–54; population, 14; procedure rates, 87; research, 79–80; risk adjustment, 53, 56–59; study, 64–65; subjective health status, 55
Outpatient services, 150
Output, 110–11, 118–19

Panakeia, 73
Pareto, Vilfredo, 112

Pareto optimum, 112–13, 272
Patient: characteristics, 49; counseling, 109–10; dumping, 191; education, 109–10; origin studies, 199; satisfaction, 217–18; self-protection legislation, *ix*; surveys, 61
Patient judgment system, 198
Patient-level analysis, 12–14, 49; cross-sectional study, 61; data, 198–99; distributive justice, 180; effectiveness study, 66; framework, 53; outcome measures, 55; risk adjustment, 56–57
Patient outcome research teams, 122
Patient Protection Act, 297
Payment arrangements, 28–29
PCCM, 33, 97
Performance evaluation, 262
Performance monitoring, 75, 76, 79; effectiveness, 90–91; improvement, 94; state initiatives, 299–300, 301, 303; system, 80
Performance standards, 157–58
Personal healthcare, 30, 218–19
Personal health services, 3, 138–39
Pew Foundation, 16
Pharmacoeconomics, 122
PHC, 30, 218–19
Physical activity, 21, 41
Physical environment, 19
Physician: availability, 25; group practice, 26, 149–50; organizations, 26–27; payment arrangements, 28–29, 136, 150; services, 149–50
Point-of-service plans, 26, 216
Police power, 17, 176
Policy: allocative efficiency

concerns, 108–10; alternatives, 258–61, 266–69; consequences, 259–62; effectiveness considerations, 74–80, 9; efficiency assessment, 156–58; equity considerations, 180–81, 185, 187–88, 229, 230; goal, 180–81; government's role, 17–19; health service research relationship, *xiv*; medical versus non-medical alternatives, 108; objectives, 257; participation, 185, 187–88; preventive services, 109; reform, 93–94; treatment, 109–10

Policy analysis: comparisons, 8; definition, 5–7; equity considerations, 208; framework, 16–32; health services research role, 262–73; informational needs, 248–51; models, 251–55; objectives, 5–7, 247–51; policymaking, 6–7, 255–62

Policymaking process: alternatives, 258–61; consequences, 261–62; problem definition, 256–58

Policy strategies: efficiency, 131–38; equity, 207–9, 268; evidence, 84–93

Political model, 253–54

Population effectiveness, 2; assessment, 52, 54–66; criteria, 93–94, 269; evidence, 84–90, 91–92; focus, 11, 46–48, 271–72; framework, 48–50, 53; policy strategies, 74–78; problem definition, 263; research, 208

Population health: indicators, 81; outcomes, 14, 54–55; strategy, 75–76

Population information system. *See* POPULIS

Population-level analysis, 196

POPULIS, 75, 76, 93

PORT, 122

POS plans, 26, 216

PPO, 26, 216, 218

PPRC, 259

PPS, 29, 133, 136, 151–52

Practice guidelines, 79–80, 91, 94

Preferred provider organization. *See* PPO

Prenatal care, 22, 42

Prescriptive information, 248

Preventable hospitalizations, 90

Prevention, 4, 140

Preventive services, 22–23, 42, 76; allocative efficiency, 109; cost-effectiveness, 190; effectiveness, 84–85; efficiency evidence, 139–40

Primary care case management, 33, 97

Private insurance, 30, 218–19, 282–83, 291–93

Private market, 117–18

PRO, 79

Problem: definition, 256–58, 263–64; redefinition of, 262

Procedural equity, 2, 181; criteria, 185–95; evidence, 209; focus, 11; indicators, 185–95; policy, 227, 230

Process, 10, 11; analysis, 12–14; effectiveness, 49–50, 88–89, 269; variables, 49–50, 51, 88

Production efficiency, 2, 110–11; assessment, 118–23; definition, 107; evidence, 148–55, 164; focus, 11; Medicaid managed care, 160–61; policy, 156–58, 264–65; state health reform, 306

Production function, 118–19, 139

Production possibility frontier, 110–11
Professional review organization, 79
Professional standards review organization, 79, 90
Prospective analysis, 255, 261
Prospective payment system. *See* PPS
Provider: availability, 189, 213–15; characteristics, 49; demand influence, 117–18; Medicaid involvement, 32–33; organization, 215–18; payment arrangements, 135–37; safety-net, 34, 173, 216; survey, 62
PSRO, 79, 90
Public benefits, 282, 289–91
Public coverage, 281
Public health, 3–4; clinical trials, 60; concerns, 208; effectiveness, 84; expenditures, 28; federal grant programs, 17, 18; goals, 20; interventions, 17; policy, 265; services, 27–28;state government's responsibility, 18; strategies, 74–77
Purchasing pools, 296

QALY, 120–21
Qualitative analysis, 132–33, 260
Quality: assessment, 50, 52; attributes, *ix*; definition, 50, 51, 52; improvement, 284–85, 296–98; indicators, 47, 49; outcome relationship, 91–92
Quality-adjusted life year. *See* QALY
Quality Compass, 80
Quantitative analysis, 260, 261
Quantity, 50, 51

Questionnaires, 55–56

Race, 24
Radical planning model, 254
Radon, 22
RAND Health Insurance Experiment, 16, 89; copayment, 140–41, 219–20; HMO impact, 154–55, 161; patient satisfaction, 217–18; policy consequences, 270; study design, 60
Randomized clinical trial. *See* RCT
Rational discourse, 185
Rational model, 251–52, 254–55, 273
Rawls, John, 193
RBRVS, 29, 135, 150, 259
RCT, 59–60, 85, 96
Reasonableness, 249–50
Regionalization, 151, 295
Regional Medical Program, 77–78
Reinhardt, U.E., 149, 310
Relevance, 249
Reliability, 54
Relman, A., 216
Renaud, M., 74
Report cards, *ix*
Resource: availability, 213–14; misallocation, 109–11, 141
Resource allocation, 107; criteria, 111–14; needs-based approach, 134; problems, 112; process, 111
Resource-based relative value scale. *See* RBRVS
Retrospective analysis, 255, 261
Rice, T., 116–17
Rimer, B., 84
Risk: adjustment, 53, 56–59, 64–65; assessment, 57; factors, 23–24; ratios, 24
Risk Adjustment for Measuring Health Care Outcomes, 57
Rissel, C., 184

Robertson, A., 184
Robinson, J.C., 153
Roos, N.P., 9
Rosenbaum, S., 226
Rural hospitals, 215
Russell, I.T., 91

St. Leger, A.S., 86
Satisfaction, 268; indicators, 244–45;
    questionnaires, 198; surveys,
    224–25
Schwartz, F.W., 152
Seatbelt use, 22
SEER, 62
Self-insurance, 30
Sensitivity, 54, 56
Severity-of-illness measures, 58
Sexually transmitted disease, 23,
    28, 42
SF-36, 55–56, 65
Shortell, S.M., 88, 93–94, 183
Showstack, J., 229
SHS, 55–56
Siu, A.L., 141
Smith, K.R., 149
Smoking, 21, 41
Social conditions, 248
Social environment, 83
Social justice: criteria, 186–93;
    equity considerations, 209–13,
    227, 229, 266; indicators, 186–93;
    paradigm, 176, 178–81, 183, 201;
    policy, 265
Social Security Act, 18, 76–77
Social systems accounting, 261
Social welfare, 112, 265
Social welfare function, 112
Socioeconomic status, 19–20, 24,
    211–12, 223
Specialists, 25
Spending down, 189
Staff-model HMO, 25, 109, 161

Standards, 257
Stano, M., 139
State health reform, 277–79;
    cost-containment strategies,
    283–84, 293–96; dimensions, 280;
    effectiveness criteria, 299–303;
    efficiency criteria, 299, 303–7;
    equity criteria, 299, 307–12;
    evaluation, 298–312; private
    coverage, 282–83, 291–93; public
    benefits, 282, 289–91; public
    coverage, 281, 285–89; quality
    improvement, 284–85, 296–98
Stoddard, G.L., 106
Stress-related problems, 21
Stroke, 22–23, 24, 42, 43
Structure, 10–11; analysis, 12–
    14; effectiveness, 49, 51, 269;
    variables, 88
Subjective health status. *See* SHS
Substantive equity, 2, 181, 233;
    criteria, 186, 193–95; evidence,
    209; focus, 11; indicators, 186,
    193–95; policy, 227, 230
Suicide, 21
Supplier-induced demand, 117–18
Supply, 114–15
Supply curve, 115, 116
Surveillance epidemiology and end
    result system, 62
Surveys, 61, 62, 196, 198
Survivor analysis, 149–50
System-level analysis, 49; cross-
    sectional study, 61; data,
    197–98; effectiveness study,
    64–65; framework, 53; outcome
    measures, 55; risk adjustment, 57

Technology, 119
Teen pregnancy, 21
TennCare, 285–312
Thacker, S.B., 85

Treatment: allocative efficiency, 109–10; efficiency evidence, 140–42; similar, 190–92, 310–11
Tuberculosis screening, 27
Turnock, B.J., 84

Ultimate outcome, 10, 11
Underinsured population, 221–22
Uninsured population, 30, 173, 221
Unintentional injury, 22, 24, 41
U.S. Constitution, 17
U.S. Department of Health and Human Services. See HHS
U.S. Health and Nutrition Examination Survey, 86
U.S. Vital Statistics, 62
Use variation. See Utilization
Utilitarian theory, 189–90
Utilization: copayment effect, 140–41; definition, 50, 51; efficiency strategies, 137–39; enabling factors, 221–22; health relationship, 112; HMO impact, 154–55; indicators, 243–44; international comparisons, 146; issues, 14; need assessment, 222; patterns, 214–15; predisposing factors, 220–21; rates, 50, 89; realized access, 222–24; study, 64

Validity, 54, 249
Value, ix, 105
Veatch, Robert, 191
Vertical integration, 27
Veterans Administration, 16
Violent behavior, 41

Vulnerable population, 33–34, 45, 213; access, 213–20, 243; distributive justice, 220–22; equity issues, 190–92; realized access, 222–25; social justice, 183
Wallerstein, N., 184
Wallet biopsies, 191
Ware, J.E., 55
Welfare loss, 141
Well-baby care, 28
Wennberg, J.E., 31, 47, 64
White, K.L., 48
Whiteis, D.G., 20
WHO, 11–12, 62, 183, 193, 195, 228
WIC, 28
Wickizer, T.M., 154
Williams, A.H., 134
Williams, T.F., 48
Women, Infants, and Children Program, 28
Woolf, S.H., 91
Work-related injury, 22
World Health Organization. See WHO

X-inefficiency, 119

Year 2000 Objectives for the Nation, 183, 194, 208; environmental indicators, 193; health protection, 192–93; indicators, 210–13; preventive services, 190; progress, 227

Zwanziger, J., 151, 152, 153

About the Authors

Lu Ann Aday, Ph.D., is Professor of Behavioral Sciences and Management and Policy Sciences at the University of Texas School of Public Health. She received her doctorate in sociology from Purdue University, and was formerly Associate Director for Research at the Center for Health Administration Studies of the University of Chicago. Dr. Aday's principal research interests have focused on indicators and correlates of health services utilization and access. She has conducted major national and community surveys and evaluations of national demonstrations and published extensively in this area, including eleven previous books dealing with conceptual or empirical aspects of research on equity of access to healthcare.

Charles E. Begley, Ph.D., is Associate Professor of Management and Policy Sciences at the University of Texas School of Public Health and a member of the adjunct faculty in the Department of Economics at Rice University. He received his doctorate in economics from the University of Texas at Austin and has been on the faculty of Illinois State University and Southern Illinois University School of Medicine in Springfield, Illinois. Dr. Begley's research and teaching interests include health policy, health services research, and health economics. He has directed or consulted on numerous health services and policy research projects at the national, state, and local levels.

David R. Lairson, Ph.D., is Professor of Health Economics on the faculty of the University of Texas School of Public Health and a member of the adjunct faculty in the Department of Economics at Rice University. This revision was begun while he was on leave as

Visiting Professor on the Faculty of Health, School of Public Health, Queensland University of Technology, in Brisbane, Australia. He was a doctoral fellow at the Kaiser Center for Health Research in Portland, Oregon, and received his PhD from the University of Kentucky in Lexington, Kentucky. Dr. Lairson's major research and teaching interests include the economic evaluation of healthcare.

Carl H. Slater, M.D., is Associate Professor of Health Services Organization on the faculty of the University of Texas School of Public Health. He is a graduate of the University of Colorado School of Medicine, and was a Fellow at the Center for the Study of Medical Education, University of Illinois, School of Medicine in Chicago. Dr. Slater's research interests are in assessing the quality and effectiveness of health services, with a special emphasis on outcomes research. Dr. Slater has developed and taught courses in health services effectiveness, quality assessment, and outcomes research; and published in the area of ambulatory care quality.